Clinical Study Guide
for the
Oral Boards in Psychiatry

Third Edition

Clinical Study Guide
for the
Oral Boards in Psychiatry

Third Edition

Nathan R. Strahl, M.D., Ph.D.
Consulting Associate
Department of Psychiatry and Behavioral Sciences
Duke University Medical Center
Durham, North Carolina

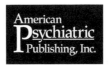

American Psychiatric Publishing, Inc.

Washington, DC
London, England

Manufactured in the United States of America on acid-free paper
12   11   10   09   08   5   4   3   2   1
Third Edition

American Psychiatric Publishing, Inc.
1000 Wilson Boulevard
Arlington, VA 22209-3901
www.appi.org

Library of Congress Cataloging-in-Publication Data
Strahl, Nathan R.
    Clinical study guide for the oral boards in psychiatry / Nathan R. Strahl.—3rd ed.
        p. ; cm.
    Includes bibliographical references and index.
    ISBN 978-1-58562-293-1 (alk. paper)
    1. Psychiatry—Examinations—Study guides. 2. Psychiatrists—Examinations—Study guides. 3. Oral examinations. I. Title.
    [DNLM: 1. Mental Disorders—diagnosis—Outlines. 2. Diagnosis, Differential—Outlines. 3. Mental Disorders—therapy—Outlines. WM 18.2 S896c 2009]
    RC343.5.S77   2009
    616.89′0076—dc22

                                                        2008018668

British Library Cataloguing in Publication Data
A CIP record is available from the British Library.

To my grandchildren
Kaitlyn Strahl, born September 10, 1999;
Emily Strahl, born September 22, 2000;
Kyle Strahl, born September 29, 2004;
Brayden Petzold, born April 14, 2006

With the treasured love of family and friends,
we give thanks for the gift of life,
for a new generation,
for four beautiful and healthy grandchildren,
and for a wonderful new day.

CONTENTS

■ List of Figures

■ List of Tables

PREFACE
TO THE THIRD EDITION

C*linical Study Guide for the Oral Boards in Psychiatry* enters into its third edition. Editing the vast and ever increasing clinical database to provide a practical guide for you to prepare effectively for the oral boards has been a greater challenge than ever. I began the editing process in November 2007, and the final version of the revised text finally went to press in late July 2008. What I found daunting during the editing period were the many new U.S. Food and Drug Administration approvals and warnings as well as updated treatment recommendations, resulting in my continually revising recently edited material.

The challenges in preparing this new edition represent an important caveat for future reference. The increase in the database of knowledge for evidenced-based psychiatry seems to be reaching exponential proportions. Surely, with adequate preparation, you have a good chance of passing the Board examination, having studied to gain a solid clinical grounding. However, passing the exam only represents the beginning. I have found that it is imperative for me to regularly provide study time to update my knowledge base so that I can remain on the forefront of the most current clinical treatment guidelines. This does require allocating additional (and hard to find) time, but knowing that I am well prepared to provide the best care for my patients is a tremendous reward for the effort. In short, what you are now doing to prepare for the Board examination should represent a behavior that you will continue throughout the remaining years of your clinical practice.

I find the newer clinical and scientific findings to be intriguing. Perhaps one of the most important is the genetic basis of response to psychotropic medication in regard to therapeutic and side effects. We are learning that the failure of a medication to provide an adequate response may not be the fault of the medication but rather may be due to genetically determined metabolic behavior or to the patient's genetically determined receptor activity.

There is also, in the current literature, a significant emphasis toward the diagnosis and treatment of bipolar disorder. Some welcome the change that the increased prevalence of this disorder has been poorly appreciated in the past. Others have cautioned that the pendulum has perhaps swung too far, in that nearly everyone who has occasional mood shifts or a history of substance abuse is preferentially labeled as "bipolar." Further studies will tease out these differences. Considerations for the utilization of atypical antipsychotic medications, the reemergence of the recognition of the significant value of lithium, and concerns that some of the antiseizure medications may not have antimanic properties are rapidly coming to the forefront.

As a consequence, psychiatry now truly presents an evidenced-based discipline, and to ensure standard of care, you are expected to provide treatment based on these principles.

Because of the rapidly expanding database for newer clinical material, I have been forced to reduce, but not eliminate, clinical information related to older "tried and true" medications. For example, tricyclic antidepressants are still important entities, especially from the standpoint of their potential toxic cardiovascular effects and their inherent dangers when combined with alcohol. A recent finding that tricyclic antidepressant medications pose a significant cardiovascular risk in the elderly represents an important clinical consideration.

In all, I find the practice of psychiatry to be exciting, refreshing, and invigorating. I look forward to the changes yet to come while at the same time appreciating that our current state of knowledge is of tremendous value to enable us to provide the best treatments possible for our patients.

Finally, I wish you the best, not only for passing the Board examination but also for your future practice of psychiatry in an ever-changing and complex world.

Nathan R. Strahl, M.D., Ph.D.
Consulting Associate
Department of Psychiatry and Behavioral Sciences
Duke University Medical Center
Durham, North Carolina

Please pass along your comments and suggestions regarding this manual and your experience taking the oral boards to me at nathan_strahl@yahoo.com. This will help with future revisions.

PREFACE
TO THE SECOND EDITION

*T*he past 3½ years since publication of the first edition of *Clinical Study Guide for the Oral Boards in Psychiatry* have witnessed a tremendous influx of new information relevant to the practice of psychiatry. Important areas of research have yielded improved diagnostic procedures—in particular, positron emission tomography (PET), functional magnetic resonance imaging (fMRI), and single photon emission computed tomography (SPECT), which allow direct views of brain functioning in health and illness. Armed with these techniques and a greater emphasis on research, our fundamental knowledge base continues to increase. As a consequence, newer and safer treatments (e.g., vagal nerve stimulation for the treatment of depression) are emerging.

However, these developments place a greater burden on the examinee for adequate preparation for the oral exam. Candidates are expected to be familiar with both older and newer treatments, and the wealth of information that can be explored by the examiners continues to grow, perhaps exponentially. Adequate time to prepare for the examination is perhaps your best ally for a successful outcome.

As of 2004, the American Board of Psychiatry and Neurology (ABPN) requires recertification every 10 years through a written, proctored, computer-based examination. I successfully completed this recertification examination in August 2004. I found the examination to be clinically grounded rather than theoretically based. Questions were directly relevant to the everyday practice of clinical psychiatry. At least on my examination, there was minimal emphasis on neurology. In addition to its stated purpose of preparation for the oral boards, this second edition of the *Clinical Study Guide for the Oral Boards in Psychiatry* will also provide an excellent review for the recertification examination.

Psychiatry is a wonderful profession. We have unprecedented access to the conscious and unconscious thinking of our patients, and I never cease to be amazed by what I hear and what I learn. My only sad commentary on psychiatry is the overwhelming emphasis today on medication rather than psychotherapeutic treatments. Certainly, our patients need our medications; however, even more, they need us to invest in them through the therapeutic milieu to foster appropriate changes that truly serve to improve outcomes.

Good luck on the exam.

PREFACE

*C*linical Study Guide for the Oral Boards in Psychiatry emerged from my experience studying for and passing the oral boards in psychiatry. When preparing for Part II of the boards, I found the process of studying for the examination by reviewing the standard textbooks and clinical journals of psychiatry arduous and time-inefficient. That experience prompted me to outline the clinical material into chapters dealing with the major mental health disorders. *Clinical Study Guide for the Oral Boards in Psychiatry* is the product of that effort.

This manual should be a distinct advantage for your review and study in that the pertinent clinical material is collected in one place. You will find a great deal of material here; there are no wasted words or irrelevant information. Each area reviewed focuses on the pertinent clinical information candidates should know and may be asked about by the examiners.

The oral examination is a measure of your clinical (not theoretical) knowledge of psychiatry. You are expected to conduct (or view) a clinical interview, present your findings in a concise yet thorough manner, provide a differential diagnosis, and provide a provisional diagnosis. You are expected to be knowledgeable about DSM-IV-TR diagnostic criteria, epidemiology, etiology, comorbidity, differential diagnosis, workup, and accepted treatments for the major psychiatric disorders.

Adequate preparation is essential. However, your practice may be limited in the type of patients you typically see. If you work at a state hospital, you will likely be more familiar with the diagnosis and treatment of psychotic and substance abuse disorders. If you work in private practice, you most likely will see patients with mood, anxiety, substance abuse, and personality disorders. Yet the patient you interview (or see interviewed) can present with any mental health disorder or combination of disorders. This study guide is intended to help fill in the gaps, recognizing that there is no substitute for sound clinical knowledge gained from your own clinical experience.

Many candidates believe that the essence of the oral examination is to demonstrate their proficiency in accurately diagnosing the patient they interview or see interviewed. Actually, in part, you, as the candidate, are being tested on your ability to *differentially diagnose.* Within reason, the examiners do not really care if your diagnostic opinion agrees or disagrees with theirs. They want to assess how you reason in providing your differential and provisional diagnoses and to ensure that you recognize, based on a short interview, that many diagnoses are possible. In many ways, a short interview is a blessing, since it offers the opportunity to provide a broad differential diagnosis. In that regard, the patient merely serves as a catalyst to open the discussion that will test your overall competency and clinical skills. If, for example, your patient presents with paranoid thinking, you demonstrate your competence not by definitively diagnosing paranoid schizophrenia, but by listing the many possible disorders (e.g., psychiatric, physical, medication-induced, substance-induced) that may present with paranoid thinking. This is a formidable task and will take effort on your part to sharpen your skills to assess patients in a differentially diagnostic mode.

You should be thoroughly familiar with any item or topic you mention. If, for example, you state that gabapentin (Neurontin) might be a good medication for the patient, you should be very familiar with its indications, dosage range, therapeutic effects, and side effects. If you state that the depressive symptoms you observe can potentially be caused by several physical illnesses, you will likely be asked to list those physical disorders. If you state that cognitive-behavioral therapy would be a helpful treatment, you should be familiar with the nuances of this treatment modality.

In addition to reviewing the clinical basis of psychiatry, mock examinations with knowledgeable mentors can be especially helpful. Like everything in life, practice makes perfect, and the more experienced you are in taking the examination, the better your chances for passing. For the mock examination(s) to serve its purpose, you must be open to criticism, listening carefully to deficiencies that may be evident, and then working to correct those deficiencies. Additional helpful aids include videotaped interviews of the examination process and the text *Boarding Time: The Psychiatry Candidate's New Guide to Part II of the ABPN Examination,* Third Edition, by James Morrison and Rodrigo A. Muñoz (American Psychiatric Publishing, Inc., 2003).

It is also important to demonstrate to the examiners your ability to show empathy for your patient. As psychiatrists, more than any other medical specialists, we are expected to show compassion and concern for the welfare of our patients, and the examiners look for this. However, because of the short time for the interview, there is a natural tendency to "push" the patient for more and more clinical information. The error in this approach, once again, is that you are not expected to provide a definitive diagnosis, but rather a differential diagnosis. You can always state to the examiners that with more time you would explore a particular area more fully. Spend some time (if even only a minute or two) building rapport with the patient. For example, provide a comment that is reassuring to the patient (e.g., "It sounds like the last couple of years have been very difficult for you"), or compliment the patient in some way (e.g., "I can see you are working very hard to get better"). Ignoring these issues could result in a failing grade even if your performance on other elements of the examination is satisfactory.

Your relationship with the examiners also is important. Although your knowledge of clinical psychiatry is clearly relevant, how you relate to the examiners may have a significant impact on the outcome. Adverse factors include having noticeable candidate anxiety (greater impact for men than for women), being excessively guarded or defensive, and taking on an adversarial rather than collegial relationship with the examiners. You should be open to suggestions for alternatives and criticism, just as if you were discussing a patient on rounds or with colleagues.

Clinical Study Guide for the Oral Boards in Psychiatry is designed to provide useful clinical information regarding the assessment and treatment of the types of patients most likely to present for the oral boards. It is not intended as a manual for the treatment of patients in clinical practice or as a textbook of psychiatry. Diagnoses are based on DSM-IV-TR criteria. DSM was designed to provide uniformity between psychiatrists with different backgrounds and training to "speak the same language," and nowhere is this more important than with the oral boards. You will see algorithms for treatment protocols. Clearly, the best treatment protocol is based on the individual needs of the patient and is founded on your experience in treating similar types of patients. However, the algorithms provided are "middle of the road" treatment protocols that will be helpful, especially if your experience with a particular patient group is limited.

I can say with confidence that adequate preparation will improve your chances for passing. I recommend providing at least 6 months for thorough review and preparation. Some sacrifices will likely be needed, since time demands are likely quite heavy before you start your review. Dedication, diligence, and a goal-directed study approach, reviewing over and over all elements of the examination process, will likely result in a better outcome. Nonetheless, certain variables, such as the individual expectations of the reviewers, play a role in determining the final outcome. However, these factors are true for every candidate. Your best arsenal for successfully passing the examination rests on your level of preparedness. Candidates who successfully passed the examination tell me that when they took the oral boards, they felt at the peak of their knowledge and level of confidence as psychiatrists.

In summary, it is essential to have an understanding of the nature of the examination process, to prepare thoroughly for the examination through in-depth study, to show empathy for the patient, and to develop a collegial relationship with the examiners. Passing the examination is not based on luck; rather, it is founded on solid preparation manifest in your presenting as a caring yet clinically competent psychiatrist. Rumor has it that if an examiner would feel comfortable referring one of his or her patients to you, you have met that examiner's criteria for passing that portion of the examination.

Prepare well.

1

SCHIZOPHRENIA AND OTHER PSYCHOTIC DISORDERS

Principal DSM-IV-TR Psychotic Disorders

Schizophrenia
Brief psychotic disorder
Schizophreniform disorder
Schizoaffective disorder
Delusional disorder
Shared psychotic disorder
Psychotic disorder due to a general medical condition
Substance-induced psychotic disorder
Psychotic disorder not otherwise specified

SCHIZOPHRENIA

DSM-IV-TR Diagnostic Criteria

A. *Characteristic symptoms:* Two or more of the following symptoms, each present for a significant portion of time during a 1-month period (or less if effectively treated):
1. Delusions.
2. Hallucinations.
3. Disorganized speech (e.g., frequent derailment or incoherence).
4. Grossly disorganized or catatonic behavior.
5. Negative symptoms (i.e., affective flattening, alogia, or avolition).
   Note. Only one Criterion A symptom is required if delusions are bizarre or hallucinations consist of a voice keeping up a running commentary on the person's behavior or thoughts, or two or more voices conversing with each other.

B. *Social/occupational dysfunction:* For a significant portion of the time since the onset of the disturbance, one or more major areas of functioning, such as work, interpersonal relationships, or self-care, are markedly below the level achieved prior to the onset (or when the onset is in childhood or adolescence, failure to achieve expected level of interpersonal, academic, or occupational achievement).

C. *Duration:* Continuous signs of the disturbance persist for at least 6 months. This 6-month period must include at least 1 month of symptoms (or less if effectively treated) that meet Criterion A (i.e., active-phase symptoms) and may include periods of prodromal or residual symptoms. During these prodromal or residual periods, the signs of the disturbance may be manifested by only negative symptoms or by two or more symptoms listed in Criterion A present in an attenuated form (e.g., odd beliefs, unusual perceptual experiences).

D. *Schizoaffective and mood disorder exclusion:* Schizoaffective disorder and mood disorder with psychotic features have been ruled out because either 1) no major depressive, manic, or mixed episodes have occurred concurrently with the active-phase symptoms; or 2) if mood episodes have occurred during active-phase symptoms, their total duration has been brief relative to the duration of the active and residual periods.

E. *Substance/general medical exclusion:* The disturbance is not due to the direct physiological effects of a substance (e.g., a drug of abuse, a medication) or a general medical condition.

F. *Relationship to a pervasive developmental disorder:* If there is a history of autistic disorder or another pervasive developmental disorder, the additional diagnosis of schizophrenia is made only if prominent delusions or hallucinations are also present for at least 1 month (or less if successfully treated).

Clinical and Diagnostic Issues

Definitions of psychosis:

➤ *Psychosis* can be defined:
  ✔ Psychiatrically as:
    ■ A gross impairment in reality testing.
    ■ An inability to distinguish what is real from what is not real.
    ■ A loss of contact with reality.
    ■ A loss of ego boundaries.
  ✔ Legally as:
    ■ "Insane" when the person who committed the crime could not distinguish between right and wrong at the time the crime was committed.
    ■ *Non compos mentis* (not of sound mind, memory, or understanding).

✔ In lay terms (at times pejoratively) as:

- Crazy, mad, lunatic, "psycho," maniac.

✔ In DSM-IV-TR (Schizophrenia and Other Psychotic Disorders) by the presence of:

- Delusions, prominent hallucinations, disorganized speech, disorganized behavior, or catatonic behavior (for schizophrenia, schizophreniform disorder, schizoaffective disorder, and brief psychotic disorder).

- Delusions (for delusional disorder and shared psychotic disorder).

- Delusions or prominent hallucinations that are not accompanied by insight and delusions (for psychotic disorder due to a general medical condition and for substance-induced psychotic disorder).

"Associated features" of schizophrenia:

➤ DSM-IV-TR includes disturbances in cognition and mood as "associated symptoms" of schizophrenia. (In reality, they are likely core symptoms.) Other "associated symptoms" listed in DSM-IV-TR include:

✔ Inappropriate affect (e.g., laughing when discussing a sad event).

✔ Lack of interest in eating or refusal to eat secondary to paranoid beliefs.

✔ Anhedonia (loss of interest or ability to experience pleasure).

✔ Lack of insight as to the nature of the disorder or to the irrationality of psychotic symptoms.

✔ Unusual psychomotor activities (e.g., grimacing, ritualistic or stereotypic movements, posturing, pacing, rocking, aimless behavior).

✔ Unusual somatic concerns (e.g., brain is missing, having several heart attacks daily).

✔ Depersonalization (feeling detached from one's body) and derealization (feeling detached from one's environment).

Diagnostic considerations:

➤ Schizophrenia:

✔ Is a psychotic disorder manifested by *two or more* symptoms from Criterion A (the active phase) lasting for a significant portion of time during a 1-month period (or less if treated), marked social and/or occupational dysfunction (Criterion B), and continuous signs of the illness lasting at least 6 months (Criterion C):

- The 1-month and 6-month exclusions help to distinguish schizophrenia from brief psychotic disorder and schizophreniform disorder, respectively.

- A prodromal or residual phase may be present (part of Criterion C) but is not absolutely required. During the prodromal and residual phases, the predominant features are negative symptoms and/or attenuated (i.e., nonpsychotic) positive symptoms.

✔ Is diagnosed only after schizoaffective disorder/mood disorder with psychotic features (Criterion D), substance-induced psychotic disorder/psychotic disorder due to a general medical condition (Criterion E), and autistic disorder/pervasive developmental disorder (Criterion F) have been ruled out. All six criteria (Criterion A–Criterion F) must be met to satisfy DSM-IV-TR diagnostic requirements.

✔ Is manifested in the active phase by:

- Positive symptoms:
  - Include delusions, prominent hallucinations, disorganization of speech, and disorganization of behavior.
  - Are reflective of an excess of normal functioning.
  - Are often linked to dysfunction of the temporal lobes (the "interpretive cortex," comprising the brain region involved in the processing and interpretation of language, vision, and sound).
  - Classified by Criteria A1–A4.

- Catatonic symptoms:
  - Are characterized by a marked reduction in or marked excess of psychomotor activity.
  - Are poorly understood in terms of etiology.
  - Are classified by Criterion A4.

- Negative symptoms:
  - Include affective flattening, alogia, and avolition.
  - Are reflective of a loss of normal functioning (i.e., "deficit" symptoms).
  - Are linked to dysfunction of the prefrontal cortex (the cortical brain region involved in organization, planning, and judgment).
  - Are classified by Criterion A5.

✔ Does not necessarily require the presence of delusions or hallucinations. Because DSM-IV-TR requires only two symptoms from the active phase, some combination of disorganization, catatonia, and negative symptoms (Criteria A3–A5) can fully satisfy Criterion A without the presence of either delusions or hallucinations (an unlikely scenario).

✔ Is not necessarily the correct diagnosis if delusions and hallucinations are present. Many disorders (e.g., medical disorders, substance-related disorders, psychiatric disorders other than schizophrenia) present with delusions and hallucinations. These possibilities must be explored and ruled out prior to assigning a diagnosis of schizophrenia.

✔ Requires only a single symptom from Criterion A under two specific circumstances:

- If delusions are bizarre (more the rule than the exception), Criterion A is fully satisfied.
- If hallucinations consist of a voice detailing a running commentary on the person's behavior or thoughts, or two or more voices conversing with each other, Criterion A is fully satisfied.

✔ Can be viewed as a group of related illnesses of differing etiologies but with similar clinical characteristics (i.e., "schizophrenia spectrum disorder").

✔ Is a multisymptomatic (i.e., heterogeneous, complex, multidimensional) disorder. For this reason:

- When a patient presents with psychotic or psychotic-like symptoms, a broad differential is expected, given that there are a multitude of disorders that can present with symptoms similar to schizophrenia. In this regard, you should consider schizophrenia to be a diagnosis of exclusion.
- Individuals with schizophrenia are "ideal" test subjects for the oral board examination. "To know schizophrenia is to know psychiatry."

Symptom Domains in Schizophrenia—The Seven "Pillars"

➤ Various combinations of symptoms from the five domains described by Criterion A (delusions, hallucinations, disorganization, catatonia, and negative symptoms), together with symptoms from two associated domains (cognitive deficits and depressed mood), form the foundation (i.e., the "pillars") of the schizophrenic process.

Delusions (Pillar 1):

➤ Are a prominent feature of the paranoid type of schizophrenia, but can also be present in other types of schizophrenia and in a wide range of psychiatric, medical, and substance-related disorders.

➤ Are categorized by Criterion A1.

➤ Are defined as false beliefs to the extent that there is an impairment in reality testing (i.e., psychosis). By definition, the belief is not true, cannot be corrected by reasoning or by presenting proof to the contrary, and is not culturally based.

➤ In schizophrenia can take virtually any form:

✔ Bizarre delusions:

- Are incomprehensible and therefore totally unbelievable (e.g., being spied on by Martians).
- Will, in themselves, fully satisfy Criterion A.

✔ Nonbizarre delusions:

- Are plausible and therefore possibly believable (e.g., being spied on by neighbors or believing one's spouse is having an affair).
- Are more difficult to assess in terms of being true or false.
- Are a cardinal feature of delusional disorder but are also present in other psychotic disorders.

✔ Systematized delusions are centered around a theme (e.g., religious, sexual, jealous, somatic).

✔ Nonsystematized delusions incorporate multiple themes (e.g., combined religious and somatic).

Delusions with distinct themes:

➤ *Grandiose*—delusion that the person is special or has special powers (e.g., the person believes he or she is the President or has a special mission to save the world).

➤ *Paranoid*—delusion that one is being persecuted (e.g., the person believes that the FBI has implanted a microphone in her brain so that her thoughts can be heard and used against her).

➤ *Somatic*—delusion that a bodily part or function is missing or impaired (e.g., the person believes that his heart or brain is missing or is not functioning).

➤ *Sexual*—delusion involving sexual themes (e.g., the person believes he has fathered more than 10,000 children).

➤ *Nihilistic*—delusion that one is dead or is dying or that the world is nonexistent.

➤ *Religious*—delusion involving a religious theme (e.g., God will punish those who enjoy pornography), at times with punitive ramifications (e.g., self-enucleation for watching pornography).

Delusions of reference:

➤ Belief that the behavior or words of others have a special meaning (e.g., a message on the radio about storms and lightning is interpreted as a signal from God that the world is coming to an end).

➤ Differ from ideas of reference, where the interpretation does not reach psychotic proportions (somewhat of a gray area of distinction).

Delusions of thought:

➤ *Thought insertion*—delusion that thoughts can be implanted in one's brain.

➤ *Thought withdrawal*—delusion that thoughts can be withdrawn from one's brain.

➤ *Thought control*—delusion that one's thoughts can be controlled by another person.

➤ *Thought broadcasting*—delusion that one's thoughts can be heard or recognized by others without being spoken.

Delusional syndromes (not all are associated with schizophrenia):

➤ *Capgras' syndrome*—delusion that someone, usually emotionally close to the person, has been replaced by an impostor ("delusion of doubles").

➤ *Fregoli's syndrome*—delusion that a familiar person is actually manifested in several other people ("delusion of disguises").

➤ *Cotard's syndrome*—delusion in which a person believes that he or she is dead, does not exist, or that the world does not exist (a nihilistic delusion).

➤ *Van Gogh syndrome*—dramatic self-mutilation. Perhaps delusional in nature.

➤ *Othello syndrome* (conjugal paranoia)—delusion of infidelity of a spouse or sexual partner.

➤ *Folie a deux* (shared psychotic disorder)—the same delusion is shared by two people with close attachments.

➤ *de Clérambault's syndrome (erotomania)*—delusional syndrome in which a person falsely believes that another person, often of higher social status, is passionately in love with him or her.

➤ *Anton's syndrome*—denial of the loss (anosognosia) of sight in a person with occipital lobe damage. Other types of denials can occur with other types of brain damage. Anosognosia is found in psychiatry as a lack of insight to the presence of mental illness (e.g., schizophrenia).

➤ *Prison psychosis*—paranoid delusions as a consequence of long-term isolation in jail or prison.

➤ *Paraphrenia*—poorly defined term reflecting the onset of systematized paranoid delusions and/or hallucinations starting late in life. Paraphrenia can be classified in many ways, including *late-onset schizophrenia with a good prognosis*. Overall functioning is usually good, and the disorder is not considered a consequence of dementia.

➤ *Koro*—delusion that one's penis is becoming smaller and will disappear, resulting in death ("penis panic"); prominent in Asian cultures.

➤ *Windigo*—delusion of being possessed by a cannibalistic monster (prominent in Canada).

➤ *Susto*—delusional syndrome in which a person believes a magical substance has entered their body; a common syndrome in Latin America.

Hallucinations (Pillar 2):

➤ Are a prominent feature of the paranoid type of schizophrenia, but also can be present in other types of schizophrenia and in a wide range of psychiatric, medical, and substance use disorders.

➤ Are categorized by Criterion A2.

➤ Are defined as sensory perceptions in the absence of external stimuli or sources.

➤ In schizophrenia:

✔ Are perceived as originating externally (33% of persons), internally (33% of persons), or a combination of both (33% of persons).

✔ Are most often auditory. Can take the form of intelligible voices (possibly command in nature) or unidentifiable sounds. Auditory hallucinations involving a running commentary on the person's behavior or thoughts, or two or more voices conversing with one another, will fully satisfy Criterion A.

✔ Can additionally involve the other four senses. However, if visual, olfactory, gustatory, or tactile hallucinations are present in the absence of auditory hallucinations, a medical ("organic") or substance-related cause is more likely. Some examples of organic etiologies include:

■ Temporal lobe epilepsy (olfactory hallucinations and religious delusions).

■ Migraine headache aura (visual hallucinations).

■ Alcohol intoxication (visual hallucinations).

■ Alcohol withdrawal (tactile hallucinations [formication]).

■ Hallucinogen intoxication (visual and olfactory hallucinations).

✔ May or may not be accompanied by insight as to their validity:

■ DSM-IV-TR does not fully clarify this issue for schizophrenia, except to say that persons with insight have a better prognosis. Most often, auditory hallucinations occur in the absence of insight into their pathological nature. Therefore, the person comes to believe that they are real.

■ In substance-induced psychotic disorder and psychotic disorder due to a general medical condition, insight regarding the validity of the hallucination is, by DSM-IV-TR definition, impaired.

✔ Must occur in a clear sensorium, not on awakening (hypnopompic hallucinations) or on going to sleep (hypnagogic hallucinations).

✔ Can occur in the absence of psychopathology. For example, highly religious individuals may, as a normal occurrence, experience hallucinations (e.g., seeing the Virgin Mary).

✔ Are not well understood mechanistically:

■ Increased activation (blood flow) to the auditory and visual cortices is associated with their corresponding hallucination.

■ Dopamine (DA) and serotonin (5-HT) excess are likely a factor in that the mechanism of action of antipsychotic medications is to block these neurotransmitters.

Hallucination syndromes:

➤ *Charles Bonnet syndrome*—visual hallucinations in a visually impaired individual.

➤ *Peduncular hallucinosis*—Lilliputian hallucinations (visual hallucinations of small people) secondary to midbrain lesions.

➤ *Formication*—tactile hallucinations typically involving the sensation of bugs crawling on or under the skin in a person undergoing alcohol or benzodiazepine withdrawal.

➤ *Oneiroid schizophrenia*—an older formulation of schizophrenia with a dreamlike state and perceptual disturbances.

➤ *Alice in Wonderland syndrome*—perceptual distortion in size and shapes of objects (e.g., a car appears the size of a cat).

Disorganized thinking and/or grossly disorganized behavior (Pillar 3):

➤ Are prominent features of the disorganized type of schizophrenia.

➤ Are categorized by Criteria A3 and A4.

➤ Can also be a presentation in other types of schizophrenia and in a wide range of psychiatric, medical, and substance use disorders.

➤ Represent an extreme disturbance in the person's ability to think or behave rationally:

✔ Disorganized thinking ("formal thought disorder") is manifested by:

■ Loose associations (nonsensical speech or writing, thoughts not logically connected, "derailment").

■ "Word salad" (totally incoherent speech or writing).

■ Tangentiality (jumping from one topic to another). Although commonly associated with mania, is often a presentation in schizophrenia.

■ Perseveration of speech (repeating the same oral or written statements over and over).

■ Neologisms (coining of new words).

■ Clang associations (connecting or rhyming of words by sound rather than by meaning).

✔ Disorganized behavior can be characterized by:

■ Childlike silliness.

■ Aimless, compulsive, or bizarre behaviors (e.g., collecting pieces of string, wearing multiple coats in summer, public masturbation).

■ Unpredictable and possibly aggressive behavior.

■ Perseveration of behavior (repeating the same behavior over and over).

Catatonic symptoms (Pillar 4):

➤ Are the predominant feature of the catatonic type of schizophrenia.

➤ Are categorized by Criterion A4.

➤ Present with significant psychomotor disturbance involving either excessive excitement or significant immobility.

➤ Can also develop as a consequence of medical illness (e.g., delirium, meningitis) or a mood disorder (e.g., major depressive disorder with catatonic features; bipolar I disorder with catatonic features). Because of the wide range of serious and life-threatening medical illnesses associated with catatonia, rapid medical intervention is mandatory.

Negative symptoms (Pillar 5):

➤ Are typically predominant features of the disorganized type, residual type, and prodromal phase of schizophrenia, but can be associated with all types of schizophrenia.

➤ Are categorized by Criterion A5.

➤ Constitute intrinsic deficits secondary to the schizophrenic process (i.e., are primary deficits).

➤ Are postulated to be due to one or more of the following:

✔ Dopaminergic hypoactivity in the mesocortical pathway.

✔ Dopaminergic/serotonergic imbalance in the prefrontal cortex.

✔ Decreased blood flow to the prefrontal cortex.

✔ Structural brain changes in the prefrontal cortex caused by errors in cell migration during fetal development.

➤ Are specifically characterized by DSM-IV-TR as:

✔ Affective flattening ("flat affect")—lack of discernible facial emotion, poor eye contact, lack of body movements (i.e., "no one home" presentation).

✔ Blunted affect—less severe than flat affect.

✔ Thought blocking—train of thought suddenly stops.

✔ Alogia (poverty of speech)—restriction in initiation and production of speech.

✔ Avolition (poverty of movement)—restriction in initiation and production of goal-directed behavior.

✔ Anhedonia (poverty of joy)—inability to experience pleasure (as opposed to *hedonism* [the pursuit of pleasure]).

➤ Additionally can include:

✔ Abulia (poverty of motivation)—restriction of will or motivation, often characterized by an inability to make decisions or set goals.

✔ Asociality (poverty of socialization)—restriction of social interactions, with little interest in developing relationships, friendships, or intimacy (including sexual).

➤ Are responsible for much of the long-term morbidity of schizophrenia.

➤ Typically intensify over time. For the paranoid type of schizophrenia, negative symptoms may progressively intensify while positive symptoms diminish.

➤ Are often overlooked because of their insidious onset and slow progression and the much greater volatility of positive and catatonic symptoms.

➤ May represent the preponderance of the presentation in a minority of patients (historically described as "deficit schizophrenia").

➤ Are significantly more refractory to treatment than are positive symptoms:

✔ Atypical antipsychotic medications (i.e., second-generation antipsychotic medications [SGAs[1]]) typically improve negative symptoms by approximately 10%–25% (somewhat controversial).

✔ Typical antipsychotic medications (i.e., first-generation antipsychotic medications [FGAs[2]]) are unlikely to improve negative symptoms and may actually worsen negative symptoms (somewhat controversial).

✔ A minority of patients dramatically respond to SGAs with a 60% or greater improvement in negative symptoms. These patients have been described as "awakenings" in that they demonstrate a dramatic response to medication treatment such that they are capable of leading productive lives, holding down jobs, and sustaining rewarding relationships.

➤ Are easily confused with "secondary" negative symptoms (i.e., negative-like symptoms not directly related to the neuropathology of schizophrenia): Examples of secondary negative symptoms include:

■ Antipsychotic-induced extrapyramidal side effects (EPS) (e.g., akinesia [absence of motor activity], bradykinesia [reduced level of motor activity]).

■ Environmental deprivation (e.g., living alone, absence of meaningful relationships, inability to sustain employment).

---

[1]SGAs include clozapine (Clozaril), olanzapine (Zyprexa), risperidone (Risperdal), quetiapine (Seroquel), ziprasidone (Geodon), aripiprazole (Abilify), and palperidone (Invega).

[2]FGAs include chlorpromazine (Thorazine), thioridazine (Mellaril), mesoridazine (Serentil), perphenazine (Trilafon), loxapine (Loxitane), trifluoperazine (Stelazine), thiothixene (Navane), haloperidol (Haldol), fluphenazine (Prolixin), and pimozide (Orap).

Cognitive deficits (Pillar 6):

➤ Are now recognized as a core component of the schizophrenia process as originally formulated by Kraepelin ("dementia praecox"). However, DSM-IV-TR does not give diagnostic weight to cognitive deficits, although consideration of cognitive impairments are described under Associated Features and Disorders.

➤ Involve impairments in memory, attention, learning, visual skills, verbal skills, and executive functioning. Executive functioning comprises elements of planning, organization, and problem solving.

➤ Include impairments in the ability to effectively filter and interpret external stimuli (a major deficit in schizophrenia).

➤ Are related to dysfunction of the prefrontal cortex (highly involved with cognition).

➤ Increase the likelihood of greater functional impairment and a poorer prognosis.

➤ Are a prominent feature of the disorganized type but not the paranoid type of schizophrenia. DSM-IV-TR states that the paranoid type presents with "little or no impairment on neuropsychological or other cognitive testing." (American Psychiatric Association 2000, p. 314).

➤ Can be further impaired by adding medications with anticholinergic properties (e.g., benztropine [Cogentin] to reduce EPS, tricyclic antidepressants [TCAs] to improve depression). Cognitive impairments not due to the neuropathology of schizophrenia are described as "secondary" cognitive deficits.

Depression (Pillar 7):

➤ Is gaining recognition as a core symptom of schizophrenia (controversial).

➤ Is described by DSM-IV-TR (Associated Features and Disorders) that mood symptoms can be comorbid with schizophrenia.

➤ Develops in 25%–50% of individuals with schizophrenia and can be associated with suicidal thinking and behaviors.

➤ Significantly contributes to the long-term morbidity of schizophrenia.

➤ Can easily be mistaken for a negative symptom.

➤ Is described as "secondary" depression when symptoms are not secondary to the neuropathology of schizophrenia .

Schizophrenia Subtypes

➤ DSM-IV-TR defines a hierarchical structuring for assigning the type of schizophrenia:

✔ Catatonic type is assigned whenever prominent catatonic symptoms are present, regardless of the presence of other symptoms.

✔ Disorganized type is assigned whenever disorganization or flat or inappropriate affect is prominent, unless the catatonic type is also present.

✔ Paranoid type is assigned when there is preoccupation with one or more delusions or hallucinations, unless symptoms characteristic of the catatonic or disorganized type are present.

✔ Undifferentiated type is a residual category in which active-phase symptoms do not satisfy another type of schizophrenia.

✔ Residual type is assigned when there are continued signs of the illness but the criteria for the active-phase symptoms are no longer met.

Schizophrenia, paranoid type:

DSM-IV-TR diagnostic criteria (both of the following criteria are met):

➤ Preoccupation with one or more delusions or frequent auditory hallucinations.

➤ None of the following is prominent: disorganized speech, disorganized or catatonic behavior, or flat or inappropriate affect.

Clinical and diagnostic issues:

➤ Requires either delusions or auditory hallucinations, although both are likely to be present. (Note: Hallucinations must be auditory.)

➤ Has an onset later in life, a more stable presentation, greater preservation of cognitive functioning, less pronounced flat or inappropriate affect, and a better prognosis than the disorganized type of schizophrenia.

➤ Delusions:

✔ Are not required to meet diagnostic criteria if frequent auditory hallucinations are present.

✔ Typically involve themes of persecution or grandiosity and are most often bizarre and systematized. If delusions are nonbizarre, it can be difficult to assess if the statements are fact or fiction (e.g., a somewhat mentally slow individual claims to be both a doctor and a lawyer). It is therefore important to assess if a questionable belief is a delusion. Ask: "Does anyone ever tell you that what you believe is not true?" By definition, a person with a delusion cannot be convinced that the belief is untrue, even with proof to the contrary.

✔ Can be either persecutory or grandiose.
Note. Given that DSM-IV-TR allows for both persecutory and grandiose delusions, *schizophrenia, delusional type* is a more appropriate description than s*chizophrenia, paranoid type.*

➤ Hallucinations:

✔ Are a predominant feature of paranoid type of schizophrenia (i.e., frequent auditory hallucinations) but are not necessary to meet diagnostic criteria if delusions are present.

✔ Can also occur in the other four senses. However, if visual, olfactory, tactile, or gustatory hallucinations are the *only* perceptual changes, a diagnosis of paranoid schizophrenia cannot be made. Instead, strongly consider neurological or substance-related causes for the hallucinations.

✔ Are often related to the delusional theme(s).

Schizophrenia, disorganized type:

DSM-IV-TR diagnostic criteria (all of the following are prominent):

➤ Disorganized speech.

➤ Disorganized behavior.

➤ Flat or inappropriate affect.

➤ Criteria are not met for the catatonic type.

Clinical and diagnostic issues:

➤ A combination of disorganized speech, disorganized behavior, and flat or inappropriate affect (all three) are essential diagnostic criteria.

➤ Characteristic findings include a flat, childlike, or silly affect. Individuals are usually active, but in an aimless, nonconstructive manner. Speech may be nonsensical, having meaning only to the person talking, possibly misinterpreted as Wernicke's aphasia (expressive aphasia with nonsensical speech).

➤ There is a relative absence of hallucinations and delusions. If present, they are superficial and poorly formed. However, DSM-IV-TR does allow for hallucinations and/or delusions as long as the other criteria are met.

➤ The disorganized type is the most disabling form of schizophrenia, was historically classified as "hebephrenic schizophrenia," and is now seen much less frequently than the paranoid type.

➤ An insidious onset usually before age 25 years, poor premorbid functioning, a disorganized active-phase course without significant remissions, poor overall functioning, significant progressive cognitive impairment (dementia praecox), and a poor long-term prognosis are characteristic of the disorganized type.

➤ Importantly, the disorganized and paranoid types present in dynamically opposite ways. Individuals with the disorganized type present with disorganization, flat or inappropriate affect, and cognitive deficits without prominent delusions or hallucinations, whereas individuals with the paranoid type present with delusions and/or frequent auditory hallucinations without prominent disorganization, flat or inappropriate affect, or cognitive deficits.

Schizophrenia, catatonic type:

DSM-IV-TR diagnostic criteria (at least two of the following are present):

➤ Motoric immobility, as evidenced by catalepsy (including waxy flexibility) or stupor.

➤ Excessive motor activity (that is apparently purposeless and not influenced by external stimuli).

➤ Extreme negativism (an apparent motiveless resistance to all instructions or maintenance of a rigid posture against attempts to be moved) or mutism.

➤ Peculiarities of voluntary movement, as evidenced by posturing (voluntary assumption of inappropriate or bizarre postures), stereotyped movements, prominent mannerisms, or prominent grimacing.

➤ Echolalia or echopraxia.

Clinical issues:

➤ Psychomotor disturbance is the defining feature of the catatonic type. Types of psychomotor disturbance include:

  ✔ Catatonic excitement (agitated, purposeless motor activity, not influenced by external stimuli).

  ✔ Catatonic restriction, immobility, or stupor:

    ■ Catatonic stupor—complete unawareness of the environment and surroundings.

    ■ Catatonic rigidity—voluntary assumption of a rigid posture, resisting efforts to move.

    ■ Catatonic posturing—voluntary assumption of an inappropriate or bizarre posture.

    ■ Catalepsy—cerea flexibilitas (waxy flexibility); the person can be molded into a position that is then maintained.

    ■ Catatonic mutism—purposeless refusal to speak; speechlessness.

    ■ Catatonic echo phenomena:

      • Echolalia—repetition of words spoken by another person.

      • Echopraxia—repetition of movements of another person.

➤ A protective hospital environment is usually necessary for catatonic states.

➤ Because of the similarities of the catatonic type to neurological illness (e.g., meningitis, neuroleptic malignant syndrome, serotonin syndrome), substance use (cocaine, alcohol withdrawal), and mood disorders (e.g., major depression with catatonic features, bipolar depression with catatonic features), a thorough medical workup is essential.

➤ Treatment with high-dose benzodiazepines or electroconvulsive therapy (ECT) are well-recognized treatment modalities.

➤ The catatonic type is now rarely seen in industrialized nations.

Schizophrenia, undifferentiated type:

DSM-IV-TR diagnostic criteria:

➤ Active-phase symptoms are present, but the criteria are not met for the paranoid, disorganized, or catatonic type.

Clinical issues:

➤ Typically, there is a mix of active-phase symptoms that do not fit any one type of schizophrenia (e.g., the presence of both delusions and disorganized behavior), or there is an unusual active-phase symptom (e.g., all the criteria for the paranoid type are met except that the hallucinations are olfactory).

Schizophrenia, residual type:

DSM-IV-TR diagnostic criteria:

➤ Absence of prominent delusions, hallucinations, disorganized speech, and grossly disorganized or catatonic behavior.

➤ Continuing evidence of the disturbance, as indicated by the presence of negative symptoms or two or more symptoms listed in Criterion A for schizophrenia, in an attenuated form (e.g., odd beliefs, unusual perceptual experiences).

Clinical issues:

➤ Much of the long-term morbidity of schizophrenia is associated with the residual phase manifested by negative symptoms and/or attenuated (milder) positive symptoms. DSM-IV-TR seems to imply that attenuated positive symptoms are "subpsychotic," using examples of odd beliefs or unusual perceptual experiences.

Phases of Schizophrenia

General considerations:

➤ The phases of schizophrenia potentially include a premorbid phase (few, if any, signs of the disorder), a prodromal phase (attenuated positive symptoms; developing negative symptoms), an acute phase (psychosis; active-phase symptoms [Criteria A1–A5]), a residual phase (resolution of active-phase symptoms; attenuated positive symptoms; negative symptoms), and a relapse phase (recurrence of active-phase symptoms [Criteria A1–A5]).

➤ DSM-IV-TR indicates that both the prodromal and residual phases of schizophrenia:

✔ Can present with similar features, especially with features of schizotypal, schizoid, or paranoid personality disorder (the "A cluster" of personality disorders).

✔ Can be diagnosed by the presence of either:

- ■ Two or more attenuated positive symptoms, such as:
  - ● Ideas of reference (but not delusions of reference), paranoid ideation (but not paranoid delusions), or magical thinking (but not delusions of thought).
  - ● Unusual perceptions (but not hallucinations).
  - ● Digressive speech (but not disorganized speech) or unusual behaviors (but not grossly disorganized behavior).
- ■ A predominance of negative symptoms.

Premorbid phase:

➤ The premorbid phase is the first recognized phase and leads to the prodromal phase. Although not addressed by DSM-IV-TR, the premorbid phase is critically important as a potential marker for the future development of early treatment interventions in hopes of preventing the illness from developing or for reducing morbidity. The Premorbid Assessment Scale (PAS) is a measure of progression of deterioration during the premorbid phase.

➤ Multiple impairments are evident during the premorbid phase, including:

- ✔ Deficits in cognitive functioning (including lower IQ) and difficulty in sequencing complex tasks.
- ✔ Neurological soft signs:
  - ■ Refers to neuromotor changes such as:
    - ● Alterations of smooth-pursuit eye movement (the eye does not move at the speed the tracked object moves; the most widely studied neurological soft sign).
    - ● Poor overall motor coordination.
    - ● Impaired sensory integration.
    - ● Decreased ability to recognize objects by touch and feel or to complete finger–thumb opposition.
  - ■ Are associated with greater cognitive impairment, prominent negative symptomatology, and a poorer outcome.
- ✔ Odd or unusual personality traits, especially schizoid, avoidant, and paranoid. These have been termed the *premorbid personality*.
- ✔ Physical anomalies (e.g., high arched palate, malformed ears).
- ✔ Delayed developmental milestones, often accompanied by a tendency to:
  - ■ Withdraw from friends and family.
  - ■ Have difficulty showing warmth and developing intimacy.

Prodromal phase:

➤ The prodromal phase, lasting from days to years, presents with attenuated positive and/or negative symptoms. A prodromal phase is seen in approximately 75% of schizophrenic patients. The individual may:

  ✔ Feel tense, have difficulty with concentration, complain of poor sleep and/or depressed mood, and function poorly at work or school.

  ✔ Further withdraw from family and friends.

  ✔ Present with eccentric ideas and erratic behavior (e.g., angry outbursts, unusual premonitions).

  ✔ Pay less attention to personal hygiene.

➤ Closer to the time active-phase symptoms develop, attenuated positive symptoms and/or negative symptoms become more pronounced.

Acute phase:

➤ Active-phase symptoms (Criterion A symptoms) emerge, perhaps after a serious stressor, after abuse of a substance, or for no discernible reason.

➤ Depending on the type of schizophrenia, the person will experience some combination of frank psychotic symptoms (e.g., auditory hallucinations, delusions, catatonia, disorganized thinking, disorganized behavior) possibly accompanied by negative symptoms. This constitutes the "first break."

➤ The person is usually hospitalized (an accepted modality for first-episode psychosis), and aggressive treatment based on a biopsychosocial model is instituted.

Residual phase:

➤ Assuming full resolution of active-phase symptoms (unlikely, but even less likely for the disorganized type of schizophrenia), the residual phase is established, and it is maintained until (and if) there is a relapse.

➤ The patient once again presents with attenuated positive symptoms and/or negative symptoms, similar to the prodromal phase.

➤ The long-term outcome often correlates with the magnitude and type of symptom presentation in the residual stage. Cognitive impairment, depression, and negative symptoms correlate with a poorer outcome. However, the degree of response to antipsychotic medications, extent of compliance to medications, presence or absence of substance abuse, and quality of the therapeutic alliance with treatment providers will also greatly influence outcome.

➤ Suicidal behavior tends to be more prominent early in the course of the illness, when patients are able to conceptually understand the damage the illness can cause, become actively psychotic, or become depressed.

Relapse phase:

➤ Involves the return of active-phase symptoms (Criterion A symptoms).

➤ Is more common with the paranoid type, resulting from poor medication compliance, from a relapse into substance abuse, from the experiencing of a stressor, or for no discernible reason.

➤ The disorganized type tends to have a chronic, unrelenting course without acute relapses or significant remissions.

➤ Requires the same considerations for management as the acute phase. Prognosis worsens with subsequent relapses.

Characteristic Findings in Schizophrenia

➤ Individuals with schizophrenia:

  ✔ Most often present with the paranoid or undifferentiated type of schizophrenia. The disorganized and catatonic type are less frequently seen in industrialized nations.

  ✔ Have been described over the years with what is now archaic terminology:

    ■ Latent schizophrenia—less ill patients, more consistent with schizoid or schizotypal personality disorder than with schizophrenia.

    ■ Oneiroid schizophrenia—dreamlike state, coupled with a strong hallucinatory component.

    ■ Simple schizophrenia—dysfunctional presentation without prominent psychotic features.

    ■ Pseudoneurotic schizophrenia—symptomatology consistent with a severe anxiety disorder that later develops into or manifests as a mild form of schizophrenia.

➤ In comparison with the general population, individuals with schizophrenia:

  ✔ Are more likely to develop HIV infection, breast cancer, obesity, poor exercise habits, and diabetes (before consideration of medication).

  ✔ Have higher mortality rates from cardiovascular disease, emphysema, infections, accidents, and suicide.

  ✔ Are three times as likely to smoke cigarettes (58%–88% smoke).

  ✔ Are more likely to abuse alcohol and illicit substances (particularly marijuana and cocaine).

  ✔ Must first be assessed for having a substance use disorder (e.g., cocaine), medical disorder (e.g., hyperthyroidism), or other psychiatric disorder (e.g., delusional disorder) before a diagnosis of schizophrenia can be made.

✔ Must have a dysfunctional course to satisfy DSM-IV-TR diagnostic criteria. Therefore, treatments for schizophrenia must not only reduce symptoms but should also be directed at improving functioning.

✔ Are likely to have a 10- to 15-year reduction in life from accidents, suicide, substance abuse, and the consequences of a poor life style (e.g., smoking, obesity, physical inactivity).

✔ Have an increased risk of suicide:

■ Ultimately, 20%–40% of persons with schizophrenia attempt suicide, and 5%–10% will eventually commit suicide (a more recent analysis puts the figure at ~ 6%).

■ Risk factors for suicide in schizophrenia include depression (a very high risk factor), male gender, multiple prior psychiatric hospital admissions, and prior suicide attempts. The risk does not appear to be related to the core psychotic or negative symptoms of the disorder. Suicide is more likely to occur during the early course of the illness.

✔ May eventually be protected from developing schizophrenia through early recognition and intervention programs (controversial; a developing area of research).

✔ Prognosis is poorer if treatment of the first psychotic episode is delayed 6 months or more (somewhat controversial). This delay has been quantified as the *duration of untreated psychosis* and typically averages about 12 months.

✔ Have inherently lower fertility rates:

■ Lower fertility rates coupled with a relatively constant prevalence of 1% establish that factors other than genetics may be operative with regard to the etiology of schizophrenia. Theoretically, lower fertility rates should, over successive generations, decrease the percentage of the population afflicted with schizophrenia. This premise has been termed the *schizophrenia paradox* and suggests that other factors (e.g., protective genes, environmental factors) also contribute to or protect against the development of schizophrenia.

■ Fertility rates are potentially further lowered by antipsychotic medications that increase prolactin levels (e.g., FGAs and risperidone). Patients switched from FGAs or risperidone to other SGAs may have an increased risk of pregnancy because prolactin levels are now lowered.

✔ Who commit violent acts often receive media attention. However, a definitive association between violent behavior and schizophrenia has not been proven and is a matter of considerable debate. Nonetheless, active psychosis from any cause (including schizophrenia) is a risk factor for violent behavior.

✔ Are often described as having a "formal thought disorder." However, this terminology should be used with caution, since it can have multiple definitions, including:

■ A synonym for disorganized thinking (the preferred definition described by DSM-IV-TR), manifested by loose associations, tangentiality, and word salad. DSM-IV-TR characterizes disorganized thinking as perhaps the single most important feature of schizophrenia.

■ The presence of any psychotic process (including psychotic disorders unrelated to schizophrenia).

■ A process reflective of Criterion A.

■ A synonym for schizophrenia itself.

✔ Must be assessed for the possibility that cultural factors, not schizophrenia, are responsible for the "psychotic" symptoms. What is considered a reality in one culture (e.g., witchcraft) might be considered a delusion in another, and an accepted experience in one culture (e.g., seeing the Virgin Mary) might be considered a hallucination in another. Failure to understand these cultural differences has likely led to a tendency to overdiagnose schizophrenia in minority groups, especially African American and Asian cultures.

✔ Have an increased (but poorly understood) tendency to compulsively drink fluids (polydipsia). Disorders of water homeostasis include compulsive water drinking, the syndrome of inappropriate antidiuretic hormone secretion (SIADH), and the syndrome of self-induced water intoxication (SIWI). Treatment is to enforce fluid restriction. Clozapine may be helpful as well.

✔ Have an increased propensity for compulsive behaviors (e.g., hoarding food, collecting garbage).

✔ Have an increased propensity for comorbid psychiatric disorders, including:

■ Depressive symptoms and depressive disorders (e.g., major depressive disorder, dysthymic disorder).

■ Substance-induced mood disorders.

■ Anxiety disorders (e.g., panic disorder, posttraumatic stress disorder [PTSD], social anxiety disorder, obsessive-compulsive disorder [OCD]).

✔ Present with dysfunction of the prefrontal cortex, as evidenced by:

■ Primary negative symptoms.

■ Cognitive impairment.

■ Perseverative errors (repetition of the same response despite being directed to change responses).

✔ Present with motor abnormalities related to:

- Frontal circuit dysfunction (e.g., poor eye tracking, poor sequencing).
- Cerebellar dysfunction (e.g., poor coordination, past pointing [poor ability to point correctly to a moving object]).

✔ Are typically poorly compliant with long-term use of antipsychotic medications, thus promoting high relapse rates (see the findings from the CATIE study in Chapter 9, "Miscellaneous Topics").

✔ Have a high propensity to become progressively dysfunctional ("downward drift") with time and with relapses.

✔ Have a higher propensity to have relatives with "schizophrenia-spectrum personality disorders," comprising schizotypal, schizoid, and paranoid personality disorders.

✔ Are appropriately characterized as having a "chronic relapsing illness." Even with rapid intervention and effective treatments, relapse rates are high. Twenty percent to 40% of schizophrenic patients who are appropriately taking antipsychotic medications continue to experience some measure of psychotic symptoms.

Historical Evolution of the Diagnosis

➤ Schizophrenia was first actively studied in the late 1800s. Kraepelin used the term *dementia praecox*. Bleuler coined the term *schizophrenia* as representative of a split of cognition from affect ("fragmented mind"), Schneider defined *first-rank symptoms,* and DSM standardized definitions and diagnostic criteria:

Kraepelin (1887):

➤ The disorder starts early in life ("praecox") as opposed to a late-life dementia. Over time, the disorder produces a pervasive and persistent impairment in many aspects of cognitive and behavioral functioning, eventually resulting in "dementia." Thus, Kraepelin believed that the disorder was a brain disease eventually leading to dementia in younger individuals. Kraepelin differentiated dementia praecox from manic-depressive illness (a less deteriorating course).

➤ A classic distinction between bipolar disorder and schizophrenia is that in bipolar disorder there is a return to normal functioning after resolution of a manic or depressive episode, whereas in schizophrenia there is progressively worsening impairment with repeated relapses (i.e., "downward drift"). However, recent studies are supportive of interepisode depression or depressive symptoms as a more common clinical manifestation of bipolar disorder, rather than symptom-free interepisode periods.

➤ In addition to being the first to characterize schizophrenia and bipolar disorder, Kraepelin was the co-discoverer (with Alois Alzheimer) of the recognition of Alzheimer's disease.

Bleuler (1911):

➤ Emphasized fragmentation and loose associations (thought disorder) as foundations of the disorder and renamed it *schizophrenia*. Lay individuals often inappropriately refer to the disorder as "split personality" rather than the more appropriate translation "shattered personality."

➤ Described "a group of schizophrenias" to reflect the diversity of illness presentations. He focused on negative symptomatology as being characteristic of the disorder, believing that delusions and hallucinations could be found in other disorders and therefore were not pathognomonic for schizophrenia.

➤ Recognized that some patients improve while others progressively worsen.

➤ Described what has now come to be known as the "four A's": loose Associations, Autism, Affective flattening, and Ambivalence.

Schneider (1957):

➤ Defined first-rank symptoms, focusing on positive symptomatology as the best indicators of schizophrenia. He emphasized an early age at onset, a generally poor outcome, and substantial cognitive impairment. Schneider's first-rank symptoms:

   ✔ Are intended to be more specific for psychosis associated with schizophrenia than for psychosis due to other disorders.

   ✔ Include:

      ■ Auditory thoughts (hallucinations).

      ■ Voices arguing or commenting on one's behavior.

      ■ Thought withdrawal, thought insertion, thought interruption, and thought broadcasting.

      ■ Somatic passivity.

      ■ Delusional perceptions.

      ■ Feelings or actions experienced as caused or influenced by external factors.

      ■ Experiencing of feelings or influences not originating with the individual.

The Diagnostic and Statistical Manual of Mental Disorders (American Psychiatric Association; first edition 1952):

➤ Was developed to improve reliability of diagnostic criteria for schizophrenia and other psychiatric disorders so that treatment providers could reliably diagnose psychiatric disorders on the basis of uniform sets of criteria and terminology.

➤ Is now in its fourth edition (DSM-IV), with publication of a text revision (DSM-IV-TR) in 2000.

Prognosis

➤ Typically, 15% of schizophrenic persons have a good outcome, 30% have an intermediate outcome, and 55% have a poor outcome. Assuming the most pure delineations, outcomes would range as follows:

✔ For the 15% of schizophrenic individuals with a *good outcome,* positive and negative symptoms gradually dissipate after the first or few psychotic episodes, possibly never to recur. This is more likely (but not guaranteed) to occur with:

■ Putting in place an early-recognition program to provide the best interventions before the first break.

■ Initiating aggressive treatment (based on a biopsychosocial model) immediately after the first break.

■ Developing and sustaining a healthy lifestyle (e.g., avoidance of alcohol and illicit substances, obtaining a job to improve self-esteem, regular exercise, healthy diet) with a goal of independent living.

■ Strict adherence to all treatment guidelines.

✔ For the 30% of schizophrenic individuals with an *intermediate outcome:*

■ The severity of the illness may plateau over time, with occasional psychotic exacerbations (relapses) followed by long periods of remission or partial remission (residual phases). During the prolonged residual phases, the individual may continue to experience attenuated positive and/or negative symptoms without a recurrent active phase. Eventually, negative symptoms become the predominant presentation (sometimes referred to as "deficit schizophrenia"), with lack of initiative, poor motivation, little social interest, anhedonia, and few emotional ties. These individuals can lead somewhat productive lives, especially if they are compliant with their treatment program and do not abuse substances.

✔ For the 55% of schizophrenic individuals with a *poor outcome,* one of two scenarios (with examples) is likely:

■ Paranoid type:

● Multiple cycles of psychotic relapses (with hospitalizations) followed by remissions (residual phases) or partial remissions, with a progressively dysfunctional, worsening, and chronic course ("downward drift"). The person may complain of extreme and irrational fearfulness or may manifest grandiosity. Poor treatment compliance, active substance abuse, depression, and suicidal behavior are common. Each psychotic relapse further propagates the downward course of the illness. Cognitive processes may be preserved. Poverty, placement in a group home or prison, and homelessness are possible outcomes. Life expectancy is approximately 10%–15% lower than that of the general population.

■ Disorganized type:

• A chronic active-phase course, typically without marked remissions, characterized by significant disorganization of thinking and behavior, negative symptomatology, and the progressive development of cognitive deficits. Inappropriate or flat affect is common. The person may act odd or bizarre, become disruptive, act silly, and use words or sentences inappropriately (e.g., word salad, clang association). Poor treatment compliance, active substance abuse, depression, and suicidal behavior are frequently present. Poverty, placement in a group home or prison, and homelessness are possible outcomes. Life expectancy is approximately 10%–15% lower than that of the general population.

➤ Table 1–1 presents the prognostic indicators for schizophrenia.

■ **Table 1–1   Schizophrenia prognostic indicators**

Factors	Good prognosis	Poor prognosis
Gender	Female	Male
Prodromal functioning	Good	Poor
Symptom onset	Acute	Gradual
Precipitating stressor	Present	Absent
Symptom profile	Predominantly positive symptoms	Predominantly negative symptoms
Presence of mood symptoms	Yes	No (blunted affect)
Family history of mood disorders	Yes	No
Family history of schizophrenia	No	Yes
Type of schizophrenia	Paranoid, catatonic	Disorganized
Onset	Later in life	Earlier in life
Interepisode functioning	Good	Poor
Duration of active-phase symptoms	Short	Long
Residual symptoms	Minimal	Many

■ **Table 1–1   Schizophrenia prognostic indicators** *(continued)*

Factors	Good prognosis	Poor prognosis
Insight into having an illness	Good	Poor
Support system	Good	Poor
Antipsychotic medications	Early use after illness starts and consistent compliance	Later use after illness starts and poor compliance
Response to antipsychotic medications	Good	Poor
Cognition deficits/ neurological soft signs	Clear/absent	Confused/present
Ventricular enlargement/ cerebral atrophy	Absent	Present
Substance abuse	Absent	Present

Epidemiology

➤ Lifetime prevalence is approximately 1.0% and is relatively stable worldwide. However, the prevalence of the type of schizophrenia is not constant. In the United States, the paranoid type is the most common presentation. The disorganized type can be found more commonly in Asian and African countries.

➤ Age considerations:

✔ Average age at onset (defined as the age at the first psychotic episode) is 21 years for men and 27 years for women, although signs of the illness (prodromal phase) may have been present for years prior to the first psychotic break. Ninety percent of individuals with schizophrenia fall into this category.

✔ The onset of schizophrenia before 18 years of age is less common, and before 10 years of age is rare (although symptoms are usually severe).

✔ The onset of schizophrenia after 45 years of age is classified as *late-onset schizophrenia.* Late-onset schizophrenia is more common in females, is often accompanied by prominent paranoid delusions, and responds reasonably well to antipsychotic medications.

✔ The onset of schizophrenia after 60 years of age (classified as *very-late-onset schizophrenia*) is very uncommon, occurs more often in women, and is typically accompanied by sensory losses (especially hearing). Kraepelin coined the term *paraphrenia* to reflect persecutory or grandiose delusions in patients with "well-preserved intellect and personality" (i.e., a relative absence of negative symptoms and cognitive impairment).

➤ Gender considerations:

✔ Schizophrenia (not late-onset or very-late-onset) occurs in younger men and women with equal frequency (although DSM-IV-TR indicates that the incidence is slightly greater in men).

✔ Men typically have a more severe form of the illness, more prominent negative symptoms, an earlier age at onset, a poorer prognosis, a poorer response to antipsychotic medications, and a greater potential for suicide than women.

✔ Women typically have more prominent mood symptoms, hallucinations, and delusions; better premorbid functioning; a later onset; better social functioning; a better response to antipsychotic medications; and a better prognosis than men.

➤ Cultural considerations:

✔ Cultural "pockets," in which schizophrenia is found at a greater frequency than the usual 1%, possibly occur secondary to:

■ "Downward drift," in which more severely impaired individuals progress toward lower socioeconomic status, congregating in poorer urban areas. Compared with the general population, migrants have an almost twofold risk of developing schizophrenia.

■ Genetically close relatives with schizophrenia may intermarry, thereby producing a higher proportion of offspring with schizophrenia.

Etiological Formulations

General considerations:

➤ Etiological formulations are multifactorial, complex, and intertwined. Thus, schizophrenia may best be characterized as a syndrome rather than a disorder. The phrase "risk architecture" reflects the complexity of the etiological considerations related to schizophrenia.

➤ By the early 1980s, several facts regarding the etiology of schizophrenia were well established:

✔ Schizophrenia is a brain disease, and the brain damage occurs relatively early in life.

✔ The limbic system and its connection are involved.

✔ DA is a key neurotransmitter in the expression and treatment of the illness.

✔ Schizophrenia runs in families.

➤ Despite the vastness of ongoing research, definitive knowledge regarding the etiology of schizophrenia has been slow to develop, because:

✔ There is a lack of uniformity in the type or extent of brain lesions or changes seen on brain imaging. New findings are frequently reported.

✔ The degree and types of clinical impairment vary greatly from one individual to another and, as the illness progresses, within the same individual.

✔ Multiple genetic etiologies, gene expressions, and protective genes may be present, with varying degrees of penetrance. New genetic presentations are consistently forthcoming.

✔ Environmental, developmental, and obstetrical factors are strongly suspected but are not firmly proven or universally accepted.

✔ No one theory adequately explains why the disorder usually first appears in late adolescence or early adulthood.

✔ The development of animal models to provide a research tool to help study the illness has been slow.

Overview of etiological hypotheses:

Stress–diathesis hypothesis:

➤ A stressor coupled with a diathesis (genetic susceptibility) translates into "changes" leading to the development of schizophrenia. As examples, a significant stressor (e.g., physical abuse, first move from home, death of a parent) coupled with low genetic susceptibility or a low-level stressor coupled with high genetic susceptibility can both lead to the development of schizophrenia.

Genetic hypothesis:

➤ Schizophrenia is an inherited illness encompassing one or more genes ("schizophrenia genes") coding for the illness.

➤ Genetic association is postulated to account for 50%–70% of the risk of developing schizophrenia:

✔ The risk of developing schizophrenia increases with closer genetic associations (two parents with schizophrenia > identical twin with schizophrenia > fraternal twin with schizophrenia > children from a schizophrenia parent adopted into a nonschizophrenic family >> general population):

✔ Concordance in identical twins is approximately 40% and for dizygotic twins approximately 10%–15%. If genetic expression were the only causative factor, concordance would be 100%. Thus, other protective factors must be operative.

➤ Abnormal genetic encodings linked to an increased risk of developing schizophrenia include (a very partial listing):

✔ Catechol-*O*-methyltransferase (*COMT*).

✔ Dysbindin.

✔ Neuregulin.

✔ Disrupted-In-Schizophrenia 1 (*DISC-1*).

- ✔ Regulator of G-protein signaling 4 (*RGS-4*).
- ✔ *G72.*
- ✔ *22Q11* deletion syndrome.
- ➤ The abnormal encoding:
  - ✔ May provide clues as to why there is a delay in the onset of psychotic symptoms of schizophrenia until early adulthood (just as there is a delay in the development of the symptoms of Huntington's disease).
  - ✔ Is more likely to alter the structure and functioning of the hippocampus and prefrontal cortex.
  - ✔ Leads to the possibility of utilizing novel medications directed toward preventing the abnormal genes from encoding abnormal proteins.
- ➤ The genetic hypothesis proposes that genetic errors may:
  - ✔ Produce defects in monoamine (e.g., DA, 5-HT) utilization and metabolism.
  - ✔ Produce defects in the development of the myelin sheath surrounding axons.
  - ✔ Promote errors in neuron cell migration in the fetus during pregnancy.
- ➤ Schizophrenia and bipolar disorder may share some of the same genetic expressions.

Dopamine hypothesis:

- ➤ A *hyper*dopaminergic state in the mesolimbic pathway is responsible for the positive symptoms of schizophrenia:
  - ✔ The increased hyperdopaminergic state may originate from one or more of the following:
    - ■ Increased DA[3] synthesis.
    - ■ Defective DA regulatory mechanisms.
    - ■ Upregulation of D_2 receptors (i.e., become more responsive to DA).
  - ✔ Agents that promote DA excess in the mesolimbic pathway (e.g., cocaine, amphetamine, apomorphine) can acutely produce psychotic symptoms indistinguishable from those observed during the active phase of schizophrenia.
  - ✔ Agents that block D_2 receptors (FGAs and SGAs), deplete DA stores (e.g., reserpine), or modulate DA activity (e.g., aripiprazole [Abilify]) in the mesolimbic pathway reduce psychotic symptoms.

---

[3]By convention, *dopamine* is abbreviated as *DA,* but the individual dopamine receptors (e.g., D_1, D_2) are abbreviated with only the *D.*

✔ If the antipsychotic medication blocks D_2 receptors to an excessive level (e.g., too high a percentage of the medication binds to the D_2 receptor, the medication binds too tightly to the D_2 receptor, the medication is released too slowly from the D_2 receptor), adverse side effects (e.g., EPS, consequences of elevated prolactin) can develop.

✔ An ever increasing number of DA receptors are being uncovered. D_2 receptor activity is of particlular importance. An increased density of D_2 receptor activity is found in the brains of schizophrenics, and effective medications to treat schizophrenia have potent D_2 receptor blockade activity.

➤ A *hypo*dopaminergic state in the mesocortical pathway (with projections to the prefrontal cortex) is responsible for negative symptoms. The prefrontal cortex is involved with higher cognitive functioning, such as working memory, attention, motivation, filtering stimuli, and emotional expression.

Serotonin hypothesis:

➤ An excess of serotonin (5-hydroxytryptamine [5-HT]) can induce psychotic symptoms. Supporting this hypothesis is the finding that hallucinogens acting as partial 5-HT_{2A} receptor agonists (e.g., lysergic acid diethylamide [LSD], psilocybin, mescaline) can produce florid psychotic symptoms indistinguishable from those of the active phase of schizophrenia.

➤ Blocking 5-HT_{2A} receptors (e.g., SGAs but not FGAs) purportedly has the added benefit of improving negative symptoms, reducing EPS, and reducing or eliminating prolactin increases. Additionally, the SGAs may improve depression and cognitive dysfunction, but more research is needed to formally accept this purported finding.

➤ SGAs (except aripiprazole) generally block 5-HT_{2A} receptors more than D_2 receptors.

Neurodevelopmental hypotheses (noninclusive list):

➤ There is an increased frequency of winter births (seasonality effect) and births further from the equator (latitude effect) among individuals with schizophrenia, possibly implicating a prenatal viral infection during the second trimester of pregnancy (e.g., influenza, rubella, toxoplasmosis, herpes simplex II).

➤ Nutritional deficits in pregnant mothers (e.g., calories, vitamin D, folic acid) are associated with an increased risk of schizophrenia in offspring (e.g., the famine ["Hungerwinter"] that occurred in The Netherlands near the end of World War II).

➤ Obstetrical complications at birth (e.g., hypoxia from prolonged labor, excessive maternal bleeding, forceps delivery) can lead to structural brain damage (particularly in the hippocampus) that may later result in the development of schizophrenia.

➤ Low birth weight and a shortened gestational period increase the risk of developing schizophrenia.

➤ During World War II, pregnant women were more likely to bear children who later developed schizophrenia if they learned of their husband's death during the pregnancy rather than before or after the pregnancy.

➤ Errors in neuronal cell migration in utero can lead to the development of schizophrenia later in life.

➤ Older males are more likely to father children who later develop schizophrenia.

➤ Thyroid abnormalities in the mother while pregnant may promote the later development of schizophrenia in the offspring.

Neurodegenerative hypothesis:

➤ Degenerative changes in brain structure of schizophrenic individuals progress over the life span.

➤ Elderly persons with a history of schizophrenia develop cognitive deficits virtually identical to those found in Alzheimer's disease, but without pathology consistent with Alzheimer's disease.

Autoimmune hypothesis:

➤ Schizophrenia shares many of the properties of the "autoimmune" disorders (e.g., multiple sclerosis, amyotrophic lateral sclerosis, systemic lupus erythematosus) in that both:

✔ Have a delayed onset of presentation.

✔ Have a progressively dysfunctional course.

✔ Are characterized by cycles of relapses and remissions.

Immune functioning hypothesis:

➤ Reduced immune functioning (e.g., immunoglobulin M [IgM], IgG, IgA) can be found in some individuals with schizophrenia.

Membrane hypothesis:

➤ Membrane impairments related to a deficit in unsaturated fatty acids and a decrease in the enzyme phospholipase A2 result in impaired signal transmission, thereby producing schizophrenia. Recent studies supporting the therapeutic benefits of augmentation of antipsychotic medications with high doses of fish oils rich in eicosapentaenoic acid (EPA) may involve this mechanism.

Glutamate/NMDA receptor hypothesis:

➤ Glutamate, the major excitatory neurotransmitter in the brain, naturally binds to the NMDA receptor. Drugs that block the NMDA receptor (e.g., phencyclidine [PCP], ketamine) can produce psychotic, cognitive, and negative symptoms indistinguishable from those of schizophrenia.

➤ This finding suggests that chronic glutamatergic underactivity and/or NMDA dysfunction can lead to the development of schizophrenia. This hypothesis is compelling, in that PCP can generate both positive and negative symptoms indistinguishable from those of the active phase of schizophrenia. Clozapine reverses the psychosis-inducing effects of PCP.

➤ Agents that augment NMDA receptor activity (e.g., D-cycloserine, glycine) purportedly improve negative symptoms in schizophrenia.

Structural and functional brain changes:

➤ Brain imaging demonstrates subtle structural changes, altered blood flow patterns, and metabolic changes in persons with schizophrenia. The most common findings are:

✔ Enlarged lateral and third ventricle spaces—a relatively consistent finding.

✔ Cortical gray matter atrophy (i.e., flattened cortical sulci)—a relatively consistent finding.

✔ Reduced size of the temporal lobes, frontal lobes, and prefrontal cortex.

✔ Reduced brain volume in the basal ganglia, amygdala, hippocampus, and olfactory bulb (reflective of alterations in the sense of smell).

✔ Reduced blood flow and decreased metabolic activity in the prefrontal cortex ("hypofrontality"), thereby purportedly promoting negative symptoms and cognitive deficits.

✔ Increased blood flow to Broca's area during auditory hallucinations and to the visual cortex during visual hallucinations.

✔ Increased density of DA receptors (from postmortem studies).

Infectious hypothesis:

✔ Infections from parasites (e.g., *Toxoplasma gondii*) and viruses (e.g., cytomegalovirus) can induce schizophrenia or psychotic symptoms.

Environmental hypothesis:

➤ Toxic chemicals in the environment, perhaps more prominent in poorer communities, cause brain damage that ultimately causes schizophrenia.

Mostly discounted hypotheses:

➤ Double-bind theory (no longer recognized as valid):

✔ Proposed that schizophrenia was caused by repeated contradictory patterns of interaction during early developmental years by a "schizophrenogenic" parent. For example, a parent tells the child to play outside while it is raining but not to come back wet. This becomes an unsolvable dilemma for the child, who will later, as a consequence of repeated contradictory patterns of interactions, develop schizophrenia.

➤ Expressed emotion (EE) theory:

✔ "High–expressed emotion" families (i.e., those in which family members shout at, are critical of, or are hostile to the schizophrenic person):

■ Do not contribute to the development of schizophrenia.

■ Do contribute to more frequent psychotic relapses.

➤ Sociocultural, social selection, "downward drift," and socioeconomic theories:

✔ Schizophrenia is found more often in immigrants, divorced or unmarried persons, persons living in urban centers, and persons of low socioeconomic status.

✔ These findings are suggestive of "downward drift," in that such living patterns are more likely the result of having schizophrenia than the cause of schizophrenia.

➤ Psychodynamic theories (no longer accepted as valid):

✔ Psychotic symptoms have meanings, and interpretations of these meanings are important for effective psychotherapeutic treatment.

Considerations in Differential Diagnosis

➤ Do not assume that psychosis is synonymous with schizophrenia. Psychotic symptoms also develop as a consequence of other psychiatric, medical, and substance use disorders. When providing a differential diagnosis, compile an extensive list of disorders that can be associated with psychotic or psychotic-like symptoms.

➤ Consider, as an example, a 30-year-old, never-married man who presents with anxiety and nonbizarre paranoid-like thinking in a clear sensorium. He is not working or going to school, receives Social Security disability benefits for a "nervous disorder," and has always lived with his parents. He denies a past or present history of alcohol or illicit substance abuse but reports smoking two packs of cigarettes daily. There is a history of a traumatic head injury at a young age, although cognitive abilities appear near normal or perhaps somewhat below normal. He notes compulsive tendencies, complains of a long history of depressed mood, refers to "Xanax" as having been helpful with his nerves, denies a history of manic or hypomanic episodes, and presents with restricted or perhaps blunted affect and poor eye contact. At one time he had a thyroid problem, but he is not currently taking any prescribed medications. However, he is taking a medication he found on the Internet to lose weight. A broad differential diagnosis for this patient would include the following:

✔ Psychiatric disorders:

■ Schizophrenia (paranoid vs. undifferentiated type), brief psychotic disorder, schizoaffective disorder, schizophreniform disorder, and delusional disorder, persecutory type. Although brief psychotic disorder seems unlikely, he could be recovering. The undifferentiated type of schizophrenia seems unlikely in this case, but you might choose to include it as well.

■ Mood disorder with psychotic features (e.g., major depressive disorder, bipolar I and II disorders), and dysthymic disorder. The fact that the patient denies a history of manic or hypomanic episodes does not rule out bipolar disorder, given that patients may not recall these episodes or feel that they are abnormal.

■ Anxiety disorders (e.g., generalized anxiety disorder, obsessive-compulsive disorder). The anxiety can appear to be paranoid-like and the hoarding can be consistent with obsessive-compulsive disorder.

■ Paranoid, schizoid, avoidant, and schizotypal personality disorders. These disorders, although not psychotic in nature, can present with symptoms sufficiently similar to those of a psychotic disorder and should be included in your differential. The patient's paranoid-like thinking, reclusiveness, and compulsive behaviors are consistent with these possibilities.

✔ Psychotic disorder due to a general medical condition:

■ A frontal lobe head injury could have led to blunted affect and psychosis, and thyroid disease could lead to a mood disorder with psychotic features (hypothyroidism) or to frank psychosis (hyperthyroidism). Also consider neurosyphilis and HIV infection ("the great imitators").

■ Even if there is no clear indication of a medical disorder causing psychosis, always include this possibility in your differential.

✔ Substance-induced psychotic disorder:

■ Despite a patient's denial of substance use, always include substance abuse as a potential cause of psychosis in your differential.

■ The medication this patient is taking to lose weight could contain ephedrine (e.g., ma huang) or other stimulant, which at high-enough doses can cause psychosis.

■ Prescribed medications can induce psychosis when administered:

  ● At higher-than-normal doses (e.g., digoxin, ephedrine).

  ● At normal doses in the elderly.

  ● To patients who are naturally slow metabolizers of medications (e.g., genetically slowed hepatic metabolism).

  ● To patients with renal or hepatic impairment.

  ● Along with other medications that inhibit their metabolism.

  ● To medically ill individuals.

- For all patients, always consider the possibility that prescribed or over-the-counter medications can be the cause of psychosis.

✔ Malingering:

- The individual is not working or going to school, lives at home, and is supported by Social Security.

➤ After providing a broad differential, offer a provisional diagnosis that you feel is best representative of the history and presentation. The clients chosen for the board and the short time for presentation generates tremendous ambiguity into your ability to provide *the* correct diagnosis. This is, then, the essence of the oral board—to see if you can provide a broad differential and then to support your position.

➤ A provisional diagnosis can be anything you choose *that you can support.* My list of potential provisional diagnoses supported by the information provided includes schizophrenia, schizoaffective disorder, obsessive-compulsive disorder, a mood disorder with psychotic features, and malingering, but you may see others. I might choose schizophrenia as my provisional diagnosis, because it provides the broadest possible considerations for discussion and seemingly best fits the information provided.

Psychological Screening Tools

➤ Utilize psychological screening to assess for the presence and severity of psychotic symptoms and the response to treatment:

✔ Structured Clinical Interview for DSM-IV-TR (SCID)—can help elucidate the presence of psychotic symptomatology (hallucinations, delusions) in patients who do not readily volunteer information. Example questions include:

- "Has it ever seemed like people were talking about you or taking special notice of you?"

- "Did you ever feel that someone or something outside yourself was controlling your thoughts or actions against your will?"

- "Did you ever hear things that other people couldn't hear, such as noises or the voices of people whispering or talking?"

✔ Brief Psychiatric Rating Scale (BPRS)—an 18-item scale measuring positive symptoms, general psychopathology, and affective symptoms. Higher numbers are indicative of more severe psychosis.

✔ Positive and Negative Symptom Scale (PANSS)—a 30-item rating instrument evaluating the presence and severity of positive, negative, and general psychopathology of schizophrenia. Higher numbers are indicative of more severe psychosis or greater negative psychopathology.

✔ Scale for the Assessment of Positive Symptoms (SAPS) and Scale for the Assessment of Negative Symptoms (SANS).

✔ Clinical Global Impression (CGI)—a three-item scale used to assess treatment response in psychiatric patients (Severity of Illness, Global Improvement, Efficacy Index).

✔ Minnesota Multiphasic Personality Inventory–II (MMPI-II)—composed of 567 self-report items answered either "true" or "false" by the respondent. Usually employed as a personality inventory, the MMPI-II includes paranoia and schizophrenia scales as well. Scoring can be done by computer. Clinical scales are:

■ Scale 1: Hypochondriasis

■ Scale 2: Depression

■ Scale 3: Hysteria

■ Scale 4: Psychopathic Deviate

■ Scale 5: Masculinity–Femininity

■ Scale 6: Paranoia

■ Scale 7: Psychasthenia

■ Scale 8: Schizophrenia

■ Scale 9: Hypomania

■ Scale 10: Social Introversion

✔ Projective testing (to assess for psychosis):

■ Rorschach ("inkblot") test.

■ Thematic Apperception Test (the patient develops stories related to black-and-white pictures).

Overview of Somatic Treatments for Schizophrenia

FGAs:

➤ Are also referred to as typical antipsychotic medications. Historically, FGAs have been described as "neuroleptics" and "major tranquilizers" because of their potential to cause extrapyramidal side effects (EPS) and tranquilization/sedation, respectively. Neither term is suitable for today's classification of antipsychotic medications.

➤ Include all antipsychotic medications introduced before clozapine in 1990.

➤ Listed in order of increasing relative potency in reducing psychotic symptoms (i.e., low potency is indicative of higher doses):

✔ Low potency—chlorpromazine (Thorazine), thioridazine (Mellaril), and mesoridazine (Serentil).

✔ Medium potency—perphenazine (Trilafon), loxapine (Loxitane), trifluo-perazine (Stelazine), and thiothixene (Navane).

✔ High potency—haloperidol (Haldol), fluphenazine (Prolixin), and pimo-zide (Orap).

➤ Achieve their therapeutic effects and derive some of their side effects from D_2 blockade in specific neural pathways:

✔ Mesolimbic pathway (origin of positive symptoms):

■ D_2 receptor blockade is expected to confer antipsychotic activity (i.e., reduce positive symptoms).

✔ Mesocortical pathway (origin of negative symptoms):

■ D_2 receptor blockade is expected to worsen negative symptoms (on the basis of a hypodopaminergic model).

✔ Nigrostriatal pathway (includes the substantia nigra, neostriatum, globus pallidus, and subthalamic regions of the brain; origin of basal ganglia movement disorders and EPS):

■ D_2 receptor blockade is expected to induce EPS and, over a longer period of time, TD.

✔ Tuberoinfundibular pathway (originates in the hypothalamus, with pro-jections to the pituitary; modulates prolactin release):

■ D_2 receptor blockade is expected to increase serum prolactin levels, possibly resulting in sexual side effects (e.g., reduced libido, orgas-mic dysfunction, impotence), galactorrhea, amenorrhea, "menstrual chaos," gynecomastia, decreased fertility in females, and decreased bone density.

✔ Brain stem chemoreceptor trigger zone:

■ D_2 receptor blockade is expected to confer antiemetic effects.

➤ Have an overall less-favorable side-effect profile than the SGAs (except for clozapine):

✔ Weight gain, EPS, anticholinergic side effects, and sexual side effects:

■ Are the most common patient complaints.

■ Adversely affect compliance.

■ Typically increase with increasing dose and may produce significant or intolerable side effects at doses required for efficacy.

➤ Are a viable choice for:

✔ Acute management of psychosis when agitation and aggressiveness are emergent concerns (e.g., nondepot intramuscular formulations of halo-peridol, fluphenazine, chlorpromazine).

✔ Maintenance therapy under some circumstances (e.g., patient preference, prior robust response, poor compliance with oral medications [depot formulations of haloperidol and fluphenazine], absence of troubling [e.g., anticholinergic side effects from chlorpromazine; EPS from haloperidol] or serious side effects [e.g., TD]). Choosing an FGA on the basis of lower cost is controversial.

SGAs:

➤ Are also referred to as *atypical antipsychotic medications. Atypical* can be defined in two ways:

✔ *Atypical* confers the ability to effectively treat positive symptoms, significantly improve (but not totally reverse) negative symptoms, minimize or eliminate the development of EPS, have little to no impact on increasing serum prolactin, and provide efficacy for patients refractory to the FGAs and other SGAs. Under this strict definition, only clozapine is atypical.

✔ *Atypical* confers the ability to effectively treat positive symptoms with minimal impact on inducing EPS. Under this less-strict definition:

■ Clozapine and quetiapine are the most atypical (i.e., least potential for causing EPS).

■ Olanzapine, ziprasidone, and aripiprazole are mostly atypical.

■ Risperidone and paliperidone are mostly atypical at lower doses but become typical as the dosage increases.

➤ Include clozapine (1990), risperidone (1994), olanzapine (1996), quetiapine (1997), ziprasidone (2001), aripiprazole (2002), and paliperidone extended release (2006).

➤ Listed in order of increasing relative potency in reducing psychotic symptoms:

✔ Quetiapine (Seroquel).

✔ Clozapine (Clozaril).

✔ Ziprasidone (Geodon).

✔ Aripiprazole (Abilify).

✔ Olanzapine (Zyprexa).

✔ Risperidone (Risperdal).

✔ Paliperidone extended release (Invega).

➤ Are considered first-line medications for the treatment of schizophrenia (clozapine is an exception; it is *not* a first-line choice unless suicidal ideation or behaviors are present).

➤ Are postulated to reduce positive symptoms by:

✔ Blocking both 5-HT$_{2A}$ and D$_2$ receptors in the mesolimbic pathway (all SGAs except aripiprazole).

✔ Acting as a partial agonist at D_2 and 5-HT_{1A} receptors and antagonist at 5-HT_{2A} receptors (aripiprazole) in the mesolimbic pathway. Evidence is mounting that 5-HT plays an important role in the pathogenesis and treatment of schizophrenia because:

- All SGAs block 5-HT_{2A} receptors.
- SGAs provide greater blockade of 5-HT_{2A} than D_2 receptor blockade.
- Aripiprazole is the first antipsychotic medication to effectively reduce positive symptoms without blocking D_2 receptors.
- Clozapine is not a strong antagonist of D_2 receptors.

➤ Are postulated to reduce or eliminate EPS by what is termed the *fast-off theory* (i.e., the tightness of SGA binding to D_2 receptors is sufficiently low to prevent the development of EPS).

➤ Are less likely than the FGAs to cause:

✔ Clinically significant drug interactions.

✔ Anticholinergic side effects (except for clozapine).

✔ Seizures (except for clozapine and, to a much lesser extent, olanzapine).

✔ EPS (except for both risperidone and paliperidone at higher doses).

✔ Tardive dyskinesia.

✔ Sexual side effects (except for risperidone and paliperidone).

➤ Are more likely than the FGAs to:

✔ Improve negative symptoms (somewhat controversial).

✔ Improve depression and the cognitive deficits (two of the seven pillars) inherent in schizophrenia (very controversial).

✔ Have antisuicidal properties (clozapine, possibly olanzapine).

✔ Have mood-stabilizing properties (except for chlorpromazine).

✔ Increase financial costs to the patient.

Amoxapine (Asendin):

➤ Is a heterocyclic antidepressant with strong norepinephrine but weak 5-HT reuptake inhibition. A metabolite, 7-hydroxyamoxapine, has D_2 receptor blockade activity additionally conferring antipsychotic activity.

➤ Significantly blocks the cholinergic, histaminic, and alpha$_1$-adrenergic receptors, possibly leading to a multitude of side effects (e.g., dry mouth, urinary hesitancy, dizziness, sedation, weight gain).

➤ Has a high potential for seizures and suicide in overdose.

➤ Dosage is 200–300 mg/day for outpatient treatment and as high as 600 mg/day in inpatient settings. No single dose should exceed 300 mg.

Alternative and experimental treatments:

➤ Numerous alternative and experimental treatments for schizophrenia have been proposed over the years. Examples are high-dose benzodiazepines, mood stabilizers, glycine (may reduce negative symptoms), D-cycloserine, high-dose propranolol, reserpine (depletes DA but can induce depression), megavitamins (vitamine E, C, and B), alpha lipoic acid, omega-3 fatty acids, dietetic measures, herbal remedies, sleep management, chewing betel nut, alternating cold and hot baths, "creative arts therapies" (e.g., music, art, dance), aromatherapy, and acupuncture.

Electroconvulsive therapy:

➤ Can be an effective treatment for medication-refractory schizophrenia:

✔ Effectiveness is improved when ECT is combined with an antipsychotic medication.

✔ ECT is especially effective for schizophrenia, catatonic type, and for catatonia in general.

Side-Effect Profiles of Antipsychotic Medications

Side effects secondary to D_2 receptor blockade:

Acute EPS:

➤ Develop secondary to dose-dependent D_2 receptor blockade within the basal ganglia when 80% or more of D_2 receptors are bound by the antipsychotic medication. The SGAs, by virtue of their loose binding to D_2 receptors, have less potential to induce EPS than do FGAs.

➤ The relative ordering of the antipsychotic medications with regard to their propensity to induce EPS (from higher to lower) is as follows:

✔ High-potency FGAs > risperidone/paliperidone (at high doses) > low-potency FGAs/ziprasidone/olanzapine > clozapine/quetiapine.

➤ Encompass the following:

✔ Pseudoparkinsonism (also referred to as parkinsonism):

■ Symptoms can be identical to those observed in Parkinson's disease:

● Akinesia (absence of movements).

● Bradykinesia (slowness of movements).

● Rigidity in arms and shoulders

● Hypersalivation.

● Masklike facies.

● Cogwheel rigidity.

● Postural difficulties (e.g., shuffling gait).

- In lay terms, described as the "Thorazine shuffle" (dull-eyed stare and stiff-legged walk).
- "Rabbit syndrome" (perioral tremor) of the lips. Develops late in antipsychotic therapy. Easily mistaken for early tardive dyskinesia.

✔ Acute akathisia (motor restlessness; inability to sit still):

- Typically seen early in treatment or with dosage increases of high-potency FGAs/high-dose risperidone/paliperidone.
- Is the most common antipsychotic-induced movement disorder.
- Symptoms increase in severity with increasing antipsychotic dose.
- Are a major cause of poor compliance to antipsychotic medications.
- Can be assessed with the Barnes Akathisia Scale (four-item rating scale).
- May be referred to as "pseudoakathisia" when there is an inner feeling of restlessness.

✔ Acute dystonia (involuntary spasms or stiffness):

- Can be terrifying to the patient.
- Risk is higher in males and at younger age.
- Are often described by the patient as an "allergy" to the antipsychotic medication.
- Include:
  - Laryngospasm and swelling of the tongue (can close the airway).
  - Bruxism (grinding of teeth).
  - Spasmodic torticollis (spasm of cervical muscles of the neck).
  - Trismus (spasms of the muscles of mastication).
  - Oculogyric crisis (eyes rolled back in a locked position).
  - Blepharospasm (spasm of the eyelid).
- Can be assessed with the Extrapyramidal Symptom Rating Scale (a 62-item rating scale that detects EPS and TD) or the Simpson-Angus Scale (10-item rating scale).
- Is more likely to develop in patients:
  - Treated with high-potency FGAs with inherently low anticholinergic activity (e.g., haloperidol, fluphenazine) and the SGA risperidone at dosages greater than 4–6 mg/day.
  - Who are of younger age.
  - Who are of African American and Asian races (possibly secondary to genetically slower metabolism).
  - With a prior history of EPS.
- Typically begins within hours or days of starting or increasing the dose of the antipsychotic medication.

■ May correlate with low serum iron in some patients. Correcting the anemia may reduce or eliminate the EPS.

■ Can be treated with a variety of approaches, including:

- Waiting for tolerance to develop (a poor choice in that the patient remains in discomfort, pain, or, in the worst-case scenario, a life-threatening situation if laryngeal muscles are involved).

- Reducing the dosage of the antipsychotic medication (can compromise therapeutic effectiveness).

- Switching from a high-potency FGA to a low-potency FGA or to an SGA (effective for parkinsonism and dystonia).

- Adding an anticholinergic agent (effective for parkinsonism and dystonia):

  ▸ Useful medications include:

    ✓ Benztropine mesylate (Cogentin) 1–2 mg orally bid–tid or 1–2 mg intramuscularly on an as-needed basis.

    ✓ Trihexyphenidyl (Artane) 5 mg orally bid–tid.

    ✓ Procyclidine (Kemadrin) 5 mg orally bid–tid.

    ✓ Diphenhydramine (Benadryl) 25–50 mg orally bid or 50–100 mg intramuscularly on an as-needed basis (provides anticholinergic and sedative activity).

  ▸ Anticholinergic medications should be limited to short-term use because:

    ✓ Long-term use may lead to TD (somewhat controversial).

    ✓ Abuse is possible (e.g., to promote anticholinergic delirium).

    ✓ The need for anticholinergic agents usually diminishes 7–14 days after starting or increasing an antipsychotic medication.

- Adding amantadine (a dopaminergic agent) 100 mg orally bid (effective for parkinsonism and dystonia).

- Adding a beta-blocker (effective for akathisia):

  ▸ Propranolol 20–40 mg bid.

  ▸ Nadolol up to 80 mg/day.

  ▸ Metoprolol up to 100 mg/day.

- Adding clonidine 0.1 mg bid–tid (purportedly effective for akathisia).

- Utilizing botulinum toxin (inhibits acetylcholinesterase; effective for dystonia).

- Adding a GABAergic medication (e.g., benzodiazepine, baclofen; effective for akathisia and dystonia).

➤ Table 1–2 lists the various types of acute EPS and their corresponding treatment options.

■ **Table 1–2   Acute extrapyramidal side effects and treatment options**

Type	Clinical description	Treatment options
Pseudoparkinsonism ("parkinsonism")	Presents with the classic symptoms of Parkinson's disease.	Oral anticholinergic agents. Amantadine. Switch to SGAs.
Acute akathisia	Presents with motor restlessness and may become intolerable.	Propranolol 20–40 mg bid. Clonidine 0.1 mg bid–tid. Benzodiazepines. Switch to SGAs.
Acute dystonias	Presents with sustained muscle contractions occurring within hours or days of starting or increasing the dose of an antipsychotic medication.	Intramuscular benztropine mesylate 1.0–2.0 mg or intramuscular diphenhydramine 50–100 mg provides immediate symptom resolution and confirms the diagnosis. Oral anticholinergic agents. GABAergic medications (benzodiazepines, baclofen). Botulinum toxin. Switch to SGAs.

TD:

➤ Literally means late-appearing *(tardive)* abnormal involuntary movements *(dyskinesia).*

➤ Is purported to be due to long-term D_2 receptor blockade in the nigrostriatal pathway leading to receptor supersensitivity (somewhat controversial).

➤ Is more likely to develop in patients who have experienced EPS.

➤ Is an ominous development, secondary to an insidious (i.e., easily overlooked) onset and progression, lack of reliable treatments, and potential to persist in two-thirds of patients despite discontinuation of the antipsychotic medication.

➤ Presents with involuntary movements characterized by a mix of orofacial dyskinesia, tics, chorea (jerking movements), and athetosis (writhing movements):

✔ Orofacial dyskinesia is the most common presentation and includes rhythmic movements of the lips (e.g., puckering, smacking), tongue (e.g., undulations, rolling motions, protrusions, "fly catching" movements), jaw (e.g., chewing, side-to-side movements, biting), and face (e.g., involuntary blinking, grimacing).

✔ Tongue fasciculations and periorbital movements are common early signs.

✔ Involuntary movements of the extremities are less common. Involvement of the esophagus, pectoral muscles, and diaphragm is rare but can be life-threatening.

➤ Incidence/prevalence:

✔ The risk of TD increases by approximately 5% per year for FGAs and 0.5% per year for SGAs. TD eventually develops in approximately 25%–50% of patients treated on a long-term basis with FGAs.

✔ TD does not usually develop before 2–6 months of treatment with FGAs but can develop much sooner in the elderly.

✔ Risperidone may have a higher risk of TD than other SGAs due to its greater potential to cause EPS.

✔ Clozapine has only rarely been reported to cause tardive myoclonus (jerklike movements) after long-term use.

➤ Course:

✔ TD may first emerge when the dose of the antipsychotic medication is reduced, exposing the underlying TD that was suppressed by the antipsychotic medication ("covert dyskinesia").

✔ If antipsychotic medications are discontinued very soon after the initial presentation of TD, dyskinetic movements may diminish or disappear. However, they may also continue unabated or progressively worsen. Generally, the earlier TD is diagnosed and the antipsychotic medication withdrawn, the greater the likelihood for partial or complete reversal of TD.

✔ Short-term (reversible) *withdrawal dyskinesia* can develop after abrupt discontinuation of an antipsychotic medication. A gradual rather than an abrupt medication withdrawal is always preferred.

✔ Movements similar or perhaps identical to those of TD have been reported in schizophrenic patients who had never been treated with antipsychotic medications.

➤ TD movements are:

✔ Involuntary, with patients usually unaware or not bothered by the movements.

✔ Exacerbated by emotional stress, volitional motor activity, attempts to inhibit the movements, low-dose anticholinergic medications (surprisingly, high doses may improve TD), and withdrawal of antipsychotic medications.

✔ Absent in sleep, reduced with sedation, suppressed by dose increases of the antipsychotic medication, and improved or clinically reversed with clozapine or olanzapine.

✔ Usually least severe in the morning and worse in the afternoon.

➤ Risk factors (vary from one report to another):

✔ Most agreed upon include advancing age (the most consistent risk factor), increasing duration of antipsychotic use, cumulative dose of antipsychotics, early emergence of EPS, and use of antipsychotic medications in patients with mood disorders, negative symptoms of schizophrenia, or brain damage.

✔ Additional risk factors may include female gender, dependence on alcohol or nicotine, long-term psychiatric institutionalization, schizophrenia, diabetes, African American race, depot formulations, and on–off ("drug holidays") rather than continuous use of antipsychotic medications. Studies are equivocal as to these factors being causative for TD.

✔ Anticholinergic agents are not felt to increase the risk of TD. However, low-dose anticholinergic agents (acting peripherally) can exacerbate TD movements, whereas higher-dose anticholinergic agents (acting centrally) may reduce TD movements.

➤ Differential diagnosis of tardivelike movements:

✔ TD (requires treatment with an agent that blocks D_2 receptors).

✔ Short-term withdrawal dyskinesia (when stopping or reducing an antipsychotic medication) possibly secondary to dopaminergic rebound, cholinergic overactivity, and/or DA–actetylcholine imbalance.

✔ EPS, especially akathisia.

✔ Basal ganglia movement disorders (e.g., Parkinson's disease, Huntington's chorea).

✔ Autoimmune diseases (e.g., multiple sclerosis).

✔ Neurological damage from:

■ Toxins (e.g., lead, mercury).

■ Infectious diseases (e.g., HIV, neurosyphilis).

■ Illicit drugs promoting neurodegeneration, with symptoms similar to Parkinson's disease (e.g., methamphetamine, Ecstasy, *N*-methyl-4-phenyl-1,2,3,6-tetrahydropyridine [MPTP]).

✔ Unusual or bizarre mannerisms associated with schizophrenia itself (disorganized type, catatonic type).

✔ Idiopathic dyskinesia (incidence increases with age); may be indistinguishable from TD.

✔ Substance intoxication (e.g., tremors secondary to lithium) and substance withdrawal (e.g., tremors secondary to alcohol withdrawal).

- ✔ Rabbit syndrome (a variant of EPS with oro-facial movements, but without tongue involvement).
- ✔ Poorly fitting dentures (easily mistaken for early TD).

➤ Variants of TD (treatment is like that of TD):
- ✔ Tardive akathisia (treat with beta-blockers, reserpine).
- ✔ Tardive dystonia (e.g., blepharospasm, torticollis). More painful and disabling than TD. Temporarily improved with anticholinergic agents, clozapine, and botulinum toxin.
- ✔ Tardive myoclonus (shock-like muscle contractions; reported (rarely) with clozapine). Treat with clonazepam or carbamazepine.
- ✔ Tardive tics and tardive Tourette's disorder (facial tics, vocal tics).

➤ Nonpsychotropic medications that can cause TD:
- ✔ Metoclopramide (Reglan).
- ✔ Prochlorperazine (Compazine).
- ✔ Promethazine (Phenergan).

➤ Prevention (the best "treatment"):
- ✔ TD may or may not be reversible; prevention and early recognition are therefore especially important.
- ✔ Assess the risk–benefit ratio prior to initiating or raising the dose of an antipsychotic medication.
- ✔ Use the lowest dose possible for the shortest time possible. If long-term use is likely, an SGA would be a prudent choice.
- ✔ Attempt to reduce the total cumulative antipsychotic dose by augmenting the antipsychotic medication with other agents that can help control symptoms (e.g., divalproex for agitation, diphenhydramine for sleep).
- ✔ Complete the Abnormal Involuntary Movement Scale (AIMS) at the start of therapy and every 3–6 months thereafter. The AIMS is a 12-step observer assessment for involuntary movements involving the lips, tongue, face, arms, legs, and trunk. Obtain a neurological consultation if the AIMS score becomes positive.
- ✔ Patients must be advised relatively early of the potential for developing TD. Document that the patient understood the risks (not just signed a form) for developing TD.

➤ Treatment:
- ✔ No single treatment is universally effective, although a multitude of options have been reported.
- ✔ Provide a trial of a medication or treatment reported to reduce TD movements: beta-blockers, clonidine, ECT, acetazolamide, bromocriptine (a DA agonist), amantadine (a DA agonist), vitamin E 1,600 IU/day, botu-

linum toxin, vitamin B_6, choline, insulin, GABAergic agents (e.g., baclofen, valproic acid, carbamazepine, benzodiazepines [particularly clonazepam]), lithium, melatonin, buspirone, amino acids (phenylalanine, tyrosine, tryptophan), high-dose anticholinergic medications, calcium channel blockers (e.g., verapamil), manganese (prevention and treatment), gamma-hydroxybutyrate, lecithin, opiates, DA depleters (e.g., reserpine [can induce depression]).

✔ Switch to clozapine or olanzapine. Both have been shown to reduce TD movements.

Hyperprolactinemia:

➤ Occurs when an excess of prolactin is secreted from the anterior pituitary gland.

➤ Develops (at least in part) when blockade of D_2 receptors reaches approximately 70% in the tuberoinfundibular pathway. The exact mechanism(s) are not fully elucidated.

➤ Is most prominent with FGAs and risperidone.

➤ Can lead to numerous side effects, including:

✔ Menstrual irregularities ("menstrual chaos"), galactorrhea, breast engorgement, hirsutism, decreased libido, anorgasmia, and infertility in women.

✔ Decreased libido, gynecomastia, erectile dysfunction, decreased spermatogenesis, and anorgasmia in men.

✔ Increased risk of osteoporosis secondary to reduced estrogen and reduced testosterone levels.

✔ Increased risk of cardiovascular disease (controversial).

✔ Increased risk of breast cancer and/or the spread of breast cancer in women with prolactin-sensitive tumors (controversial).

✔ Depression (controversial).

➤ Is a major cause of poor medication compliance.

➤ Is treated by:

✔ Reducing the dose of the antipsychotic medication (if possible).

✔ Switching to an SGA (except higher-dose risperidone).

✔ Adding a dopaminergic agent (e.g., amantadine, bromocriptine).

Side effects secondary to blockade of postsynaptic cholinergic, alpha$_1$-adrenergic, and histaminic receptors:

Side effects secondary to postsynaptic cholinergic (muscarinic [M_1]) blockade:

➤ Should be distinguished from muscarinic M_2 and muscarinic M_4 receptor blockade, which can lead to release of acetylcholine.

➤ Are prominent with the lower-potency FGAs (e.g., chlorpromazine, thioridazine) and the SGA clozapine.

➤ Can cause central and peripheral anticholinergic side effects:

  ✔ Central anticholinergic side effects:

    ■ Include cognitive impairment and confusion.

    ■ Are more common in the elderly.

    ■ In severe cases can lead to anticholinergic delirium from intentional overuse, unintentional overdose, or use in the elderly.

  ✔ Peripheral anticholinergic side effects affect multiple systems:

    ■ Gastrointestinal—dry mouth, delayed gastric emptying, and constipation, possibly leading to obstipation, megacolon, or paralytic ileus.

    ■ Genitourinary—urinary hesitation, urinary retention, delayed and retrograde ejaculation.

    ■ Visual—blurred vision (pupillary dilation), aggravation of narrow-angle glaucoma, and greater sensitivity to sunlight.

    ■ Cardiovascular—increased heart rate, hypotension, and quinidine-like arrhythmias.

    ■ Dermatological—decreased sweating, possibly leading to an increase in body core temperature and heat stroke.

    ■ Otolaryngological—nasal congestion.

➤ Can be treated by:

  ✔ Waiting for tolerance to develop (a poor choice).

  ✔ Lowering the antipsychotic dose (may compromise therapeutic effectiveness).

  ✔ Switching to a higher-potency FGA (at the expense of increasing the risk of EPS) or to an SGA.

  ✔ Reducing or eliminating adjunctive medications that also have anticholinergic properties (e.g., benztropine, diphenhydramine).

  ✔ Increasing fluid intake; adding bulk laxatives; utilizing sugarless gum, artificial tears, and artificial saliva; wearing sunglasses (pupils are dilated); avoiding situations where natural sweating is impaired.

  ✔ Adding bethanechol (a cholinergic medication) 10–25 mg bid or tid orally or sublingually (especially helpful for urinary hesitancy or urinary retention).

  ✔ Administering physostigmine intramuscularly to counteract central anticholinergic side effects or delirium.

Side effects secondary to alpha$_1$-adrenergic blockade:

➤ Include dizziness, postural hypotension (possibly leading to falls or syncope), reflex tachycardia, retrograde ejaculation, urinary incontinence (unusual), sedation, and weight gain.

➤ Are prominent with lower-potency FGAs and clozapine, and mildly to moderately prominent with olanzapine, risperidone, and quetiapine. Minimally present for ziprasidone and aripiprazole.

➤ Can be further aggravated by concomitant use of medications with alpha$_1$-adrenergic antagonist properties to treat hypertension or benign prostatic hypertrophy (e.g., prazosin [Minipress], tamsulosin [Flomax], terazosin [Hytrin]).

➤ Can be treated by:

  ✔ Lowering the antipsychotic dose (possibly compromising therapeutic effectiveness).

  ✔ Switching to a higher-potency FGA with inherently less alpha$_1$-adrenergic blockade (e.g., haloperidol, fluphenazine) or to the SGAs aripiprazole or ziprasidone.

  ✔ Dividing doses over the day.

  ✔ Using support stockings.

  ✔ Ensuring adequate salt and fluid intake.

  ✔ Reducing or eliminating other alpha$_1$-adrenergic receptor antagonists.

  ✔ Adding fludrocortisone (0.1–0.2 mg/day).

  ✔ Adding alpha$_1$-adrenergic agonists (e.g., phenylephrine, norepinephrine). However, beta-adrenergic agonists (e.g., epinephrine) should be avoided because they can further lower blood pressure.

  ✔ Adding sustained-release phenylpropanolamine (25–100 mg bid) or pseudoephedrine (15–60 mg tid).

Side effects secondary to histamine 1 (H$_1$) receptor blockade:

➤ Are prominent with lower-potency FGAs and the SGAs clozapine, olanzapine, and quetiapine.

➤ Include sedation and increased appetite (with possible associated weight gain). Appetite increase:

  ■ Is often associated with carbohydrate craving.

  ■ Is mediated through H$_1$, 5-HT$_{2C}$, and alpha$_1$-adrenergic receptor blockades (controversial).

  ■ With associated weight gain can lead to an increased potential for insulin resistance, increased leptin levels, hyperlipidemia, glucose intolerance, metabolic syndrome, and diabetes mellitus type 2:

- A genetic component may also be operative regarding glucose intolerance, in that a minority of patients may develop diabetes in the absence of weight gain.

- U.S. Food and Drug Administration (FDA) labeling changes regarding the possible link between SGAs and diabetes mellitus type 2 were announced in September 2003. Also noted was an increased background (i.e., nonmedicated) potential for schizophrenic patients to develop diabetes mellitus type 2. All SGAs carry this warning (not a black box warning).

- The relative ordering of the SGAs with regard to their potential to cause weight gain (from highest to lowest) is as follows:
  - Clozapine > olanzapine > risperidone/paliperidone/quetiapine > ziprasidone/aripiprazole.

- The risk of developing diabetes must be weighed against the risks inherent in not adequately treating the psychosis. Psychotic patients are less likely to adequately manage their diabetes or other medical problems.

- As per recommendations of the American Diabetes Association, for all patients prescribed an SGA, check:
  - Weight at baseline, at 1, 2, and 3 months, then every 3 months.
  - Fasting blood glucose and blood pressure at baseline, at 3 months, then at least annually.
  - Lipids at baseline, at 3 months, at 1 year, and every 5 years thereafter if normal.

■ May be prevented or treated by:

- Early intervention. Olanzapine, the most-studied SGA with reference to weight changes, causes the majority of weight increase within the first 12 weeks of use.

- Proactively dealing with the potential for weight gain by instituting a program of increased exercise and decreased caloric intake (behavioral modification) for all patients on any antipsychotic medication. For example, switching from sugar-laden soft drinks to water or diet soft drinks and developing an exercise program (as little as an additional 2,000 steps per day) can substantially protect from weight gain and facilitate weight loss. If weight gain continues to be problematic (i.e., greater than 5%–7% of base weight), consider:
  - Switching to another SGA (e.g., ziprasidone or aripiprazole).
  - Adding medications that are FDA approved for weight loss (orlistat [Xenical] 120 mg tid, sibutramine [Meridia]) 10–15 mg/day) or medications (off-label) that may promote weight loss (e.g., his-

tamine H_2 blockers [nizatidine] 150 mg bid, amantadine 100 mg bid, bupropion 75–150 mg bid, topiramate [Topamax] 25–100 mg bid, modafinil [Provigil] 50–200 mg/day, metformin [Glucophage] 500 mg bid–tid).

Cardiovascular side effects:

➤ Nonspecific electrocardiographic changes (clozapine and thioridazine).

➤ Cerebral vascular accidents are more likely in elderly patients treated with SGAs for dementia-related psychosis (FDA black-box warning for all SGAs).

➤ QTc interval prolongation:

✔ Is potentially dangerous. Manifestations may be brief and self-limiting, may manifest with syncope, or may progress to life-threatening polymorphous ventricular tachycardia (torsades de pointes). Intervals exceeding 500 msec could lead to death.

✔ In milliseconds: thioridazine (35.8), ziprasidone (20.6), quetiapine (14.5), paliperidone (12.3), risperidone (10.0), olanzapine (6.4), and haloperidol (4.7).

✔ Can be further increased by adding medications with inherently long QTc intervals (e.g., thioridazine + ziprasidone) or through drug interactions involving the cytochrome (CYP) 2D6 isoenzyme system (e.g., amitriptyline inhibits metabolism of thioridazine).

✔ Should be minimized:

■ Monitor ziprasidone for QTc interval prolongation at the start of therapy and then on a regular basis (not mandated by the FDA).

■ Avoid thioridazine and mesoridazine (use only as a last resort as recommended by the FDA).

Seizures:

➤ Are more likely to occur:

✔ With the low-potency FGAs (especially chlorpromazine and loxapine) and clozapine.

✔ As the antipsychotic dosage increases.

➤ Can be prophylactically treated with divalproex.

Neuroleptic malignant syndrome:

➤ Can conceptually be characterized as "severe EPS (i.e., extreme rigidity) with fever."

➤ May be part of the EPS spectrum of side effects (possibly secondary to dopaminergic receptor blockade in the substantia nigra producing rigidity and fever).

➤ Presents with symptoms easily recalled with the acronym *FARGO* (formulated by A. McLean):

✔ F   Fever.

✔ A   Autonomic dysregulation (e.g., hypertension, tachycardia, urinary incontinence, diaphoresis).

✔ R   Rigidity ("lead-pipe").

✔ G   Granulocytosis (as well as increased lactic dehydrogenase, liver function tests, creatine phosphokinase [CPK], and myoglobinemia).

✔ O   Orientation changes (confusion, coma).

➤ Can additonally present with acute renal failure (due to myoglobinuria), proteinuria, deep vein thrombosis, respiratory distress, and dehydration.

➤ Can develop within hours, days, or the first few weeks after initiating (or increasing the dosage of) an antipsychotic medication. Symptoms usually progress insidiously over 1–3 days and typically last 5–10 days after the antipsychotic medication is discontinued. For depot formulations, symptoms can last a month or longer. Ninety percent of cases occur within 30 days of starting or raising the dosage of the antipsychotic medication.

➤ Etiology is thought to be due to DA blockade in the basal ganglia. DA depletion from sudden discontinuation of amantadine (an indirect DA agonist) or stopping anticholinergic agents (cholinergic rebound induces DA deficit) can also precipitate neuroleptic malignant syndrome (NMS).

➤ Additionally reported (albeit rarely) with antidepressants, lithium, metoclopramide (Reglan) and prochlorperazine (Compazine).

➤ The incidence is difficult to quantitate due to differing diagnostic criteria, but likely ranges from .02%–2%. The fatality rate is 5%–12%.

➤ Risk factors are not clearly defined, but purportedly include FGAs > SGAs, high potency > low potency, prior NMS, male, age between 20 and 40 years, and rapid antipsychotic dose escalation.

➤ Treatment (mostly supportive) includes:

✔ Discontinuation of antipsychotic and anticholinergic medications.

✔ Hospitalization on a medical intensive care unit and provision of hydration and fever-reduction measures (e.g., cooling blanket, antipyretic medications).

✔ Trials of DA agonists (e.g., bromocriptine, amantadine, L-dopa), muscle relaxants (e.g., dantrolene, baclofen, benzodiazepines), carbamazepine, or botulinum toxin. The two most often-recommended medications are bromocriptine and dantrolene.

✔ ECT (ventricular fibrillation and cardiac arrest have rarely been reported).

➤ Rechallenging after recovery:

✔ Rechallenging with the same antipsychotic medication at the same dose has a high likelihood of again inducing NMS.

✔ Rechallenging with an SGA (particularly olanzapine, risperidone, or clozapine) with gradual dosage increases is likely a safer approach.

✔ Wait at least 2 weeks after symptom resolution before restarting an antipsychotic medication. Extreme caution is advised.

Hematological side effects:

➤ Transient benign leukopenia (~3% of patients).

➤ Agranulocytosis:

✔ Can lead to severe, life-threatening infections (e.g., pneumonia, sepsis).

✔ Is most prevalent with clozapine and chlorpromazine.

✔ Can be monitored by assessing the white blood cell (WBC) count:

■ Order a WBC count for any patient on an antipsychotic medication who develops a sore throat or other signs of an infection.

■ Routine WBC testing is mandated for clozapine.

Less prominent side effects:

➤ Hypersalivation (clozapine).

➤ Hyperthermia (secondary to anticholinergic side effects; developing NMS).

➤ Syndrome of inappropriate antidiuretic hormone secretion (SIADH).

➤ Retrograde ejaculation (thioridazine).

➤ Hepatic effects:

✔ Transient increases in transaminase levels (FGAs and SGAs), sustained increases in transaminase levels (rare), and reversible cholestatic jaundice with chlorpromazine.

➤ Ocular effects:

✔ Retinitis pigmentosa (lenticular pigmentation) with thioridazine at doses greater than 800 mg/day.

✔ Cataract formation with quetiapine.

➤ Circulatory effects:

✔ Venous thrombosis, possibly leading to pulmonary embolism (clozapine).

➤ Dermatological effects:

✔ Skin rash, abnormal pigmentation, and photosensitivity (chlorpromazine, thioridazine, trifluoperazine, fluphenazine, and perphenazine).

➤ Urological effects:

✔ Priapism (thioridazine), likely secondary to alpha$_1$-adrenergic blockade.

✔ Urinary incontinence (FGAs, clozapine), likely secondary to alpha$_1$-adrenergic blockade.

✔ Urinary retention (e.g., chlorpromazine, thioridazine, clozapine) secondary to anticholinergic side effects.

➤ Hypersensitivity reactions at injection sites (e.g., Haldol Decanoate).

➤ Fetal toxicity secondary to teratogenic effects or systemic neonatal effects just after birth (e.g., chlorpromazine).

➤ Loss of gag reflex or difficulty swallowing (FGAs and SGAs).

➤ Bronchopneumonia.

➤ Sudden death:

✔ Often unexplained. Some reported causes include ventricular fibrillation secondary to QTc interval prolongation, cardiac conduction delays, paralytic ileus with megacolon-induced shock, and NMS. However, a true cause-and-effect relationship between antipsychotic medications and sudden death has not been firmly established.

Therapeutic Range and Therapeutic Index

➤ *Therapeutic range* (TR) refers to the difference between the highest and lowest effective dose. The broader the TR, the more difficult it is to establish an effective dose. For example, it is expected that it would be more difficult to find the effective therapeutic dose for quetiapine, which has a wide TR, than for risperidone, which has a narrow TR. Generally, a high TR is consistent with looser binding to D$_2$ receptors, conferring a lower risk of EPS.

➤ *Therapeutic index* (TI) refers to the ratio of the toxic dose to the therapeutic dose. Psychotropic medications with a low TI (i.e., the toxic dose and therapeutic dose are relatively close to each other) include thioridazine/mesoridazine, lithium, TCAs, and monoamine oxidase inhibitors (MAOIs).

Characteristics of the Common Antipsychotic Medications

Clozapine (Clozaril):

General considerations:

➤ Approved in 1990 for the treatment of schizophrenia refractory to other antipsychotic medications and in 2002 for schizophrenia or schizoaffective disorder accompanied by suicidal behavior.

➤ A low-potency medication with a wide TR.

➤ Unusual receptor activity, with D_1, D_3, D_4, D_5, and 5-HT_{2A} receptor blockade but little D_2 receptor blockade. D_1 and D_4 receptors are abundant in the prefrontal cortex but not in the nigrostriatal pathway (i.e., basal ganglia). This may explain why clozapine improves negative symptoms without inducing EPS. Also, clozapine alters glutamate/NMDA receptor activity and has GABAergic activity. This complex set of actions is felt, when taken together, to provide benefits for both positive and negative symptoms while reducing or eliminating EPS and sexual side effects.

➤ Moderate to high levels of blockade of cholinergic (M_1), histaminic (H_1), and alpha$_1$-adrenergic receptors confer a broad range of troubling side effects.

➤ Initiate dosing with 12.5–25.0 mg/day, and increase 25–50 mg every 1–2 days as clinically warranted to a usual therapeutic maintenance dose of 150–250 mg bid over a 2- to 4-week period. The maximum daily dose is 900 mg.

➤ Metabolism is primarily via CYP 1A2, leading to the active metabolite norclozapine. CYP 3A4 and CYP 2D6 are also involved.

Advantages:

➤ Effective for positive and negative symptoms of schizophrenia.

➤ Effective for treatment-resistant schizophrenia, as evidenced by a lowering of rehospitalization rates, aggressiveness, and suicidal behavior.

➤ Off-label use in many nonschizophrenic disorders (e.g., manic phase of bipolar disorder, mixed episodes of bipolar disorder, major depression with psychotic features, schizoaffective disorder, psychosis associated with Parkinson's disease [without aggravating underlying parkinsonism], schizoid personality disorder, aggression/regression of borderline personality disorder), psychosis associated with L-DOPA treatment, psychosis associated with Lewy body dementia, intractable insomnia.

➤ EPS risk is low but not totally absent. Mild pseudoparkinsonism and akathisia (but not dystonia) have occasionally been reported.

➤ TD risk is thought to be very low or absent. Clozapine actually suppresses TD movements.

➤ Minimal QTc interval prolongation.

➤ Low incidence of sexual side effects (i.e., little impact on serum prolactin).

Disadvantages:

➤ Requires a slow titration schedule.

➤ Optimal benefits may require 6 months to 2 years.

➤ Requires twice-daily dosing.

➤ Prominent discontinuation syndrome (e.g., cholinergic rebound leading to nausea, vomiting, and diarrhea; dopaminergic rebound leading to withdrawal dyskinesia). Discontinuation of clozapine should be undertaken gradually over 12–16 weeks.

➤ Clozapine levels are lowered by cigarette smoking, phenytoin, and pheno-barbital (via CYP 1A2 and CYP 3A4 isoenzyme induction) and increased by fluvoxamine, paroxetine, fluoxetine, grapefruit juice, and erythromycin (via CYP 1A2 and CYP 3A4 isoenzyme inhibition).

➤ Increased risk of seizures and NMS when used with lithium.

➤ Contraindicated in patients with a history of drug-induced agranulocytosis, severe granulocytopenia, or myeloproliferative disorders (especially if patient is immunocompromised secondary to HIV infection or tuberculo-sis). Clozapine should not be used concomitantly with medications known to suppress bone marrow function (e.g., carbamazepine) or in patients tak-ing benzodiazepines (increased potential for cardiac or pulmonary arrest).

➤ Increased incidence of cerebrovascular/cardiovascular events and pneumo-nia in elderly patients treated for agitation associated with dementia. Cloza-pine is not approved for this indication.

➤ Side effects found in more than 4% of patients taking clozapine include drowsiness/sedation (39%), hypersalivation (31%), dizziness/vertigo (19%), weight gain (18%), headache (7%), tremor (6%), syncope (6%), tachycardia (25%), hypotension (9%), sweating (6%), dry mouth (6%), visual distur-bances (5%), and EPS (4%–7%). Side effects also include:

✔ Strong anticholinergic activity.

✔ Urinary incontinence (more prominent than previously reported).

✔ Exacerbation of OCD symptoms (perhaps secondary to 5-HT$_{2A}$ block-ade). Adding an SSRI can be helpful.

➤ Serious side effects include:

✔ Weight gain, elevated lipids (triglycerides, cholesterol). Weight gain can reduce compliance and lead to diabetes mellitus type 2. Baseline and rou-tine assessments of weight, fasting blood glucose, and lipids are recom-mended.

✔ Venous thromboembolism, with reports of life-threatening pulmonary embolism (uncommon). Seemingly not a class effect.

✔ Plasma level increases of heavily protein-bound medications (e.g., digoxin, warfarin) secondary to their displacement from protein-binding sites by clozapine.

✔ Eosinophilia (1%). Discontinue if the eosinophil count is greater than 4,000/mm^3.

✔ Aplastic anemia (rare).

✔ Pancreatitis (rare).

✔ An atypical NMS has been reported with clozapine (elevated creatine phosphokinase [CPK] without fever or rigidity, possibly secondary to weak D$_2$ binding).

➤ Serious side effects with black box warnings:

✔ Agranulocytosis (defined as an absolute granulocyte [neutrophil] count of <500/mm^3):

■ A life-threatening side effect occurring in approximately 0.4% of monitored and 1%–2% of unmonitored patients (versus 0.1% of patients taking FGAs). Maximal risk occurs 4–18 weeks after initiation of therapy, with a peak incidence at 3 months. The risk is greater in females. The incidence increases with advancing age and decreases after the first 6 months of use. The fatality rate is extremely low (0.01%), due in part to the required rigorous monitoring of blood counts.

■ A genetic contribution leading to an increased risk has been identified. A pharmacogenetic test to measure the probability of developing agranulocytosis is now available.

■ Combining clozapine with carbamazepine is not recommended due to their combined effects on bone marrow suppression.

■ Order a WBC count for complaints of a sore throat or other symptoms suggestive of an infection (classic recommendation for all antipsychotic medications).

■ A baseline WBC count is required. Permanently discontinue clozapine if the WBC count falls to 3,000/mm^3 or lower or the absolute neutrophil count is less than 1,500/mm^3 on follow-up WBC testing.

■ Patients must be registered with the Clozapine Patient Registry (even if a generic form is used). Standard assessment is for WBC testing weekly for the first 6 months. If the patient has been stable without an "abnormal blood event" for 6 months, WBC testing every 2 weeks is allowed for the next 6 months. Thereafter, testing is once monthly. WBC testing must continue for at least 1 month after clozapine is discontinued.

■ If agranulocytosis develops:

● Immediately discontinue clozapine and consult with a hematologist.

● If the WBC count falls below 2,000 mm^3 or the absolute neutrophil count is less than 1,000 mm^3, do not rechallenge with clozapine.

✔ Seizures:

■ The risk of a grand mal (tonic–clonic) seizure is 3%–5%. The risk increases with increasing dose (especially above 600 mg/day) and rapid upward dose titration (especially more than 100 mg/day). Myoclonic jerks may be an early sign for the eventual development of a grand mal seizure. Divalproex has been recommended as a prophylactic antiepileptic medication to prevent clozapine-induced seizures in susceptible individuals. Carbamazepine should not be used with clozapine due to potential additive effects on bone marrow suppression.

✔ "Collapse, respiratory arrest, cardiac arrest":

- ■ A possible life-threatening drug interaction involving respiratory or cardiac arrest with benzodiazepines or "other psychotropic medications." Also rarely reported for clozapine monotherapy.

✔ Myocarditis:

- ■ Most likely to occur during the first month of therapy, as observed from postmarketing data. Fatalities have been reported. Do not rechallenge with clozapine.

Risperidone (Risperdal):

General considerations:

➤ FDA approved for acute (1993) and maintenance (2002) treatment of schizophrenia, manic and mixed episodes of bipolar I disorder (2003), and as a long-acting intramuscular formulation (Risperdal Consta) for the treatment of schizophrenia (2003).

➤ A high-potency agent with a low TR.

➤ Initiate dosing at 0.5–2.0 mg/day on a once-daily or twice-daily dosage regimen, and titrate upward as needed. Once-daily dosing is acceptable (FDA approved in 2003).

➤ Usual dosage range is 2–4 mg/day. Ninety percent of patients respond to risperidone at doses of 6 mg/day or less. Higher doses may be less effective at the expense of greater side effects.

➤ Metabolized by CYP 2D6 enzyme pathways.

➤ Paliperidone extended-release (Invega) is a metabolite of risperidone that is FDA approved for acute and maintenance treatment of schizophrenia. It is administered once daily at a dose of 6–12 mg. Important side effects include mild QTc prolongation, EPS (e.g., akathasia), and prolactin elevation (similar to risperidone). Weight gain is minimal at dosages up to 6 mg/day, but increases at higher dosages. Elimination is 90% by urinary excretion. Paliperidone demonstrates improvement in social functioning, as measured by the Personal and Social Performance scale.

Advantages:

➤ Effective for positive symptoms, negative symptoms, and cognitive deficits (especially verbal working memory) of schizophrenia.

➤ May be beneficial for positive symptoms refractory to FGAs.

➤ Low potential for anticholinergic side effects and QTc interval prolongation.

➤ Only SGA available in a liquid formulation.

➤ Risperdal M-Tab, a wafer with rapid disintegration properties when placed on the tongue, helps to improve compliance.

➤ Risperdal Consta 25–50 mg intramuscularly every 2 weeks is a long-acting (nondecanoate) formulation utilizing microparticle technology. Doses higher than 50 mg intramuscularly are not recommended. Patents should be started on oral risperidone or other antipsychotic medications for at least 3 weeks prior to initiating the long-acting formulation.

Disadvantages:

➤ Side effects include:

  ✔ Sedation.

  ✔ Weight gain and elevated lipids. Weight gain can reduce compliance and lead to diabetes mellitus type 2. Baseline and routine assessments of weight, fasting blood glucose, and lipids are recommended.

  ✔ Transient orthostatic hypotension at initiation of therapy.

  ✔ Increase in serum prolactin, resulting in a higher incidence of sexual dysfunction than with other SGAs. Approximately 10% of patients treated with risperidone at doses up to 6 mg/day experience hyperprolactinemia-related side effects (e.g., galactorrhea in females, impotence in males).

  ✔ Dose-dependent EPS. Anticholinergic medications may be needed for dosages greater than 4–6 mg/day.

  ✔ Increased incidence of cerebrovascular/cardiovascular events and pneumonia in elderly patients treated for agitation associated with dementia. Risperidone is not approved for this indication.

➤ Paroxetine and fluoxetine can raise risperidone blood levels secondary to CPY 2D6 enzyme inhibition.

Olanzapine (Zyprexa):

General considerations:

➤ Indicated for the treatment of schizophrenia (1996), the manic and mixed episodes of bipolar I disorder (2000), and the maintenance phase of bipolar disorder (2004).

➤ When combined with fluoxetine (Symbyax), indicated for the treatment of depression associated with bipolar disorder (2003). Five formulations (olanzapine/fluoxetine) are available: 3/25, 6/25, 6/50, 12/25, and 12/50.

➤ Indicated for the acute management of agitation of schizophrenia and bipolar I disorder as a nondepot intramuscular injection (Zyprexa IntraMuscular; 2004).

➤ Available as an oral medication, a fast-disintegrating wafer (Zyprexa Zydis; 2000), and a nondepot intramuscular formulation (Zyprexa IntraMuscular).

➤ A medium- to high-potency agent with a moderate TR. Therapeutic effectiveness established for the treatment of positive symptoms, negative symptoms, depressive symptoms, and cognitive impairment.

➤ Metabolized by CYP 1A2 (major pathway) and CYP 2D6 isoenzyme pathways.

➤ Initiate dosing at 5–10 mg/day given once daily, and titrate upward as needed. Dosage range is 5–20 mg/day. A daily dosage of 10 mg or more may be needed to adequately treat positive symptoms. Effective treatment of negative symptoms may require higher doses.

Advantages:

➤ Relatively rapid onset of action.

➤ Mechanism of action (and structure) is like that of clozapine, but olanzapine has significantly less risk of inducing agranulocytosis and seizures than clozapine.

➤ Like clozapine, olanzapine reduces aggressive and violent behavior in schizophrenic patients.

➤ Low incidence of EPS, TD, QTc interval prolongation, clinically significant anticholinergic side effects, and sexual dysfunction (olanzapine has minimal effects on prolactin).

➤ Once-daily dosing.

➤ Use of wafer oral formulation (Zyprexa Zydis; a fast-disintegrating wafer placed on the tongue) can improve compliance.

➤ Minimal drug interactions.

Disadvantages:

➤ Side-effect profile includes:

  ✔ Sedation.

  ✔ Weight gain (can be significant) and elevated lipids. Weight gain can reduce compliance and lead to diabetes mellitus type 2. Baseline assessments of weight, fasting blood glucose, and lipids are recommended.

  ✔ Transient orthostatic hypotension when initiating treatment.

  ✔ Increased incidence of cerebrovascular/cardiovascular events and pneumonia in elderly patients treated for agitation associated with dementia. Olanzapine is not approved for this indication.

  ✔ Transient increases in transaminase levels when initiating treatment.

  ✔ Occasional reports of ankle edema.

➤ The incidence of seizures (0.9%) is somewhat higher than for other SGAs (except for clozapine [3%]).

➤ Female gender confers a 30% reduction in olanzapine clearance compared with males, resulting in higher blood levels at equivalent doses.

➤ CYP 1A2 inhibitors (e.g., grapefruit juice, fluvoxamine) can raise olanzapine blood levels. Some physicians add fluvoxamine (off-label) to raise the blood level of olanzapine without the necessity of increasing the olanzapine dose.

➤ CYP 1A2 inducers (e.g., cigarette smoking) can lower blood levels.

Quetiapine (Seroquel):

General considerations:

➤ FDA approved for the treatment of schizophrenia (1997) and the manic episodes of bipolar I disorder (2004) and depression associated with bipolar disorder (2006).

➤ An extended-release formulation (Seroquel XR) is approved for the acute and maintenance treatment of schizophrenia (2007). Advantages include once-daily dosing and perhaps somewhat less sedation. Administer with a light meal. Dosage range similar to the non-extended-release formulation.

➤ Metabolized by the CYP 3A4 isoenzyme system to principally inactive metabolites.

➤ Initiate dosing at 25 mg bid, and titrate upward daily on a bid regimen as clinically indicated. The usual therapeutic maintenance dose is 200–400 mg bid, although higher doses may be needed for treatment-refractory schizophrenia. The FDA-approved dosing limit is 800 mg/day.

Advantages:

➤ Effective for positive and negative symptoms of schizophrenia. May have utility as an antidepressant based on its indication for treatment of bipolar depression.

➤ EPS and prolactin elevation are virtually absent over the entire approved dosage range. There is a low incidence of TD, QTc interval prolongation, and anticholinergic side effects.

Disadvantages:

➤ Side-effect profile includes:

   ✔ Sedation (possibly due to H_1 postsynaptic receptor blockade).

   ✔ Mild to moderate weight gain and elevated lipids. Weight gain can reduce compliance and lead to diabetes mellitus type 2. Baseline and routine assessments of weight, fasting blood glucose, and lipids are recommended.

   ✔ Dose-dependent orthostatic hypotension (possibly due to postsynaptic alpha$_1$-adrenergic receptor blockade) can be problematic at dosages greater than 300 mg/day (or lower in the elderly). The combination of a moderate level of sedation and dose-dependent increases in orthostatic hypotension can significantly increase the risk of falls.

   ✔ Cataracts have been found in patients taking quetiapine for long periods, but it is not known if they are secondary to the medication or a natural occurrence. Therefore, it is prudent to routinely screen for cataracts (slit-lamp) in patients taking quetiapine. The potential for cataract formation may be more problematic in terms of patient acceptance and compliance than to the actual event developing.

➤ Twice-daily dosing regimen is recommended (although many physicians dose once daily at night).

➤ Carbamazepine and phenytoin induce metabolism secondary to CYP 3A4 enzyme induction, lowering the blood level.

➤ Erythromycin and ketoconazole inhibit metabolism secondary to CYP 3A4 enzyme inhibition, raising the blood level.

➤ Increased incidence of cerebrovascular/cardiovascular events and pneumonia in elderly patients treated for agitation associated with dementia. Quetiapine is not approved for this indication.

Ziprasidone (Geodon):

General considerations:

➤ FDA approved for the treatment of schizophrenia (2001) as an oral medication and acute agitation of schizophrenia as a nondepot intramuscular formulation (2002).

➤ FDA approved for the treatment of manic and mixed episodes of bipolar I disorder (2004).

➤ In addition to high 5-HT_{2A} and low D_2 receptor blockade (typical for the SGAs), additional blockade of 5-HT_{1D} and agonism of 5-HT_{1A} may additionally confer antipsychotic activity as well. A medium-potency agent with a medium TR.

➤ Ziprasidone purportedly blocks the reuptake of norepinephrine and serotonin from presynaptic neurons (controversial) and may also confer antidepressant effects.

➤ Initiate dosing at 20 mg bid *with food* (significant positive impact on raising blood levels). The usual therapeutic maintenance dose is 40 mg bid, although doses as high as 160–200 mg/day may be needed. Usually at least 120 mg/day is needed for the effective treatment of acute episodes of schizophrenia. The maximum approved dosage is 160 mg/day.

➤ Metabolism is via the CYP 3A4 enzyme pathway and CYP 1A2 to a much lesser extent.

Advantages:

➤ Effective for positive symptoms and negative symptoms of schizophrenia.

➤ Low incidence of weight gain, EPS, anticholinergic side effects, and sexual dysfunction.

➤ No enzyme induction with smoking.

➤ Food improves absorption.

Disadvantages:

➤ Side-effect profile includes:

✔ Dose-dependent QTc interval prolongation. QTc interval prolongation can potentially lead to episodes of polymorphous ventricular tachycardia (*torsades de pointes*), which may be self-limiting and nonproblematic, may manifest with syncope, or may progress to ventricular fibrillation and sudden death:

■ QTc interval prolongation and the risk of sudden death secondary to ziprasidone carry a warning in the product labeling.

■ Prolongations of the QTc interval are additive to individual risk factors. The presence of multiple risk factors, each of which individually prolongs the QTc interval, cumulatively raises the overall cardiovascular risk for ventricular fibrillation.

■ There is a contraindication for concomitant use of medications that also prolong the QTc interval (e.g., thioridazine, chlorpromazine) or that inhibit the metabolism (via CYP 3A4) of ziprasidone (e.g., fluvoxamine, ketoconazole, erythromycin).

■ Ziprasidone is contraindicated in patients with a known history of QTc interval prolongation, acute myocardial infarctions, or uncompensated heart failure.

■ Pretreatment and follow-up ECGs are not required but are strongly recommended. Discontinue ziprasidone if the QTc interval is greater than 450–500 msec.

➤ Moderate (but usually transient) levels of sedation and hypotension at the initiation of pharmacotherapy.

➤ CYP 3A4 isoenzyme inhibitors (e.g., grapefruit juice, ketoconazole, erythromycin) can raise ziprasidone levels, thereby increasing the risk of QTc prolongation and related problems.

➤ Carbamazepine induces metabolism of ziprasidone via CYP 3A4, thereby lowering blood levels and possibly reducing ziprasidone's effectiveness.

➤ Twice-daily dosing is recommended.

➤ Higher doses (e.g., 120 mg/day) may be needed for optimal effectiveness.

➤ Although the potential for weight gain is low, baseline and routine assessments of weight, fasting blood glucose, and lipids are recommended.

➤ Increased incidence of cerebrovascular/cardiovascular events and pneumonia in elderly patients treated for agitation associated with dementia. Ziprasadone is not approved for this indication.

Aripiprazole (Abilify):

General considerations:

➤ Approved for the treatment of schizophrenia (2002), for the treatment of manic or mixed episodes of bipolar I disorder (2004), for the maintenance treatment of bipolar disorder (2005), and as an adjunctive treatment to antidepressants for major depressive disorder (2007).

➤ An IM injectable dosage form is approved for the treatment of agitation associated with schizophrenia or bipolar disorder (2006).

➤ An orally disintegrating formulation (Discmelt) is approved for the treatment of schizophrenia (2006).

➤ First of a new class of "modulators," aripiprazole is a partial agonist of D_2 and 5-HT_{1A} receptors and antagonist of 5-HT_{2A} receptors. *Partial agonism* refers to the ability to block a receptor if it is overstimulated and to stimulate a receptor if it is understimulated. Aripiprazole blocks 5-HT reuptake (conferring antidepressant activity) but has no activity at postsynaptic cholinergic sites.

➤ Classified as a "dopamine–serotonin system stabilizer." This unique mechanism of action is postulated to be secondary to its effects on:

✔ Decreasing DA activity in the mesolimbic pathway (secondary to blocking D_2 receptors), thereby improving positive symptoms.

✔ Increasing DA activity in the prefrontal cortex (secondary to DA agonism), thereby improving negative symptoms and cognitive functioning.

➤ Starting dose is 10–15 mg/day, with dosage increases to 30 mg/day as needed. However, the 20 mg/day or 30 mg/day dosage may not confer much added improvement. The maximum daily dosage is 30 mg.

➤ Metabolized by CYP 3A4 and CYP 2D6 isoenzyme systems.

Advantages:

➤ Effective for positive symptoms and negative symptoms of schizophrenia.

➤ Low propensity to cause weight gain, sedation, sexual dysfunction (actually lowers prolactin), EPS, TD, QTc interval prolongation, seizures, and anticholinergic side effects.

➤ Once-daily dosing.

➤ Food does not affect absorption.

➤ Side effects are minimal and often transient.

Disadvantages:

➤ Side effects include transient orthostatic hypotension, insomnia, somnolence, and nausea/vomiting at the initiation of therapy.

➤ Blood levels are elevated by CYP 2D6 isoenzyme inhibitors (e.g., fluoxetine, paroxetine) and CYP 3A4 isoenzyme inhibitors (e.g., ketoconazole, erythromycin) and lowered by CYP 3A4 isoenzyme inducers (e.g., carbamazepine, phenytoin).

➤ Some patients may experience an increase in anxiety or agitation secondary to DA agonism when starting or raising the dosage.

➤ Although the potential for weight gain is low, baseline and routine assessments of weight, fasting blood glucose, and lipids are recommended.

➤ Increased incidence of cerebrovascular/cardiovascular events and pneumonia in elderly patients treated for agitation associated with dementia. Aripiprazole is not approved for this indication.

Chlorpromazine (Thorazine), thioridazine (Mellaril), and mesoridazine (Serentil):

General considerations:

➤ Chlorpromazine was the first antipsychotic medication FDA approved for the treatment of schizophrenia (1954) and is also approved for the treatment of acute mania in bipolar I disorder (1973). Thioridazine and mesoridazine are FDA approved for the treatment of schizophrenia only after other medication treatments have failed.

➤ Low-potency medications with a wide TR.

➤ Standardization of dosages for other antipsychotic medications are often based on "chlorpromazine equivalents":

✔ Acute psychosis: chlorpromazine equivalents = 300–1,000 mg/day.

✔ Maintenance dosage: chlorpromazine equivalents = 300–600 mg/day.

➤ Historically, and inappropriately, dosages as high as 2,000 mg/day of chlorpromazine were used for "treatment refractory" schizophrenia. These higher doses likely only served to increase side effects but not effectiveness. Higher dosing was found more frequently in males, in younger individuals, and in African American, Asian, and Hispanic individuals.

➤ For thioridazine, the dosage range is 200–800 mg/day in divided doses.

➤ For mesoridazine (a metabolite of thioridazine), the dosage range is 100–400 mg/day.

Advantages:

➤ Effective for positive symptoms of schizophrenia.

➤ Low potential for EPS because of "built-in" anticholinergic properties.

➤ Intramuscular dosage forms for chlorpromazine and mesoridazine are available.

➤ Liquid formulations for chlorpromazine, thioridazine, and mesoridazine are available.

➤ Chlorpromazine is available as a suppository.

➤ Once-daily dosing is usually effective.

Disadvantages:

➤ Not effective for and may actually worsen negative symptoms, depression, and cognition in schizophrenia (controversial).

➤ For chlorpromazine, the side-effect profile includes reduction of the seizure threshold, orthostatic hypotension, prominent anticholinergic side effects, sedation, weight gain, sexual dysfunction, skin rashes, increased sensitivity to sunlight, SIADH, jaundice, cataracts, agranulocytosis, TD, NMS, and sudden death (somewhat controversial, but rare). EPS are typically low or absent.

➤ For thioridazine, the side-effect profile is very similar to that of chlorpromazine but also includes the potential for retinitis pigmentosa (at dosages greater than 800 mg/day), retrograde ejaculation, and significant dose-dependent QTc interval prolongation. Mesoridazine also causes dose-dependent increases in QTc interval prolongation. Thioridazine and mesoridazine are the most side-effect prone and dangerous of the available antipsychotic medications; for this reason, these two agents should be used (if at all) for schizophrenia, and only when other antipsychotic medications have failed.

➤ Chlorpromazine, thioridazine, and mesoridazine are metabolized by the CYP 2D6 pathway. Medications that inhibit the 2D6 pathway (e.g., paroxetine, fluoxetine, TCAs) can raise blood levels of these medications, thereby further increasing the risk of ventricular tachycardia and ventricular arrhythmias (thioridazine and mesoridazine).

Thiothixene (Navane), perphenazine (Trilafon), and trifluoperazine (Stelazine):

General considerations:

➤ Medium-potency agents with an intermediate TR.

Advantages:

➤ Effective for positive symptoms of schizophrenia.

➤ Historically, widely used because of a favorable balance between effectiveness and side effects.

➤ Perphenazine was the FGA chosen for the CATIE study (see Chapter 9 in this volume, "Miscellaneous Topics").

Disadvantages:

➤ Not effective for and may actually induce or worsen negative symptoms, depression, and cognition in schizophrenia (controversial).

➤ Often (but not always) given in divided doses to reduce side effects. However, more-frequent dosing can compromise compliance.

➤ Can induce many of the same side effects as chlorpromazine/thioridazine/mesoridazine and haloperidol/fluphenazine, although of lower frequency and lesser intensity.

➤ Intermediate potential for EPS; high potential for TD.

Haloperidol (Haldol), fluphenazine (Prolixin), and pimozide (Orap):

General considerations:

➤ High-potency medications with a low TR.

➤ Usual dosage range is highly variable, often ranging from 0.5 to 20 mg/day. Historically, oral dosages of 100 mg/day or more of haloperidol have been used for patients with "treatment-refractory" schizophrenia but are not considered more effective than 8–20 mg/day despite dramatically and unnecessarily increasing side effects (somewhat controversial).

➤ Intramuscular depot preparation (Haldol Decanoate) typically is administered once monthly at a dose range of 50–300 mg in the gluteus muscle. Use the following formula for converting from the oral to the depot preparation: haloperidol 10 mg/day orally = Haldol Decanoate 100–150 mg intramuscularly administered every 4 weeks. Prior to initiating the depot formulation, the patient should be started on the oral formulation.

➤ Intramuscular depot preparation (Prolixin Decanoate) typically is administered at a dosage of 12.5–75.0 mg every 1–4 weeks in the gluteus muscle. Use the following formula for converting from the oral to the depot preparation: fluphenazine 10 mg/day po = Prolixin Decanoate 12.5–25 mg intramuscularly administered every 1–3 weeks. Prior to initiating the depot formulation, the patient should be started on the oral formulation. The usual regimen is every 2 weeks.

➤ Pimozide (Orap) is approved when the symptoms of schizophrenia are not accompanied by agitation or hyperactivity. The usual dosage is 2–12 mg/day. Doses above 20 mg/day are associated with greater QTc interval prolongation. Pimozide serum levels can rise when it is administered with medications that inhibit CYP 3A4 (e.g., erythromycin, ketoconazole) or with citalopram (Celexa), potentially further increasing the QTc interval.

Advantages:

➤ Effective for positive symptoms of schizophrenia.

➤ Favorable side-effect profile (advantageous in emergency settings) includes a low risk of reducing the seizure threshold, a low risk of sedation (minimal H_1 blockade), a low potential to induce orthostatic hypotension (minimal alpha$_1$-adrenergic blockade), and a low potential for anticholinergic side effects (minimal M_1 blockade).

➤ Once-daily oral dosing of the oral formulation is effective.

➤ Liquid formulations of haloperidol and fluphenazine are available.

➤ Intramuscular (nondepot) dosage forms for haloperidol and fluphenazine are available for treating acutely psychotic patients.

➤ Depot dosage forms (long-acting) of haloperidol and fluphenazine are especially helpful when patient compliance is problematic.

➤ Therapeutic window of 2–12 ng/mL may be operable for haloperidol but is rarely assessed clinically.

➤ Pimozide is especially useful for the treatment of tics, Gilles de la Tourette's syndrome, and delusional disorder, somatic type (e.g., delusional parasitosis).

Disadvantages:

➤ Not effective for and may actually worsen negative symptoms, depression, and cognition in schizophrenia (controversial).

➤ Very high potential for EPS; high potential for TD.

➤ Potential drug interactions listed in the product literature for haloperidol include:

  ✔ Haloperidol + indomethacin → significant drowsiness.

  ✔ Haloperidol + high doses of lithium → encephalopathy with permanent brain damage and severe EPS. However, haloperidol and lithium are often safely used together.

  ✔ Haloperidol + TCAs → increased TCA levels secondary to inhibition of TCA metabolism.

Summary of characteristics of the common antipsychotic medications:

➤ Table 1–3 summarizes the potency, effectiveness, and side effects of the common antipsychotic medications.

Table 1–3 Characteristics of the common antipsychotic medications

Medication	Usual daily dosage range, mg	Relative potency (chlorpromazine = 100)	Efficacy for		Acute EPS	Chronic EPS (TD)	NMS	Side-effect risk				
			Positive symptoms	Negative symptoms				Sedation	Orthostatic hypotension	Anticholinergic side effects	Weight gain	Sexual dysfunction
First-generation antipsychotics (FGAs)												
Chlorpromazine (Thorazine)	200–1,000	Low (100)	Yes	No	Low	High	Medium to low	High	High	High	Medium	High
Thioridazine (Mellaril)	200–800	Low (100)	Yes	No	Low	High	Medium to low	High	High	High	Medium	High
Perphenazine (Trilafon)	8–64	Medium (10)	Yes	No	Medium	High	Likely intermediate, but not clarified	Low	Low	Low	Medium	Medium
Loxapine (Loxitane)	25–250	Medium (10)	Yes	No	Medium	High	Likely intermediate, but not clarified	Low	Low	Low	Medium	Medium
Thiothixene (Navane)	5–40	Medium (25)	Yes	No	Medium	High	Likely intermediate, but not clarified	Medium	Medium	Medium	Medium	Medium
Trifluoperazine (Stelazine)	5–20	Medium (25)	Yes	No	Medium	High	Likely intermediate, but not clarified	Medium	Medium	Medium	Medium	Medium

Table 1–3 Characteristics of the common antipsychotic medications (*continued*)

Medication	Usual daily dosage range, mg	Relative potency (chlorpromazine = 100)	Efficacy for		Acute EPS	Chronic EPS (TD)	NMS	Side-effect risk				
			Positive symptoms	Negative symptoms				Sedation	Orthostatic hypotension	Anticholinergic side effects	Weight gain	Sexual dysfunction
First-generation antipsychotics (FGAs) (*continued*)												
Haloperidol (Haldol)	0.5–20	High (2)	Yes	No	High	High	High	Low	Low	Low	Medium	Medium
Fluphenazine (Prolixin)	0.5–40	High (2)	Yes	No	High	High	High	Low	Low	Low	Medium	Medium
Pimozide (Orap)	2–12	High (2)	Yes (but not for acute management)	No	High	High	Likely high, but not clarified	Low	Low	Low	Medium	Medium
Second-generation antipsychotics (SGAs)												
Quetiapine (Seroquel)	75–800	Low (80)	Yes	Yes	Low	Low	Likely low, but not clarified	Medium	Medium	Low	Minimal	Low
Quetiapine XR (Seroquel)	75–800	Low (80)	Yes	Yes	Low	Low	Likely low, but not clarified	Medium	Medium	Low	Minimal	Low
Clozapine (Clozaril)	75–900	Low (50)	Yes	Yes	Low	Low	Low[a]	High	High	High	High	Low
Olanzapine (Zyprexa)	5–20	Medium (4)	Yes	Yes	Low	Low	Low[a]	High initially, then low	Medium initially, then low	Low	High	Low
Risperidone (Risperdal)	1–16	High (12)	Yes	Yes	Low, but increases with dose	Low, but increases with dose	Low[a]	Low	Medium	Low	Medium	Higher than with the other SGAs

■ Table 1–3 Characteristics of the common antipsychotic medications (continued)

Medication	Usual daily dosage range, mg	Relative potency (chlorpromazine = 100)	Efficacy for Positive symptoms	Efficacy for Negative symptoms	Acute EPS	Chronic EPS (TD)	NMS	Side-effect risk Sedation	Side-effect risk Orthostatic hypotension	Side-effect risk Anticholinergic side effects	Side-effect risk Weight gain	Side-effect risk Sexual dysfunction
Second-generation antipsychotics (SGAs) (continued)												
Paliperidone extended release (Invega)	6–12	High (?)	Yes	Yes	Low, but increases with dose	Low, but increases with dose	Not known	Low	Medium	Low	Medium	Higher than with the other SGAs
Ziprasidone (Geodon)	40–160	Low-medium (16)	Yes	Yes	Low	Low	Not clarified	Low	Low	Low	Low	Low
Aripiprazole (Abilify)	10–30	Medium (4)	Yes	Yes	Low	Low	Not clarified	Low	Low	Low	Low	Low

Note. Thioridazine, mesoridazine, pimozide, IV haloperidol, ziprasidone, and paliperidone extended release have notable QTc interval prolongation.
EPS = extrapyramidal side effects; NMS = neuroleptic malignant syndrome; TD = tardive dyskinesia.
[a]Lowest incidence of NMS.

General Guidelines for Antipsychotic Pharmacotherapy

Choosing an antipsychotic medication:

➤ The CATIE study puts into question the advisability of initiating treatment with an SGA when the clinical effectiveness of the SGAs and perphenazine were fairly equivalent for positive symptoms. However, the side-effect profile, over the long term, likely favors SGAs, especially with regard to the greater potential of FGAs to cause EPS and TD. Also, there is a greater likelihood that SGAs are effective for negative symptoms, whereas FGAs likely worsen negative symptoms. Nevertheless, for purposes of the oral boards, the right or wrong is not the important issue; rather, it is the understanding of the dynamics of a topic that is not yet fully resolved. Be prepared to defend your position.

➤ Based on an assumption that SGAs are normally preferred over FGAs, consider choosing or continuing an FGA for patients who:

  ✔ Require an antipsychotic medication for short-term use (e.g., emergency settings).

  ✔ Had a prior robust response to an FGA without appreciable side effects and specifically request the medication. The only exceptions may be thioridazine and mesoridazine, secondary to a generally unfavorable side-effect profile coupled with significant QTc interval prolongation, making these medications the most side-effect prone and dangerous antipsychotics in use.

  ✔ Do not present with appreciable negative symptoms or in whom negative symptoms are not exacerbated by the medication.

  ✔ Are among a minority of patients who are refractory to SGAs but responsive to one or more of the FGAs.

  ✔ Require a long-acting (depot) formulation secondary to poor compliance. However, this issue is less valid with the availability of long-acting risperidone (Risperdal Consta).

  ✔ Have been well stabilized on a depot FGA and prefer not to change to a depot SGA (Risperdal Consta).

Dosing and side-effect considerations:

➤ Adequate dosing and allowing time for therapeutic effects to develop are the rules, not the exception. Recall the axiom:

  ✔ Expect a positive response when the right drug is used at the right dose, for the right duration, for the right diagnosis.

➤ Monotherapy is preferred. Optimize the dosage to provide the best potential for a single medication to be effective, adjusting the dosage to balance effects and side effects. Allow adequate time for a therapeutic response to develop.

➤ The CATIE study demonstrated extremely high discontinuation rates for all the antipsychotics used in the trials, primarily because of lack of efficacy and secondarily because of adverse side effects.

Switching antipsychotic medications:

➤ Switching from one FGA to another FGA is not expected to produce significant benefits, since both agents work similarly through D_2 receptor blockade. Recommendations are to switch to an SGA if a trial of an FGA fails.

➤ Switching from one SGA to another SGA has merit. However, switching medications can introduce new side effects that may not have been present with the first medication. Clozapine is the most effective antipsychotic medication.

➤ When switching medications, several techniques can be utilized (physician preference):

✔ Abruptly stop the old medication and start the new medication with an upward titration. This technique is more likely to result in reemergence of psychotic symptoms and the development of a rebound withdrawal syndrome.

✔ Cross-titrate by gradually reducing the old medication while gradually increasing the new medication. This technique can also result in reemergence of psychotic symptoms secondary to neither medication being at therapeutic levels but will reduce the potential for a withdrawal syndrome.

✔ Overlap and then taper, by keeping the first medication at or near full strength while the dosage of the new medication is gradually titrated upward to full therapeutic dose. This is followed by a gradual taper of the old medication over 4–6 weeks (8–12 weeks for clozapine). This is probably the most desirable switching method although it puts the patient at the greatest risk of complications from polypharmacy.

Combining antipsychotic medications
(assuming that monotherapy has first been optimized):

➤ Combining antipsychotic medications is only recommended as a last resort, when monotherapy has failed. However, this approach may or may not be effective and carries the risk for increased medication side effects, utilizing additional medications to treat those side effects, decreased patient adherence due to increased complexity of the treatment, greater potential for drug interactions, further difficulty for the clinician to determine which medication(s) is/are helpful, and increased costs to the patient. Clozapine added to another SGA has consistently demonstrated value. Other combinations (e.g., olanzapine + risperidone) have been studied and appear effective for treatment-resistant schizophrenia.

Discontinuing antipsychotic medications:

➤ Absolute indications for discontinuing an antipsychotic medication:

✔ Agranulocytosis (most often reported with clozapine and chlorpromazine).

✔ Aplastic anemia (most often reported with clozapine, pimozide, and perphenazine).

✔ NMS (all antipsychotic medications).

✔ Polymorphous ventricular tachycardia secondary to QTc interval prolongation (potentially with thioridazine, mesoridazine, intravenous haloperidol, pimozide, paliperidone, and ziprasidone).

➤ Relative indications for discontinuing an antipsychotic medication:

✔ TD (weigh the benefit–risk ratio).

✔ Leukopenia (reduction in the circulating WBC count to below 4,500 cells/μL).

✔ SIADH (relatively rare). Compulsive water drinking is also a feature of schizophrenia.

✔ Nonventricular arrhythmias or cardiac conduction delays.

✔ Narrow-angle glaucoma or prostatic hypertrophy secondary to anticholinergic side effects (most prominent with low-potency FGAs and clozapine).

Antipsychotic withdrawal syndromes:

➤ If an antipsychotic medication is stopped abruptly, a substantial withdrawal syndrome (i.e., rebound) can develop, with symptoms dependent on the type of receptor blockade that is suddenly lost:

✔ Cholinergic rebound due to altered acetylcholine interaction with down-regulated choline receptors (low potency FGAs and clozapine). Symptoms include nausea, vomiting, diarrhea, constricted pupils, increased urination, increased salivation, increased sweating, and, in extreme cases, psychosis and/or delirium.

✔ Dopaminergic rebound due to upregulation of D_2 receptors (FGAs and SGAs). Symptoms include short-term withdrawal dyskinesia, anxiety, and insomnia.

✔ Unmasking TD due to upregulation of D_2 receptors with "emergence" of choreoathetoid movement.

Anxiety and depression:

➤ Apathy, depressive symptoms, or major depressive disorder develops in approximately 25%–50% of schizophrenic individuals. These symptoms can be attributed to:

✔ An integral part of the schizophrenic process (i.e., a "primary" negative symptom). Adequate treatment of schizophrenia may resolve the symptoms.

✔ Antipsychotic medication–induced akinesia (i.e., a "secondary" negative symptom). Treat by switching to an SGA, adding an anticholinergic medication, adding a benzodiazepine, or adding a beta-blocker.

✔ A comorbid medical disorder (e.g., hypothyroidism) or substance use disorder. Additionally, treat the underlying disorder.

✔ Major depressive disorder, a comorbid depressive disorder, or possibly a corrected diagnosis of schizoaffective disorder.

➤ Anxiety, agitation, and irritability are common findings. These symptoms can be attributed to:

✔ An integral part of the schizophrenic process. Adequate treatment of the schizophrenia may resolve the symptoms.

✔ Antipsychotic-induced akathisia. Treat by switching to an SGA other than risperidone or by adding an anticholinergic agent, benzodiazepine, or beta-blocker.

✔ A comorbid medical (e.g., hyperthyroidism) or substance use disorder. Additionally, treat the underlying disorder.

Antipsychotic medications in an emergency setting (when severe agitation or aggressiveness is a concern):

➤ Nondepot intramuscular formulations of chlorpromazine, haloperidol, fluphenazine, ziprasidone, and olanzapine are available:

✔ Haloperidol and fluphenazine have little impact on lowering the seizure threshold, minimal anticholinergic side effects, a low incidence of postural hypotension, a low incidence of excessive sedation, but a high potential for EPS. Intramuscular benzodiazepines that are evenly released from the injection site (e.g., lorazepam [Ativan], but not diazepam [Valium]) are often combined with intramuscular haloperidol or intramuscular fluphenazine.
Note. Haloperidol administered intravenously may rarely produce torsades de pointes with resultant ventricular fibrillation and possible sudden death.

✔ Ziprasidone and olanzapine have little impact on lowering the seizure threshold, minimal anticholinergic side effects, and a low incidence of postural hypotension. However, olanzapine can cause sedation (possibly desired) and ziprasidone can increase the QTc interval.

✔ Chlorpromazine is widely used but causes significant side effects, including pain at the injection site.

✔ The liquid formulation of risperidone and wafer formulations of olanzapine (Zydis) and risperidone (M-Tab) can improve compliance.

✔ Psychosis secondary to anticholinergic-induced delirium (e.g., overuse or abuse of trihexphenidyl [Artane]) is best treated with intravenous physostigmine.

Antipsychotic use during pregnancy and lactation:

➤ Assessment of benefit (e.g., sustaining antipsychotic benefit, protecting against postpartum psychosis) must be balanced against the risk to the fetus (e.g., congenital malformations, behavioral abnormalities immediately after birth).

➤ No medication can be considered absolutely safe during pregnancy. The risk of teratogenic effects is greatest during the first trimester but can persist throughout the pregnancy.

➤ Haloperidol is not highly associated with congenital malformations, whereas chlorpromazine has been associated with nonspecific congenital malformations, a "neonatal withdrawal syndrome" (e.g., sedation, tachy-arrhythmias), and an increased risk of neonatal jaundice in premature infants.

➤ The SGAs have not been adequately studied for their impact on fetal development. Therefore, their risk of causing congenital malformations is not well known.

➤ Clozapine, olanzapine, risperidone, and quetiapine carry the greatest risk of inducing maternal weight gain, thereby increasing the risk of gestational diabetes mellitus type 2. Gestational diabetes places the developing fetus at greater risk of premature birth, congenital abnormalities (e.g., neural tube defects), larger infant weight at birth (which can lead to complications during vaginal delivery or the need for cesarean section), perinatal mortality, and the future development of diabetes for both mother and child.

➤ Antipsychotic medications are excreted into breast milk to varying degrees. The benefit–risk ratio should be evaluated for each patient.

Depot intramuscular formulations:

➤ Are typically used in approximately 10%–15% of patients with schizophrenia to improve compliance or as a convenience to the patient.

➤ Are available for haloperidol (oil formulation of haloperidol; Haldol Decanoate), fluphenazine (oil formulation of fluphenazine; Prolixin Decanoate), and risperidone (microparticles of risperidone; Risperdal Consta).

➤ Are administered intramuscularly at various sites (e.g., gluteus maximus, gluteus medius, deltoid).

➤ May contribute to a greater extent than the corresponding oral formulations to the development of TD and NMS (controversial).

Guidelines for the Biopsychosocial Treatment of Schizophrenia

➤ A large body of literature providing guidelines for the treatment of schizophrenia is available. The diversity of the guidelines makes it difficult to provide a single algorithm that satisfies all potential considerations. Clearly, the knowledge base and experience of the clinician, in light of these diverse recommendations, provide the best directive for the effective management of schizophrenia. Provided in this text are general guidelines recognized as appropriate by most bodies of literature, although all recommendations are not universally accepted. All recommendations include a combination of psychosocial and somatic treatments. Prominent organizations that have issued treatment guidelines include the following:

✔ Agency for Healthcare Research and Quality.

✔ National Institute of Mental Health–sponsored Schizophrenia Patient Outcomes Research Team (http://www.ahrq.gov/clinic/schzrec.htm).

✔ Texas Medication Algorithm Project (http://www.dshs.state.tx.us/ mhprograms/ TMAPover.shtm).

✔ American Psychiatric Association Practice Guidelines (http://www. psychiatryonline.com/pracGuide/pracGuideHome.aspx).

Psychosocial Interventions in Schizophrenia

General considerations:

➤ Psychosocial treatments are an integral part of the overall treatment approach (biopsychosocial model). Early intervention aimed at building a therapeutic relationship between the patient and the treatment providers can improve outcomes.

➤ Interventions are directed at educating the patient (and family if appropriate) regarding the nature of the illness, available treatments, and issues related to living arrangements, drug or alcohol abuse, education, employment, and relationships.

➤ Psychosocial treatment can be particularly valuable for helping patients learn to deal with negative symptoms.

Types of psychosocial treatment:

➤ Social skills training is directed at helping patients learn to relate appropriately to others. This can include even the basic considerations of appropriate hygiene, keeping appointments, and respecting the rights of others.

➤ Family therapy can help to reduce relapse rates by decreasing conflicts from "high EE" families. Encourage family participation in the National Alliance for the Mentally Ill (http://www.nami.org), a nationwide support group for families of patients with psychiatric disorders. Other sources of support include The Schizophrenia Help Home Page on the World Wide Web (http:// www.schizophrenia-help.com) and the National Mental Health Association (http://www.nmha.org).

➤ Group therapy can help patients learn from one another to effectively solve problems. Led by a trained treatment-team provider.

➤ Individual psychotherapy can help facilitate a therapeutic and trusting relationship between the patient and the therapist. Supportive therapy is usually recommended, but some patients may benefit from insight-oriented psychotherapy once their mental status improves (e.g., residual stage). Educational approaches (e.g., learning to recognize early changes consistent with a relapse) can be very helpful. Psychodynamic therapy is generally considered ineffective.

➤ Vocational rehabilitation (e.g., sheltered workshop, low-stress job) can help patients develop job skills.

➤ Self-help groups provide an opportunity for patients to share ideas, discuss concerns about medications, and learn from others with similar problems.

➤ Assistance in arranging for an appropriate living environment, preferably in a structured setting (e.g., family home, foster family, halfway house), is extremely important. Independent living is a desirable (but not always obtainable) long-term goal.

➤ Long-term institutionalization is reserved for patients with severe illness, marked cognitive deficits, recurrent suicidal ideation or behavior, frequent relapses, and overall poor response to treatment. May not always be available or utilized when appropriate.

Phase-Specific Treatment Guidelines for Schizophrenia

Treatment of a first psychotic episode ("first break"):

➤ Hospitalization is recommended to determine the cause for the psychosis and to initiate treatment. Assessment for medical and substance-related causes of psychosis are mandatory prior to making a diagnosis of a primary psychiatric disorder. A brain scan is recommended for a first psychotic episode and psychological testing (e.g., MMPI-II, Rorschach test, Thematic Apperception Test) can be of great value.

➤ If a preliminary diagnosis of schizophrenia is then made, treatment should be initiated to provide rapid intervention. Nevertheless, because the patient is likely to be discharged from the hospital before an optimal therapeutic response is achieved, discharge planning begins when the patient is admitted to the hospital.

➤ Initiate a comprehensive treatment program, including antipsychotic medication, educational services, and social work intervention (based on a biopsychosocial model).

➤ Initiate somatic treatment with an antipsychotic medication. Adjust the dosage depending on the clinical response and side effects. Response to antipsychotic medications typically develops gradually, and an optimal response can take 6 months or longer to achieve (especially for clozapine).

➤ Consider adding other medications at the start of or during treatment to treat symptoms other than psychosis:

   ✔ Benzodiazepines may be helpful on a short-term basis to reduce anxiety or provide sedation. Use cautiously (if at all) in this patient group due to the increased potential for abuse. Do not use benzodiazepines with clozapine (contraindicated). Trazodone, diphenhydramine, and hydroxyzine can also be added to help with sleep and to reduce anxiety.

   ✔ Divalproex or carbamazepine can reduce excessive agitation, hostility, aggressiveness, or manic-like symptoms. Do not use carbamazepine with clozapine (additive effects on bone marrow suppression).

   ✔ Antidepressants can be added to treat depression.

➤ If the patient's symptoms remain treatment refractory, implement the OACS (Optimize, Augment, Combine, Switch) principle.

   ✔ First, *optimize* by gradually increasing the antipsychotic dose, paying close attention to developing side effects. Dosage increases above FDA-approved limits can further improve response for some of the antipsychotic medications but represent an off-label use. Medications that have demonstrated efficacy at dosages above FDA-approved limits include:

      ■ Olanzapine up to 30 mg/day (albeit with the possible development of EPS and significant sedation).

      ■ Quetiapine up to 1,200 mg/day (albeit with the possibility of significant sedation and orthostasis).

      ■ Ziprasidone up to 200 mg/day (albeit with possible further increases in QTc interval prolongation).

➤ If the patient's symptoms still remain treatment refractory (psychotic symptoms persist), consider the following options:

   ✔ *Augment* the antipsychotic medication. Anecdotal reports and small studies are suggestive that SSRIs, mood stabilizers (divalproex, carbamazepine, lithium), acetylcholinesterase inhibitors (e.g., donepezil), and ECT added to an antipsychotic medication can be helpful to improve the core symptoms of treatment-refractory schizophrenia. None (except for ECT) are well-established protocols.

   ✔ *Combine* two antipsychotic medications:

      ■ Anecdotal reports and small studies provide support that combining two SGAs can improve efficacy without incurring significantly increased side effects. Clozapine added to another SGA is perhaps the most helpful, but other combinations reported include olanzapine plus riperidone and quetiapine plus aripiprazole. However, combining two antipsychotic medications carries increased risks from drug interactions, a more complicated treatment protocol, increased costs to the patient, and lack of uniform acceptance as a routine treatment protocol. Often used as a last resort for the most impaired patients. Combining two FGAs is not recommended.

✔ *Switch* antipsychotic medications:

- From an FGA to an SGA (can be very effective).

- From an SGA to another SGA (clozapine is considered the most effective antipsychotic medication).

- From an SGA to an FGA (can result in increased side effects). Switching from one FGA to another FGA is not expected to provide much added benefit.

- From an antipsychotic medication to ECT (although ECT can be used along with an antipsychotic medication).

Treatment during remission:

➤ Maintaining remission after recovery from a psychotic episode for a patient confirmed to have schizophrenia is important to help protect against a relapse. Maintain the effective medication at a dosage equal to or perhaps somewhat lower than that used to effectively treat the psychosis.

✔ Because the magnitude of recovery is so variable, a trial off medications:

- *May* be warranted if all of the following are in place (very controversial):

  • The patient has been fully compliant with all treatment recommendations for a period of 1–2 years.

  • Response has been excellent without symptom exacerbation.

  • There are no concerns regarding aggressiveness or substance abuse.

  • There are acceptable social supports, a reasonable ability to provide self-care, and a continuing improvement in overall functioning.

  • A slow downward taper does not result in symptom exacerbation.

- Is *not* warranted if:

  • Stressors are present or likely to be present in the future.

  • Compliance with treatment recommendations is suboptimal or poor.

  • Substance abuse is active, suspected, or likely.

  • There are concerns regarding aggressiveness or adequate self-care if medications are discontinued.

Treatment of a relapse:

➤ Determine the reason for the relapse and address the underlying problem(s):

✔ Wrong diagnosis (e.g., bipolar I disorder rather than schizophrenia).

✔ Comorbid disorders conferring additional barriers to recovery:

- Substance use disorders—present in up to 50% of persons with schizophrenia and is a major precipitant of relapse.
- Depressive disorders—either comorbid with schizophrenia or an intrinsic part of the illness.
- Anxiety disorders—commonly comorbid with schizophrenia.
- Medical illness (e.g., thyroid disease) or medication side effects (e.g., digoxin, glucocorticoids)—commonly overlooked.

✔ Poor compliance due to adverse medication side effects, comorbid substance abuse, denial of illness, unwillingness to accept medication treatment, a poor patient–physician relationship, a cumbersome dosing schedule, or a desire to maintain the sick role for secondary gain. Compliance can possibly be improved by:

- Improving the physician–patient relationship.
- Ensuring that the oral medication is swallowed and is not "cheeked." A liquid (risperidone) or wafer (olanzapine, risperidone) formulation can improve compliance.
- Administering the medication in depot intramuscular form (haloperidol, fluphenazine, risperidone).
- Switching to a medication with a more favorable side-effect profile (e.g., from an FGA to an SGA).
- Switching to a medication with fewer daytime doses.
- Effectively treating substance abuse.

✔ Medication failure due to:

- Inherent lack of efficacy of a given medication (e.g., treating a patient with predominantly negative symptoms with an FGA).
- Antipsychotic blood levels below a therapeutic window secondary to too-low dosages or rapid metabolism (e.g., genetically rapid metabolizer, CYP isoenzyme induction).
- Antipsychotic blood levels above a therapeutic window due to too-high dosing or slow metabolism (e.g., renal impairment, hepatic impairment, CYP isoenzyme inhibition by another medication, genetically slow metabolizer). A therapeutic window is possibly applicable to haloperidol, fluphenazine, and clozapine but is rarely assessed clinically.

Special treatment issues and remedies:

➤ Patient fails to take prescribed medications:

✔ Education as to need for medications (e.g., more frequent visits, group therapy).

✔ Switch to a depot formulation.

➤ Problematic medication side effects develop:

✔ Lower the dosage, treat side effects, or switch to a less side effect–prone medication.

➤ There is an inherently poor response to the first trial of an FGA:

✔ Switch to an SGA (clozapine, if suicidal issues are relevant).

➤ There is an inherently poor response to monotherapy:

✔ Implement the OACS principle.

✔ Switch to clozapine or ECT.

➤ Comorbid substance abuse:

✔ Aggressively treat the substance abuse.

➤ Comorbid medical illness:

✔ Aggressively treat the medical illness.

➤ Depression emerges:

✔ If the patient is being treated with an SGA, optimize the dose. Adequate treatment of the psychosis may improve the depression if it is a core component of the schizophrenia. Alternatively, provide a trial of an antidepressant.

✔ If the patient is being treated with an FGA (which may possibly induce or aggravate depression; controversial), strongly consider switching to an SGA or providing a trial of an antidepressant.

✔ Increase the frequency of psychotherapy visits (e.g., individual, group).

➤ Cognitive impairment becomes evident:

✔ Switch from an FGA to an SGA (may or may not be helpful).

✔ Add an anticholinesterase inhibitor (may or may not be helpful).

✔ Appreciate that cognitive impairment is a natural consequence of the schizophrenic process, especially the disorganized type, and may not be highly amenable to treatment.

➤ Suicidal issues become evident:

✔ Switch to clozapine.

✔ Add an antidepressant if depression is evident.

✔ Increase the frequency of psychotherapy visits, provide day treatment, or provide hospitalization.

➤ TD emerges and an antipsychotic medication is still required:

✔ Implement the usual strategies for the treatment of TD (described earlier in this chapter).

✔ Switch to olanzapine or clozapine.

✔ Additionally coordinate care with a neurologist familiar with TD.

BRIEF PSYCHOTIC DISORDER

DSM-IV-TR Diagnostic Criteria (Summary)

A. Presence of one (or more) of the following symptoms:
1. Delusions.
2. Hallucinations.
3. Disorganized speech (e.g., frequent derailment or incoherence).
4. Grossly disorganized or catatonic behavior.
    Note. Do not include a symptom if it is a culturally sanctioned response pattern.

B. Duration of an episode of the disturbance is at least 1 day but less than 1 month, with eventual full return to premorbid level of functioning.

C. The disturbance is not better accounted for by a mood disorder with psychotic features, schizoaffective disorder, or schizophrenia and is not due to the direct physiological effects of a substance (e.g., a drug of abuse, a medication) or a general medical condition.
    Note. Specify if the disorder presents with a marked stressor, without a marked stressor, or with postpartum onset.

Clinical Issues

➤ Brief psychotic disorder:

  ✔ Is often precipitated by a stressor that would affect most people in a similar way, but can also develop without a marked stressor or within 4 weeks postpartum.

  ✔ Presents with psychotic and/or behavioral symptoms (e.g., disorganized behavior, catatonic behavior) that may be indistinguishable from symptoms of the active phase of schizophrenia. However, the rapid resolution of symptoms in brief psychotic disorder helps to differentiate the two disorders. DSM-IV-TR does not include negative symptoms as part of the diagnosis.

  ✔ Typically presents with a sudden onset of emotional turmoil and/or overwhelming confusion. Emotional turmoil can manifest as rapid shifts in affect (e.g., screaming, mutism, peculiar posturing, gibberish speech). The level of agitation, excitement, and psychotic impairment may be so severe as to result in violence and/or poor self-care. Rapid intervention in a protected environment is critically important.

  ✔ Has, by definition, symptoms that last from 1 day to less than 1 month, with full return to premorbid functioning.

  ✔ Usually occurs in the 20- to 30-year age group; therefore, maintain a high suspicion for a substance-induced psychotic disorder.

- ✔ Is more common in individuals with personality and dissociative disorders.
- ✔ Was classified in DSM-III-R (American Psychiatric Association 1987) as brief reactive psychosis when psychosis developed after a marked stressor.
- ➤ The sudden onset and relatively rapid resolution of florid psychotic symptoms with a dysfunctional course often immediately following a significant stressor, in the absence of a substance-induced psychosis, a psychosis secondary to a medical illness, or a psychosis secondary to another psychiatric disorder, is consistent with a diagnosis of brief psychotic disorder.
- ➤ Pay strict attention to time course requirements:
  - ✔ Schizophrenia—1 month (or less if treated) of active phase symptoms and at least 6 months of continuous signs of the illness coupled with a dysfunctional course.
  - ✔ Brief reactive psychosis—symptom resolution in 1 month or less without a progressively dysfunctional course.
  - ✔ Schizophreniform disorder—active phase symptoms from 1 month to 6 months with full symptom resolution without a progressively dysfunctional course.

Prognosis

- ➤ Good prognostic indicators include:
  - ✔ Sudden onset.
  - ✔ Short duration of symptoms.
  - ✔ Severe stressor.
  - ✔ Prominent mood symptoms.
  - ✔ Little affective blunting.
  - ✔ Significant confusion and perplexity at the height of the psychosis.

Differential Diagnosis

- ➤ Psychiatric disorders that can also present with a rapid onset (e.g., schizophrenia, catatonic type, schizophreniform disorder, manic phase of bipolar disorder, major depression with catatonic features).
- ➤ Substance-induced psychotic disorder or substance-induced delirium.
- ➤ Psychotic disorder due to a general medical condition (e.g., Cushing's disease).
- ➤ Borderline or schizotypal personality disorder (can present with somewhat similar symptoms under stress).
- ➤ Delirium.
- ➤ Malingering and factitious disorder.

Treatment

➤ Hospitalization is usually required to:

✔ Provide a safe environment.

✔ Rule out medical (especially neurological), medication-related, and substance-induced causes of psychosis.

✔ Initiate treatment (e.g., antipsychotic medications for psychosis, benzodiazepines or mood stabilizers for acute agitation).

SCHIZOPHRENIFORM DISORDER

DSM-IV-TR Diagnostic Criteria (Summary)

➤ Criteria A, D, and E of schizophrenia (see "DSM-IV-TR Diagnostic Criteria" at the beginning of this chapter) are met.

➤ An episode of the disorder (including prodromal, active, and residual phases) lasts at least 1 month but less than 6 months.

Clinical Issues

➤ Schizophreniform disorder and schizophrenia share nearly identical criteria except that for schizophreniform disorder:

✔ The total duration of the disorder (including prodromal phase, active phase, and residual phase) is at least 1 month but less than 6 months.

✔ Impairment in social/occupational functioning is not required.

➤ One-third of patients fully recover before 6 months and are given a final diagnosis of schizophreniform disorder. Two-thirds of patients progress with their illness and are eventually given another diagnosis (e.g., schizophrenia, schizoaffective disorder).

➤ Depression is frequently present, and there is a significant risk of suicide (~8%).

Prognosis

➤ DSM-IV-TR lists the following "good prognostic features":

✔ Onset of prominent psychotic symptoms within 4 weeks of the first change in usual behavior or functioning.

✔ Confusion or perplexity at the height of the psychotic episode.

✔ Good premorbid social and occupational functioning.

✔ Absence of blunted or flat affect.

Differential Diagnosis

➤ Basically the same as for schizophrenia, but because of the shorter duration of symptoms, there is greater emphasis on ruling out medical and substance-related causes of psychosis.

Epidemiology

➤ Lifetime prevalence is approximately 0.2% (male = female in prevalence).

Treatment

➤ Basically the same as for schizophrenia.

SCHIZOAFFECTIVE DISORDER

DSM-IV-TR Diagnostic Criteria (Summary)

A. Uninterrupted period of illness during which, at some time, there is either a major depressive episode, a manic episode, or a mixed episode concurrent with symptoms that meet the active-phase criteria for schizophrenia (Criterion A). The major depressive episode must include depressed mood.

B. During the same period of illness, there have been delusions or hallucinations for at least 2 weeks in the absence of prominent mood symptoms.

C. Symptoms that meet the criteria for a mood episode are present for a substantial portion of the total duration of the active and residual periods of the illness.

D. The disturbance is not due to the direct physiological effects of a substance, a medication, or a general medical condition.

Clinical Issues

Essential diagnostic criteria:

➤ Diagnostically, three criteria must all be met:

✔ An uninterrupted period of illness in which symptoms that meet Criterion A for schizophrenia occur simultaneously with a major depressive, manic, or mixed episode.

✔ During this period of illness, delusions or hallucinations are present for at least 2 weeks in the absence of mood symptoms.

✔ The mood symptoms are present for a substantial portion of the total duration of the illness.

Course of illness:

➤ Schizoaffective disorder may be more severe than schizophrenia because of the added burden of prominent mood symptoms. Symptoms may last for years or indefinitely.

Epidemiology:

➤ Lifetime prevalence is approximately 0.5%–0.8% and is more common in females.

Classification:

➤ There is significant debate as to how this disorder should be classified. Possibilities are that schizoaffective disorder:

✔ Is truly schizophrenia with incidental affective (mood) symptoms.

✔ Is truly a mood disorder with incidental schizophrenia-like symptoms.

✔ Lies on a continuum between schizophrenia and a mood disorder.

✔ Is a unique disorder unrelated to schizophrenia or a mood disorder.

➤ DSM-IV-TR classifies schizoaffective disorder as a psychotic disorder. Although the mood and psychotic symptoms co-occur, there must also be at least a 2-week period where significant mood symptoms are absent (Criterion B), thereby diagnostically separating schizoaffective disorder from schizophrenia and from a mood disorder with psychotic features.

➤ Because DSM-IV-TR requires a mood episode for a significant portion of the total duration of the illness (Criterion C), it may be difficult clinically to distinguish schizoaffective disorder from either schizophrenia or a mood disorder with psychotic features, especially after a short interview. Always additionally include these two disorders in your differential whenever you are considering schizophrenia as a diagnosis.

Etiology

➤ Some fundamental elements of schizophrenia are prevalent (e.g., neurological soft signs, significant suicide risk, incidence of 1% or less, a genetic component is likely).

➤ Some fundamental elements of a mood disorder are prevalent (e.g., more common in women, reduced latency of rapid eye movement [REM] sleep when depressed, a genetic component is likely).

Prognosis

➤ Prognosis is thought to be better than schizophrenia but poorer than bipolar disorder:

✔ Suicide risk is approximately 10%.

✔ Substance abuse is found in approximately 50% of patients.

✔ Homelessness prevalence is approximately 12%.

✔ Hospitalizations for relapses are common.

Differential Diagnosis

➤ Include a combined differential diagnosis inclusive of both psychotic disorders ("schizo") and mood disorders ("affective").

Treatment

General considerations:

➤ Substance abuse can complicate the differential diagnosis due to its impact on inducing or exacerbating mood changes.

➤ Treatment options vary, without a clear consensus in the literature. However, it is generally accepted that a combination of antidepressant and antipsychotic medications along with psychosocial interventions represents the best approach.

Somatic treatments:

➤ SGAs seem to be more efficacious than the FGAs. Clozapine may be the most effective antipsychotic medication for the treatment of schizoaffective disorder, especially when accompanied by manic and/or suicidal behavior.

➤ Antidepressants can be utilized for depressed mood, and mood stabilizers (e.g., lithium, divalproex) can be utilized for manic-type symptoms. The SGAs have the advantage of treating both the psychotic and manic symptoms.

➤ Anxiolytics can be helpful for the anxiety that often accompanies the disorder and to provide needed sedation when mania is prominent.

➤ ECT can be an effective treatment for patients refractory to the usual treatments or who are actively suicidal.

Psychotherapeutic approaches:

➤ Supportive psychotherapy, assertive community treatment (community outreach programs), group therapy, family therapy, and cognitive-behavioral therapy can be helpful as adjuncts to medications.

DELUSIONAL DISORDER

DSM-IV-TR Diagnostic Criteria (Summary)

A. One or more nonbizarre delusions (i.e., involving situations that occur in real life, such as being followed, poisoned, infected, loved at a distance, or deceived by a spouse or lover, or having a disease) of at least 1 month's duration.

B. Criterion A (active-phase symptoms) for schizophrenia has never been met.

C. Apart from the impact of the delusion or its ramifications, functioning is not markedly impaired and behavior is not obviously odd or bizarre.

D. If mood episodes have occurred concurrently with delusions, their total duration has been brief relative to the duration of the delusional periods.

E. The disturbance is not due to the direct physiological effects of a substance (e.g., a drug of abuse, a medication) or a general medical condition.
    Note. Specify type based on the predominant delusional theme: erotomanic, grandiose, jealous, persecutory, somatic, mixed, or unspecified.

Clinical Issues

➤ Delusional disorders:

✔ Present with one or more persistent (lasting 1 month or longer), non-bizarre (i.e., plausible) delusions that are not caused by a medical illness, a substance (e.g., medication side effect, illicit drug, alcohol), or another psychiatric disorder:

■ Nonbizarre delusions are often the only presenting symptom, marking delusional disorder as a monosymptomatic disorder (unlike schizophrenia, which is a multisymptomatic disorder [i.e., the seven pillars previously discussed]).

■ There are no prominent hallucinations. Tactile and olfactory hallucinations may be present if they are related to the delusional theme.

■ Symptoms are "compartmental" or "encapsulated" rather than "global." Most often, delusions are systematized. Behavior and thinking can be remarkably unimpaired in other areas, although overall functioning can be significantly impaired secondary to the consequence of the delusion.

✔ Are uncommonly seen in clinical practice because of their low prevalence, the absence of associated psychopathology, and patient denial of illness (a core feature of delusional disorder).

✔ Were classified as paranoid disorder in DSM-III (American Psychiatric Association 1980) and as delusional (paranoid) disorder in DSM-III-R.

➤ Common defenses include:

  ✔ Denial (avoidance of painful aspects of reality).

  ✔ Reaction formation (an unacceptable impulse is transformed into its opposite).

  ✔ Projection (unacceptable impulses are transferred to another individual or situation).

Diagnostic considerations:

➤ Delusions should be distinguished from ideation. Ideation (i.e., near-delusional thinking) does not qualify for a diagnosis of delusional disorder. Differentiation between these two can at times be difficult.

➤ A belief does not qualify as a delusion if:

  ✔ It is true.

  ✔ It is a common belief within the person's culture or religion (e.g., belief in witchcraft in Louisiana).

  ✔ The person is able to accept or be convinced that what was believed is not true.

➤ Often the patient's presentation of the delusional theme appears believable at first. However, when the validity of the belief is challenged, patient reactions can range from fervent denial to violence. Violent behavior is more likely with the jealous and erotomanic subtypes of delusional disorder.

➤ When listing a differential diagnosis for any patient with paranoid beliefs, always include a broad differential, as outlined for schizophrenia. Be sure to include both delusional disorder and paranoid personality disorder. However, clarify that you recognize that delusional disorder requires nonbizarre delusions and that paranoid personality disorder involves paranoid ideation but not frank delusions. The accurate diagnosis of disorders with delusional-type symptoms often rests on the type, intensity, and quality of the delusional or near-delusional belief. The most likely causes of persistent (duration greater than 6 months) delusional symptoms are schizophrenia, schizoaffective disorder, delusional disorders, neurological disorders (e.g., dementia, delirium, brain tumor), substance use disorders, and mood disorders.

Research considerations:

➤ Little research has been undertaken on delusional disorders, especially in comparison to the burgeoning outpouring of research on schizophrenia and bipolar disorder. This is due in part to the low prevalence of the disorder and in part to the general unwillingness of persons with the disorder to accept psychiatric treatment. As a consequence, etiological foundations, possible genetic contributions, and treatment recommendations are not as well defined as in schizophrenia, mood disorders, and anxiety disorders.

Historical significance:

➤ The current precepts of delusional disorder are based on Kraepelin's original formulations. He recognized that in addition to patients with dementia praecox, a subset of patients held rigid delusional beliefs without manifesting hallucinations, a downhill course, or impaired functioning. This subset of patients warranted a diagnosis of paranoid disorder. Kraepelin also defined persecutory, grandiose, erotomanic, and jealous subtypes.

➤ Historically, perhaps the most famous example of a delusional theme (described by Freud) was the grandiose delusion of Paul Schreber (a judge), who developed an unshakable belief that God was transforming him into a woman so that he could be impregnated to save the human race. Since this delusion is bizarre and implausible, it could not, by DSM-IV-TR criteria, be consistent with a diagnosis of delusional disorder.

Delusional Subtypes

Persecutory subtype:

➤ Persons with the persecutory subtype:

✔ Present with the most common form of delusional disorder.

✔ Believe that they are chronically treated in malevolent ways. They feel cheated, harassed, conspired against, spied on, poisoned, or drugged. Often, the delusions are elaborate and detailed. Significant anger or hostility can develop.

✔ May use the legal system or violence to correct the injustice.

Erotomanic subtype (de Clérambault's syndrome):

➤ Persons with the erotomanic subtype:

✔ Believe that another person, usually of prominence (but can be a stranger), is in love with them ("secret love" or "love from afar"). Often, a benign sign (e.g., wearing a blue tie) is misinterpreted by the believer as an offer or confirmation of love. The belief of reciprocated love can be so strong as to survive for years even when no communication occurs between the two individuals.

✔ Make strong efforts to contact the person, often by pestering, harassing, or invading the person's privacy (i.e., stalking). There may be repeated phone calls, letters, or visits. Individuals may come into repeated conflict with the law as a result of their unrelenting pursuit of the desired person despite legal intervention (e.g., failure to honor a restraining order).

✔ Often describe excitement or challenge in pursuit of the other person.

✔ Are more commonly female.

✔ Can become violent in their pursuit.

Grandiose subtype ("megalomania" or "delusions of grandeur"):

➤ Persons with the grandiose subtype:

✔ Believe that they have some great talent or insight, that they have made some important (but not as yet recognized) discovery, or believe that they have a special relationship with a prominent person. The individual may seek to become a leader of a religious cult or become a street preacher.

Jealous subtype ("Othello syndrome" or "conjugal paranoia"):

➤ Persons with the jealous subtype:

✔ Believe, without due cause, that their sexual partner is unfaithful. They may collect "evidence" (e.g., recording phone calls, following the partner) to "document" the infidelity.

✔ May take physical action against the partner (e.g., refuse to allow the partner to leave the home), the "lover," and/or themselves.

✔ Are more commonly male.

✔ Can become violent in their pursuit of the "truth."

Somatic subtype ("delusional parasitosis" or "delusions of infestation"):

➤ Persons with the somatic subtype:

✔ Firmly believe that they have a serious physical defect or disease, despite evidence to the contrary. Examples include believing that a foul odor is emanating from a body part (olfactory type), that there is an infestation of insects or parasites (infestation type; delusional parasitosis), or that certain body parts are significantly altered (body dysmorphic type).

✔ Intensively and unrelentingly seek treatment for their presumed ailments. They may produce a sample of the parasite or body fluid to support their claim. When one treatment provider does not support their belief, they seek treatment from another provider. Individuals with delusional parasitosis are much more likely to be seen by a dermatologist than by a psychiatrist.

Mixed subtype:

➤ Persons with the mixed subtype have more than one delusion from different subtypes, without a predominant theme.

Unspecified subtype:

➤ Persons with the unspecified subtype have delusional themes that cannot be clearly determined or that are not adequately described by a specific subtype.

Epidemiology

➤ Prevalence is very low (about 30 per 100,000, or 0.03%).

➤ Most often starts in midlife (ages 35–50 years) and is slightly more frequent in females.

Etiology

➤ Etiology is not well defined, but delusional disorder is not believed to be genetically related to schizophrenia or the mood disorders.

➤ Genetic transmission appears to be an important factor.

➤ Psychosocial stressors may also play a role in the etiology, as in shared psychotic disorder (folie à deux), in which the person (A) develops a delusion similar to that of another individual (B) with whom A has a close relationship. If the two are separated, A's delusion may dissipate.

➤ Head injuries or other neurological insults may precipitate or exacerbate the disorder. The relatively common occurrence of delusions in neurological illness has led to the speculation that the limbic system, basal ganglia, and neocortical associations may be involved in the development of the disorder.

Risk Factors

➤ Advancing age.

➤ Sensory deprivation (e.g., hearing loss).

➤ Social isolation (e.g., living alone).

➤ Recent immigration.

➤ Family history of psychiatric disorders.

➤ Female gender.

➤ Neurological injury

Course of Illness

➤ The course tends to be chronic, although 33%–50% of patients show substantial improvement after 10–15 years.

➤ Prognosis is better with an acute presentation and an early age at onset, and with separation of the two individuals in folie à deux.

Differential Diagnosis (Disorders That Can Present With Delusions or Near-Delusional Symptoms)

Psychiatric disorders:

➤ Brief psychotic disorder, schizophreniform disorder, schizoaffective disorder, schizophrenia, delusional disorder, shared psychotic disorder.

➤ Major depressive disorder with psychotic features (unipolar and bipolar depression).

➤ Manic phase of bipolar disorder when accompanied by psychotic features.

➤ Nonpsychotic disorders that can present with near-delusional thinking:

  ✔ Paranoid personality disorder. The person is suspicious and hypervigilant (paranoid ideation) but usually does not have frank paranoid delusions.

  ✔ Schizoid and schizotypal personality disorders can present with paranoid ideation.

  ✔ Hypochondriasis and body dysmorphic disorder (both are nonpsychotic disorders but are founded on near-delusional thinking relating to physical health or to body image, respectively).

  ✔ OCD (obsessions can easily appear to be delusional in nature).

  ✔ Anorexia nervosa (obsession with food can appear to be delusional).

Psychotic disorder due to a general medical condition:

➤ Basal ganglia disorders (e.g., Parkinson's disease, Huntington's chorea).

➤ CNS involvement (e.g., head injury, HIV infection, brain tumor, seizure disorder).

➤ Deficiency states (e.g., vitamin B_{12}, folate, thiamine, niacin).

➤ Delirium or dementia.

Substance-induced psychotic disorders:

➤ Substance intoxication (e.g., CNS stimulants, hallucinogens, large doses of digoxin).

➤ Substance withdrawal (e.g., alcohol, benzodiazepines).

Treatment

General considerations:

➤ To help distinguish between truth and delusion, review past medical records and, if possible, interview family, friends, and co-workers. Because these procedures are not possible during the oral board examination, your differential will necessarily be quite large.

➤ Persons with delusional disorder typically do not seek mental health treatment because of denial of mental illness and trust issues. They may seek help from the legal system, become violent, or relentlessly pursue medical treatment for a nonexistent physical disorder.

➤ It is difficult to build an alliance with the patient, and patients are frequently noncompliant with treatment recommendations. Even with a good alliance, psychotherapy is often only marginally effective. Even obtaining a history can be difficult (and possibly dangerous, if the validity of the delusion is challenged).

➤ Hospitalization typically is not required unless dangerousness becomes an issue.

➤ A complete medical workup is indicated to rule out medical or substance-related causes of the delusions. Also assess for comorbid depression, anxiety, agitation, and the potential for violence.

➤ Psychological testing (e.g., MMPI-II, Rorschach test, Thematic Apperception Test) can be helpful to establish the diagnosis and the extent of impairment.

Pharmacotherapy:

➤ Patients may refuse medications because of delusionally based fears of being poisoned or denial of illness.

➤ A trial of an SGA (preferred) or a high-potency FGA could be helpful. Pimozide (Orap) can be particularly effective for delusional disorder with somatic symptoms (e.g., delusional parasitosis). Antipsychotic medications may diminish the intensity of the delusion but may have little impact on the core delusional process.

➤ SSRIs have been reported to be helpful in some patients with delusional disorders (independent of their effects on depression).

Psychotherapy:

➤ Attempt to establish a strong therapeutic alliance with the patient. The therapist's unwavering reliability and willingness to listen are essential. Trust is often a major issue. Assure the patient of confidentiality (except if dangerousness becomes an issue). Over time, explore how the delusion interferes with the patient's life.

➤ Do not directly challenge the validity of the delusion. Direct challenges are likely to result in discontinuation of treatment or, in extreme cases, violent behavior. With a strong alliance, insight-oriented psychotherapy can be beneficial. Supportive and cognitive-behavioral therapies may also provide benefit.

➤ Patients typically reject group therapy because of trust issues.

➤ Family members often have a difficult time dealing with the patient's delusional belief(s).

SHARED PSYCHOTIC DISORDER

DSM-IV-TR Diagnostic Criteria (Summary)

➤ A delusion develops in an individual in the context of a close relationship with another person(s), who has an already-established delusion.

➤ The delusion is similar in content to the delusion of the person who already has the established delusion.

➤ The disturbance is not better accounted for by another psychotic disorder (e.g., schizophrenia) or a mood disorder with psychotic features and is not due to the direct physiological effects of a substance (e.g., a drug of abuse, a medication) or a general medical condition.

Clinical Issues

➤ Shared psychotic disorder:

  ✔ Is also called *folie à deux.*

  ✔ Is diagnosed when:

   ■ The delusion develops in the context of a close relationship with another person who already has the delusion.

   ■ The acquired delusion is similar in content to the established delusion held by the originating person.

   ■ The delusion is not secondary to a substance or a medical condition.

  ✔ Most commonly involves the following presentations:

   ■ Type of delusion—persecutory.

   ■ Psychiatric disorder of the primary holder of the delusion—schizophrenia.

   ■ Relationship of person acquiring the delusion—a spouse or first-degree biological relative.

  ✔ Is most likely to occur when:

   ■ The two individuals are in close and continuous physical proximity to each other.

   ■ The two individuals are poor or live in poverty.

   ■ The person who acquired the delusion sees the other person as someone in authority.

   ■ Some measure of psychological gain is derived by the person acquiring the delusion.

✔ Is of unknown etiology. A proposed mechanism is that the person originally having the delusion has authority over a more passive and dependent person who accepts the delusion. The person acquiring the delusion
would rather accept the delusion than risk losing the relationship.

Treatment Considerations

➤ Treatment must be individualized:

✔ Physical separation may reverse the delusion (*folie imposée*).

✔ Antipsychotic medications may be needed for both individuals.

✔ A new psychosis can develop in the person who acquired the initial delusion (*folie induite*).

PSYCHOTIC DISORDER DUE TO A GENERAL MEDICAL CONDITION

➤ Diagnostic criteria require the presence of prominent hallucinations or delusions that are a direct physiological effect of a medical condition. The psychotic symptoms are not caused by another psychiatric disorder, and the disturbance is not secondary to a delirium:

✔ Hallucinations can occur in any of the five senses. Recall that auditory
hallucinations are a requirement for the diagnosis of schizophrenia, paranoid type.

✔ Delusions can express any theme, but are most often paranoid.

✔ Delusions are less common than hallucinations.

➤ The diagnosis *cannot be made* if the person maintains reality testing for the
hallucination (i.e., appreciates that the perceptual experience results from
the medical condition). Therefore, the person must have lack of insight
regarding the hallucination to qualify for the diagnosis.

➤ DSM-IV-TR lists two examples of medical conditions that may involve psychosis without reality testing:

✔ *Temporal lobe epilepsy*—unpleasant olfactory hallucinations and religious delusions.

✔ *Right parietal lesions*—contralateral neglect syndrome, in which the
patient denies the existence of parts of his or her body.

➤ Psychotic disorder due to a general medical condition always belongs in the
differential diagnosis when a patient presents with psychotic symptoms.

SUBSTANCE-INDUCED PSYCHOTIC DISORDER

➤ Diagnostic criteria require the presence of prominent hallucinations (without insight as to being substance-induced) or delusions that are a direct physiological effect of a substance (e.g., a drug of abuse, a medication, a toxin). Examples include:

✔ Substance intoxication (e.g., alcohol, inhalants, opioids, cannabis, stimulants [e.g., amphetamine, cocaine]).

✔ Substance withdrawal (e.g., alcohol, benzodiazepines).

✔ Medications (e.g., corticosteroids, anticholinergic agents, disulfiram, antidepressants).

✔ Toxins (e.g., anticholinesterase inhibitors, organophosphate insecticides, nerve gases, carbon monoxide).

➤ The diagnosis *cannot be made* if the person maintains reality testing for the hallucination (i.e., appreciates that the perceptual experience results from abuse of the substance unless delusions are also present). Therefore, lack of insight regarding the hallucination is a requirement.

➤ Substance-induced psychotic disorder always belongs in the differential diagnosis when a patient presents with psychotic symptoms.

PSYCHOTIC DISORDER NOT OTHERWISE SPECIFIED

General Considerations

➤ A diagnosis of psychotic disorder not otherwise specified is assigned when psychotic symptoms are present but one of the following circumstances applies:

✔ There is not enough information to make a specific diagnosis.

✔ There is contradictory information.

✔ The psychotic symptoms do not meet the criteria for any specific psychotic disorder (e.g., tactile hallucinations are the only symptoms and are not caused by a substance or a medical disorder).

Postpartum Psychosis

➤ Is categorized by DSM-IV-TR as a psychotic disorder not otherwise specified.

➤ Is rare, affecting 1–2 in 1,000 mothers giving birth.

➤ Typically occurs within 2–4 weeks postpartum, but onset can be within hours of delivery.

➤ Is characterized by psychotic symptoms (e.g., hallucinations, delusions [often religious], disorganization) that may be coupled with suicidal and/or homicidal ideation or behavior. It is estimated that 5% of persons with postpartum psychosis will try to harm themselves or someone else (possibly the newborn infant).

➤ Is classified as a medical emergency necessitating hospitalization.

➤ Has a number of risk factors, including bipolar disorder (a powerful risk factor) and a prior episode of postpartum psychosis (a powerful risk factor). Additional risk factors include thyroid disease, schizophrenia, and a family history of bipolar disorder or thyroid disease.

➤ May actually represent a variant of bipolar disorder with manic features (controversial).

➤ Can be treated with antipsychotic medications. Olanzapine, haloperidol, risperidone, and clozapine can be of significant value in reducing psychotic symptoms. Response to treatment can be rapid.

2

MOOD DISORDERS

Principal DSM-IV-TR Mood Episodes and Mood Disorders

Major depressive episode
Major depressive disorder
Mood disorders due to a general medical condition and
   substance-induced mood disorders
Dysthymic disorder
Manic, hypomanic, and mixed episodes
Bipolar I disorder, bipolar II disorder, and cyclothymic disorder
Bipolar depression and rapid cycling (not DSM-IV-TR diagnoses)
Bipolar spectrum disorders (not a DSM-IV-TR diagnosis)
Mood disorder not otherwise specified

MAJOR DEPRESSIVE EPISODE

DSM-IV-TR Diagnostic Criteria (Summary)

➤ Two-week history of either depressed mood (most of the day nearly every day) or markedly diminished interest or pleasure in all, or almost all, activities (anhedonia), and four or more of the following:

✔ Significant change in appetite or change in weight (without dieting).

✔ Insomnia or hypersomnia nearly every day.

✔ Psychomotor agitation or retardation.

✔ Fatigue or loss of energy nearly every day.

✔ Feelings of worthlessness or excessive or inappropriate guilt (which may be delusional).

✔ Difficulty concentrating, thinking, focusing, or making decisions.

✔ Recurrent thoughts of death, recurrent suicidal ideation without a specific plan, or a suicide attempt or a specific plan for committing suicide.

➤ Symptoms do not meet criteria for a mixed episode.

➤ Symptoms cause clinically significant distress or impairment in important areas of functioning.

➤ Symptoms are not due to the physiological effects of a substance or a general medical condition.

➤ Symptoms are not due to bereavement.

Diagnostic Issues

➤ Major depressive episode (MDE):

✔ Can be characterized by some combination of:

■ Emotional and cognitive symptoms (e.g., depressed mood, tearfulness, hopelessness, anhedonia, undeserved guilt, slowed thinking, poor memory, suicidal ideation).

■ Neurovegetative symptoms (e.g., poor sleep, poor appetite, stooped posture, slowed movements, fatigue, absence of gesturing, sexual dysfunction, aches and pains, weakness).

✔ Does not necessarily require depressed mood to satisfy diagnostic criteria. Anhedonia and four additional symptoms listed in DSM-IV-TR will suffice.

✔ Requires that symptoms:

■ Are present for at least 2 weeks.

■ Do not satisfy criteria for a mixed bipolar episode, are not due to bereavement, and cause significant functional impairment.

■ Are not due to the effects of a substance (e.g., a medication side effect, alcohol, an illicit drug). A mood disorder secondary to the use of a substance is classified as a *substance-induced mood disorder.*

■ Are not the direct physiological consequences of a medical (i.e., systemic, neurological) illness. A mood disorder caused by medical illness is classified as a *mood disorder due to a general medical condition,* with the name of the illness inserted for "a general medical condition."

✔ Serves as a "building block" (i.e., provides the core diagnostic features) for:

■ Major depressive disorder (i.e., unipolar depression).

■ Bipolar depression.

■ Schizoaffective disorder.

Characteristic Findings

➤ Anhedonia is defined as a decreased ability or an inability to experience pleasure from situations or behaviors that normally would be pleasurable.

➤ Depressed mood:

   ✔ *Mood* is defined as a person's sustained emotional state ("pervasive affect") over a given period of time (e.g., a week, a month). Descriptions patients may use to describe depressed mood include s*ad, depressed, unhappy, discouraged, hopeless, "down in the dumps," "as low as I can get," "blah,"* and *empty.*

   ✔ Mood is most often assessed from the patient's perspective of their emotional state. However, such descriptions can at times be misleading. For example, a depressed individual may deny or not appreciate depressed mood, instead complaining of physical symptoms that are not found to have an organic basis (historically described as *masked depression*).

➤ Depressed affect:

   ✔ *Affect* is defined as a person's emotional state at a particular time and is assessed by the interviewer observing the person's overall reactivity, facial expression, body movements, and speech patterns.

   ✔ Affect consistent with an MDE can appear restricted (reduction in expression), depressed (sad expression), blunted (severe reduction in expression), or flat (little or no expressed emotion). In mixed bipolar episodes, affect can be labile (frequent shifts between elation and depression).

➤ Psychomotor retardation (e.g., slowed pace, retarded body movements) and psychomotor agitation (e.g., restlessness, inability to sit still) are common findings. Psychomotor retardation is more common in younger adults, and psychomotor agitation is more common in the elderly.

➤ Speech latency (long pauses between the time questions are asked and person responds) and lowered speech intensity (i.e., words are spoken softly).

➤ Frequent crying spells or frequently feeling like crying.

➤ Impaired or slowed cognitive functioning (e.g., poor memory, poor concentration), typically with the complaint that memory is poor.

➤ Social withdrawal or isolation.

➤ Decreased appetite with associated weight loss (the classic presentation) or increased appetite, usually with carbohydrate cravings, and associated weight gain (most often found in major depressive disorder with atypical or seasonal features).

➤ Insomnia (e.g., initial, middle, terminal insomnia) or hypersomnia (most often found in major depressive disorder with atypical or seasonal features). The classic presentation is early-morning awakening (i.e., middle or terminal insomnia), but initial insomnia is also a common finding.

➤ Feelings of hopelessness (high risk factor for suicide).

➤ Poor self-esteem or feelings of worthlessness.

➤ Feelings of guilt (even though undeserved).

➤ Suicidal ideation and behavior (risk factors are detailed in Chapter 7 ["Violent Behavior"]):

  ✔ Always assess for suicidal ideation and a history of suicidal behaviors:

    ■ Suicidal thinking can range from "The world would be better off if I were dead" to obsessive thoughts of suicide with a plan. Depressed individuals may have acquired materials (e.g., ropes, guns, medications) to kill themselves. If you were to have the opportunity, you would ask, in progression: "Do you have thoughts that the world would be better off if you were dead or thoughts of wishing to be dead? Do you have thoughts of harming yourself? If so, how would you do it? Do you have any past history of suicidal thinking or suicide attempts? Have you acquired the means to harm yourself? What keeps you from harming yourself?"

  ✔ Assess whether the ideation is:

    ■ Acute or chronic.

    ■ Active or passive.

  ✔ A gun is the most common and hanging the second most common means of committing suicide.

  ✔ The family should be told to remove guns or other potential weapons from the home if there is any concern for the possibility of suicide.

  ✔ For the oral boards, you will not be penalized for taking extra time to explore these issues.

➤ Homicidal ideation and behavior (risk factors are detailed in Chapter 7 ["Violent Behavior"]):

  ✔ Always assess for angry feelings, homicidal ideation, and prior history of homicidal behaviors:

    ■ Depressed individuals can become violent toward others and may have acquired materials (e.g., knives, guns) to harm others. Ask, in progression: "Do you have thoughts of wanting to harm others? If so, on whom, why, and how would you commit this act? Do you have a history of harming others? Have you acquired materials that can be used to harm others? What keeps you from harming others?"

  ✔ Assess whether the ideation is:

    ■ Acute or chronic.

    ■ Active or passive.

  ✔ According to the *Tarasoff* ruling, the clinician has both:

    ■ A duty to protect the threatened person or persons (designated as the third party) by warning the person(s) of the impending imminent danger (despite violating patient confidentiality).

- ■ A duty to prevent the patient from harming the third party, typically through psychiatric commitment or by alerting the police for legal restraint.
  - ✔ For the oral boards, you will not be penalized for taking extra time to explore these issues.
- ➤ Sexual dysfunction:
  - ✔ Includes reduced libido, erectile dysfunction, and delayed or impaired ability to achieve orgasm.
  - ✔ Should not always be assumed to be secondary to antidepressant treatment. Sexual dysfunction may:
    - ■ Have been present prior to the depression.
    - ■ Be a consequence of the depression.
    - ■ Be caused or worsened by antidepressants (the usual assumption).
- ➤ A useful mnemonic for remembering the key symptoms of depression (in addition to depressed mood) is *SIG: ECAPS:*
  - ■ S   Sleep disturbance.
  - ■ I   Interest.
  - ■ G   Guilt.
  - ■ E   Energy.
  - ■ C   Concentration.
  - ■ A   Appetite.
  - ■ P   Psychomotor retardation or agitation.
  - ■ S   Suicidal thoughts.

MAJOR DEPRESSIVE DISORDER

Major Depressive Disorder, Single Episode

DSM-IV-TR diagnostic criteria (summary):

- ➤ Requires the presence of a single MDE.
- ➤ The MDE is not better accounted for by schizoaffective disorder and is not superimposed on schizophrenia, schizophreniform disorder, delusional disorder, or psychotic disorder NOS.
- ➤ There has never been a manic, mixed, or hypomanic episode.

Diagnostic and clinical issues:

- ➤ If the MDE is secondary to schizoaffective disorder or is superimposed on schizophrenia, schizophreniform disorder, delusional disorder, or psychotic disorder NOS, a diagnosis of major depressive disorder (MDD) is not appropriate.

➤ A history of a single manic, mixed, or hypomanic episode definitively rules out a diagnosis of MDD. However, a diagnosis of MDD can be maintained if the manic, mixed, or hypomanic episode was induced by an antidepressant, although the episode itself qualifies as a "substance-induced mood disorder."

➤ Risk factors for MDD, single episode, include:

✔ Female > male, by a ratio of 2 to 1 (lifetime and point prevalence).

✔ Age between 18 and 45 years or age greater than 60 years.

✔ An underlying dysthymic disorder.

✔ A family history of MDD, especially in a first-degree relative.

✔ Chronic low self-esteem and a pessimistic outlook.

✔ Recent stressors or losses (usually of a significant nature but can be minor).

✔ The postpartum or perimenopausal period.

✔ Few social or family supports.

✔ A prior suicide attempt or family history of suicide attempts.

✔ Lower socioeconomic status (e.g., less educated, unemployed).

✔ Psychiatric illness (e.g., anxiety disorders, schizophrenia).

✔ Active substance abuse and possibly a history of substance abuse.
Note. Depression stemming from the direct physiological effects of a substance (legal, illegal) does not qualify for a diagnosis of MDD. However, the use/abuse of a substance can also increase the risk for MDD (e.g., marital issues develop, loss of job, failure in school).

✔ Medical illness (e.g., hypothyroidism, cerebrovascular accident, Cushing's disease).
Note. Depression resulting from the direct physiological effects of a medical illness does not qualify for a diagnosis of MDD. However, a medical illness can also increase the risk for MDD (e.g., realization of decreased ability to function, chronic pain).

Major Depressive Disorder, Recurrent

DSM-IV-TR diagnostic criteria (summary):

➤ Presence of two or more discrete MDEs separated by at least 2 consecutive months.

Diagnostic and clinical issues:

➤ MDD, recurrent, must satisfy the same diagnostic criteria as MDD, single episode, except that the depressive episodes must be separated by at least 2 months.

➤ As the number of depressive episodes increase:

✔ The time between successive episodes and responsiveness to treatment decreases.

✔ The duration and severity of episodes increases.

✔ The prognosis worsens.

➤ MDD eventually recurs in ~75% of previously treated individuals unless maintenance treatment (e.g., antidepressant medications, ECT, psychotherapy) is provided.

➤ Risk factors for MDD, recurrent, include many of the risk factors for MDD, single episode. Aditionally, risk factors for MDD, recurrent, include considerations related to the prior depressive episode(s):

✔ A severe index episode (e.g., MDD with melancholic features, MDD with psychotic features).

✔ Long duration of a prior episode of MDD.

✔ Incomplete recovery from a prior episode of MDD.

➤ The risk of MDD, recurrent, is reduced:

✔ The longer the patient has remained depression free (i.e., in recovery).

✔ The longer the patient has remained on maintenance therapy (antidepressants, psychotherapy).

Specifiers Applicable to Mood Disorders

Chronic:

DSM-IV-TR diagnostic criteria for chronic specifier (summary):

➤ Full criteria for MDD have been met continuously for at least the past 2 years.

Clinical issues:

➤ *Chronic* is a specifier (not a disorder) that can apply to MDD (single episode, recurrent), bipolar I disorder, and bipolar II disorder.

➤ MDD, chronic:

✔ Develops in 10%–20% of persons with MDD.

✔ Is often undertreated or remains untreated.

✔ Is associated with significant functional impairment. Antidepressants often are only partially effective and may be needed indefinitely.

➤ Risk factors include:

✔ Long duration of depression before initiating treatment.

✔ Inadequate treatment of the MDD.

✔ Recurrent episodes of MDD.

✔ Active substance abuse.

With catatonic features:

DSM-IV-TR diagnostic criteria for catatonic features specifier (summary):

➤ Presence of MDD.

➤ The clinical picture is dominated by at least two of the following:

 ✔ Catalepsy (motoric immobility).

 ✔ Excessive motor activity (purposeless; not influenced by external stimuli).

 ✔ Extreme negativism.

 ✔ Peculiarities of voluntary movement (e.g., odd posturing).

 ✔ Echolalia or echopraxia.

Clinical issues:

➤ *Catatonic features* is a specifier (not a disorder) that can apply to MDD (single episode, recurrent), bipolar I disorder, and bipolar II disorder

➤ MDD with catatonic features:

 ✔ Presents with classic features of catatonia (e.g., either immobility or excessive motor activity; odd or bizarre posturing; negativism; parroting of the words [echolalia] or actions [echopraxia] of others).

 ✔ Can easily be mistaken for a wide range of neurological disorders (e.g., delirium, carbon monoxide poisoning, head injury) and psychiatric disorders (e.g., schizophrenia, catatonic type; brief psychotic disorder).

 ✔ Often requires hospitalization because of concerns about adequacy of self-care and uncertainty of the diagnosis.

 ✔ Is typically highly responsive to ECT.

With melancholic features:

DSM-IV-TR diagnostic criteria for melancholic features specifier (summary):

➤ Presence of MDD.

➤ Either of the following, occurring during the most severe period of the episode:

 ✔ Loss of pleasure in all, or almost all, activities (pervasive anhedonia).

 ✔ Lack of reactivity to usually pleasurable stimuli (does not feel much better, even temporarily, when something good happens).

➤ Three or more of the following:

 ✔ Distinct quality of depressed mood (i.e., the depressed mood is experienced as distinctly different from the kind of feeling experienced after the death of a loved one).

 ✔ Depression regularly worse in the morning.

✔ Early-morning awakening (at least 2 hours before usual time of awakening).

✔ Marked psychomotor retardation or agitation.

✔ Significant anorexia or weight loss.

✔ Excessive or inappropriate guilt.

Clinical issues:

➤ *Melancholic features* is a specifier (not a disorder) that can apply to MDD (single episode, recurrent), bipolar I disorder, and bipolar II disorder.

➤ Melancholia ("black bile") was recognized as an ailment of the earth (one of the four humors) prior to the birth of Christ.

➤ Cardinal features of MDD with melancholic features usually include an inability to experience pleasure, even with a very desired event (i.e., "nonreactive mood"); early-morning awakening; appetite loss and/or weight loss; depression worse in the morning; and marked psychomotor retardation.

➤ Melancholic depression is:

✔ A severe form of depression.

✔ Often recurrent.

✔ Accompanied by psychotic features in 10%–15% of patients (thereby simultaneously conferring the two most severe forms of depression).

✔ More common after 50 years of age.

✔ Typically responsive to somatic therapies.

✔ Likely to have a genetic basis.

✔ *Possibly* more responsive to antidepressants with combined serotonin (5-hydroxytryptamine [5-HT]) and norepinephrine (NE) agonist activity (e.g., tertiary-amine tricyclic antidepressants [TCAs],[1] selective norepinephrine reuptake inhibitors [SNRIs],[2] mirtazapine,[2] monoamine oxidase inhibitors [MAOIs][3]) than to antidepressants with principally selective 5-HT activity (e.g., selective serotonin reuptake inhibitors [SSRIs],[4] nefazodone) or with principally selective NE activity (e.g., the secondary-amine TCAs desipramine and nortriptyline).

---

[1]TCAs include amitriptyline, desipramine, imipramine, and nortriptyline.

[2]SNRIs and atypical antidepressants (AtypANs) include bupropion, venlafaxine (Effexor), duloxetine (Cymbalta), mirtazapine (Remeron), and nefazodone (Serzone). Nefazodone is a nearly pure serotonin agonist, and bupropion is without 5-HT agonist properties.

[3]MAOIs include selegiline transdermal (EmSam), phenelzine (Nardil), tranylcypromine (Parnate), and isocarboxazid (Marplan).

With atypical features:

DSM-IV-TR diagnostic criteria for atypical features specifier (summary):

➤ Presence of MDD.

➤ Mood reactivity (i.e., mood brightens in response to actual or potentially positive events). Described as "preserved reactivity of mood."

➤ Two or more of the following features:

✔ Significant increase in appetite or weight gain.

✔ Hypersomnia.

✔ Leaden paralysis (i.e., arms and legs feel heavy, as if made of lead).

✔ Long-standing pattern of interpersonal rejection sensitivity (not limited to episodes of mood disturbance) that results in significant social or occupational impairment.

➤ Criteria are not met for "with melancholic features" or "with catatonic features" during the same episode.

Clinical issues:

➤ *Atypical* is a specifier (not a disorder) that can apply to MDD (single episode, recurrent), dysthymic disorder, bipolar I disorder, and bipolar II disorder.

➤ Often characterized as a "reverse mood pattern," with increased appetite, increased sleep, and ability to experience pleasure:

➤ Historically described as "hysteroid dysphoria."

➤ Typically find an early age at onset, chronic course, higher frequency in females, higher frequency in patients with borderline personality disorder, and an especially good response to SSRIs, bupropion, and MAOIs but not to TCAs.

➤ Chromium picolinate 600 µg/day may be helpful in reducing carbohydrate cravings and in improving mood.

Postpartum onset:

DSM-IV-TR diagnostic criteria for postpartum onset specifier (summary):

➤ Presence of MDD.

➤ Onset of major depression within 4 weeks following childbirth.

Clinical issues:

➤ *Postpartum onset* is a specifier (not a disorder) that can apply to MDD (single episode, recurrent), bipolar I disorder, and bipolar II disorder.

---

[4]SSRIs include fluoxetine (Prozac), paroxetine (Paxil), sertraline (Zoloft), citalopram (Celexa), and escitalopram (Lexapro).

➤ MDD with postpartum onset:

  ✔ Affects ~10%–15% of women giving birth.

  ✔ Is easily missed and may remain untreated.

  ✔ Is more likely to develop in women with:

    ■ A history of a mood disorder (especially bipolar disorder).

    ■ A family history of a mood disorder.

    ■ A history of thyroid dysfunction.

    ■ Significant stress (e.g., ambivalence about having a new child, lack of support to help with the new child).

Treatment considerations:

➤ Antidepressants and psychotherapy can be very helpful. Caution should be exercised for nursing mothers.

Recurrent, with seasonal pattern:

DSM-IV-TR diagnostic criteria for seasonal pattern specifier (summary):

➤ Recurrent cycles of MDEs temporally related to a particular time of the year (usually fall or winter). There is an absence of an obvious seasonal stressor precipitating the depression (e.g., being unemployed each winter).

➤ Full remission also occurs at a characteristic time of the year.

➤ In the past 2 years, two MDEs have occurred that demonstrate the temporal relationship defined in the two items above. Also, no nonseasonal MDEs have occurred during that time period.

➤ Seasonal MDEs substantially outnumber the nonseasonal MDEs that may have occurred over the individual's lifetime.

Clinical issues:

➤ *Seasonal pattern* is a specifier (not a disorder) that can apply to MDD (single episode, recurrent), bipolar I disorder, and bipolar II disorder.

➤ Synonyms include *seasonal affective disorder (SAD), winter depression, holiday blues,* and *arctic blues.*

➤ The prevalence is significantly higher in females (~4:1) in northern geographical regions with less winter light, and in persons between ages 18–40 years.

➤ Core features of MDD, recurrent, with seasonal pattern, include:

  ✔ At least a 2-year history of MDEs that occur at a particular season of the year, with complete remission between episodes.

  ✔ Absence of a stressor to explain the onset of depression.

  ✔ "Reverse neurovegetative" symptoms, secondary to an increased tendency to sleep and eat excessively (especially carbohydrates) during the depressive episode. Neurovegetative symptoms typically precede the onset of depressed mood.

✔ A regular yearly pattern for the recurrence of depression is a cardinal requirement. An alternate regular pattern (e.g., feeling better in the winter and worse in the summer) is possible.

Etiology:

➤ Possibly related to decreased availability of sunlight in winter coupled with a biological drive for "winter hibernation." Dysregulation of melatonin and decreased 5-HT are likely contributing factors.

➤ Melatonin:

✔ Release from the pineal gland is suppressed by light.

✔ Is produced in excess by animals hibernating during the winter (e.g., long periods of sleeping, lower body temperature).

✔ Is marketed as a sleeping aid and can be helpful for normalizing sleep patterns (e.g., after east-to-west long-distance flights across several time zones).

➤ Carbohydrate craving accompanying the disorder may be linked to a biological drive to replenish 5-HT.

Treatment considerations:

➤ Light therapy (phototherapy):

✔ Suppresses melatonin release and can be very effective.

✔ Can produce a switch into mania/hypomania in susceptible individuals.

➤ Antidepressants and psychotherapy are alternative treatments and can be used alone or in combination with phototherapy.

Severity of depression:

➤ Mild—few, if any, symptoms in excess of those required to make the diagnosis, resulting in only minor impairment in occupational functioning or in usual social activities or relationships with others.

➤ Moderate—symptoms of functional impairment between mild and severe.

➤ Severe—symptoms far in excess of those required to make the diagnosis, and symptoms markedly interfere with occupational functioning or with usual social activities or relationships.

Terminology and Descriptors Associated With Depression

➤ Numerous (and at times confusing) terminology and descriptors have been and are used to describe the varying nuances of depression.

The "five R's":

➤ **R**esponse—reduction of depressive symptoms by at least 50% from the initial Hamilton Rating Scale for Depression (HAM-D) score. By this definition, a severely depressed patient with an initially high HAM-D score can show a "response" to a treatment, yet still be significantly depressed.

➤ Remission—minimal or no depressive symptoms. Defined as a reduction in the HAM-D score to 7 or below.

➤ Relapse—return of depressive symptoms before recovery.

➤ Recovery—asymptomatic period lasting at least 6 months following an episode of depression. Recovery is the ultimate goal of treatment. A partial response is highly predictive of a recurrence of MDD.

➤ Recurrence—a new depressive episode with onset at least 2 months after prior full recovery.

Clinical depression:

➤ A general expression describing a depressive episode attributable to any number of causes (e.g., MDD, schizophrenia with an associated depression, bipolar depression, a medication side effect, alcohol, an illicit substance, a medical illness).

Endogenous versus exogenous (reactive) depression:

Definitions:

➤ Endogenous depression—depression develops without an obvious stressor. Genetic underpinnings are presumed.

➤ Exogenous (reactive) depression—depression develops in response to a stressor.

Clinical implications:

➤ Genetic influences (e.g., race) can provide either "vulnerability" or "resiliency" genes. Developmental and social factors (e.g., gender, age, pre/post-menopause, stressors) add an additional layer of vulnerability.

➤ Often there is a definable stressor for the first few depressive episodes. After one or more episodes of stress-induced (exogenous) depression, subsequent depressive episodes may develop autonomously (i.e., without a stressor).

➤ Despite this differentiation, it may be impossible to distinguish between exogenously and endogenously induced depressions. As noted by Hans Selye, "the absence of stress is death."

Primary versus secondary depression:

➤ Primary ("functional") depression—depression is an intrinsic illness (i.e., not due to the direct physiological effects of a medical illness or a substance).

➤ Secondary ("organic") depression—depression is due to the direct physiological effects of a medical illness or a substance.

NOTE: "Primary" versus "secondary" is also applicable to other mental health disorders when the direct physiological effects of a medical disorder or a substance can induce mental health symptoms (e.g., mania, anxiety, psychosis).

Unipolar versus bipolar depression:

➤ Unipolar depression—implies MDD, either single episode or recurrent (i.e., no history of manic, mixed, or hypomanic episodes).

➤ Bipolar depression—implies depressive episodes as part of bipolar I or bipolar II disorder.

➤ DSM-IV-TR does not distinguish between the characteristics or etiological considerations of depression associated with MDD and bipolar depression. These two depressions are felt to be genetically distinct and can be clinically expressed differently and are treated differently.

Masked depression:

➤ A somewhat antiquated term, popular in the 1970s.

➤ Somatic symptoms, rather than depressed mood, predominate in the clinical presentation.

➤ When somatic symptoms dominate the clinical picture, additional diagnostic considerations include somatization disorder, somatoform disorder, and hypochondriasis (see Chapter 9 of this volume, "Miscellaneous Topics").

Depressive spectrum disorders:

➤ A categorization of depressive disorders based on a severity continuum. Ranking from very severe to mild:

✔ MDD with melancholic and/or psychotic features > MDD > minor depressive disorder > dysthymic disorder > "sad mood."
Note. Some authorities reverse the order of minor depressive disorder and dysthymic disorder.

"Double depression":

➤ If MDD develops at least 2 years after an established diagnosis of dysthymic disorder and is superimposed on the dysthymic disorder, both diagnoses are appropriate.

➤ If MDD develops during the first 2 years of a dysthymic disorder, the diagnosis is changed from dysthymic disorder to MDD.

Treatment-resistant depression:

➤ Defined as a lack of an adequate response after two or more trials of antidepressants from different medication classes given at therapeutic dosages for an adequate period of time (4–12 weeks).

➤ Some authorities feel that a designation of treatment-resistant depression should be made only after the patient has also unsuccessfully undergone a trial of ECT.

➤ The designation *treatment-resistant depression* can easily be mistakenly applied when other causes of failure to respond to somatic treatments (e.g., wrong diagnosis, inadequate treatment duration, wrong medication, poor compliance, malingering) are instead operative.

Involutional depression:

➤ Depression in the elderly; an antiquated term.

Postpsychotic depression:

➤ Is commonly associated with schizophrenia and schizoaffective disorder.

➤ Can persist for a prolonged period, is associated with psychomotor retardation, and is often treatment resistant.

Bereavement:

➤ DSM-IV-TR provides a V Code for diagnostic classification:

✔ The loss is limited to the death of a loved one, and symptoms must develop and resolve within 2 months of the loss.

✔ The full spectrum of depressive symptoms may be present in bereavement. However:

■ The majority of symptoms should resolve within 2 months.

■ Psychomotor retardation, morbid feelings of guilt not related to the loss, morbid preoccupation with worthlessness, and marked functional impairment are more common in MDD than in bereavement and serve as a useful means to distinguish bereavement from MDD.

➤ Many clinicians feel that the 2-month limitation is far too short and that the loss should not be limited to the death of a loved one.

Significance of response versus remission/recovery:

➤ *Response* requires a 50% reduction in the HAM-D score, whereas *remission/recovery* requires an absolute reduction in the HAM-D score to 7 or less, regardless of the initial HAM-D score.

➤ Remission, but not necessarily response, confers improved measures of functioning, comparable to nondepressed individuals.

➤ Only one-third of patients achieve remission with the first trial of an antidepressant.

➤ The presence of residual depressive symptoms (i.e., incomplete recovery) dramatically increases the risk of relapse and of the development of a chronic course.

Epidemiology of Major Depressive Disorder

➤ The peak ages of incidence of MDD are 18–44 years.

➤ The average duration of a cycle of MDD is ~4–12 months.

➤ The prevalence of MDD is ~1% in preschool-age children, 2% in school-age children, and 8% in adolescents.

➤ The lifetime prevalence of MDD in adults is ~16.2% and the 12-month prevalence is 6.6%.

➤ MDD is more prevalent in females (2:1), Native Americans, middle-aged, low income, and divorced/widowed/separated individuals and less prevalent in Asian, Hispanic, and African American races.

Epidemiology of Mood Disorders Associated With Various Medical Conditions

➤ The prevalence of depression (either from the direct physiological consequences of the disorder or from the emotional stress dealing with the disorder) is significantly high in many medical disorders:

✔ Cushing's syndrome: 60%–80%.

✔ Hypothyroidism: ~40%.

✔ Cancer: ~31%.

✔ Parkinson's disease: ~29%.

✔ A recent myocardial infarction (MI): 15%–22%.

✔ A recent CVA: ~38%.

✔ Diabetes: 20%–30%.

Etiological Formulations

Neurotransmitter model (also known as the monoamine, monoaminergic, or biogenic amine model):

➤ Low brain levels of 5-HT, norepinephrine (NE), and/or dopamine (DA) in the limbic system ("mood center") are associated with depression:

✔ 5-HT:

■ 5-HT (an indoleamine) is involved in the regulation of mood, hunger, sleep, impulsivity, cognitive processes, pain, and sexual functioning.

■ Deficits of 5-HT as a cause of depression are described as the *indoleamine hypothesis* of depression.

■ Reserpine, a depressogenic antihypertensive agent associated with suicidal ideation, depletes NE, DA, and 5-HT from presynaptic vesicles.

■ Levels of the 5-HT metabolite 5-hydroxyindoleacetic acid (5-HIAA) in the cerebrospinal fluid (CSF) are lower in suicidally depressed persons.

■ Carbohydrate craving during depression may be linked to the body's desire to produce more 5-HT. Carbohydrates are a precursor for 5-HT. The increased carbohydrate craving in seasonal affective disorder may be stimulated by low 5-HT levels that develop during the winter months.

- Medications that increase 5-HT in the limbic system synaptic cleft (e.g., TCAs, MAOIs, SSRIs) invoke antidepressant effects.

✔ Norepinephrine:

- NE (a catecholamine) is involved in the regulation of mood, energy, interest, motivation, and pain.
- Deficits of NE as a cause of depression are described as the *catecholamine hypothesis* of depression.
- Levels of the NE metabolite 3-methoxy-4-hydroxyphenylglycol (MHPG) in the urine are lower in depressed persons.
- Medications that increase NE in the limbic system synaptic cleft (e.g., TCAs, MAOIs, SNRIs, some AtypANs[5]) invoke antidepressant effects.

✔ Dopamine:

- DA (a catecholamine) is involved in the regulation of mood, motivation, drive, and pleasure/reward.
- Deficits of DA as a cause of depression are described as the *catecholamine hypothesis* of depression (as is also described for NE).
- Levels of the DA metabolite homovanillic acid (HVA) in the CSF are lower in suicidally depressed persons.
- Medications that increase DA in the limbic system synaptic cleft (e.g., bupropion, possibly high-dose sertraline) invoke antidepressant effects.

Genetic transmission model:

➤ The potential to develop MDD is genetically influenced (first-degree relatives of persons with depression have two to three times the risk of developing depression); however, the genetic basis is not as strong as for bipolar disorder or schizophrenia.

➤ Persons with relatives who have a history of bipolar disorder have an increased risk of developing MDD.

➤ Clinical studies assessing the impact of genetics on the metabolism of medications for different ethnic groups is a rapidly developing discipline (pharmacogenetics).

Cholinergic-adrenergic balance hypothesis:

➤ Depression develops when NE and DA are low relative to acetylcholine, and mania occurs when the reverse develops.

➤ Scopolamine, an anticholinergic agent, provides (experimentally) rapid antidepressant effects when given IV. Cognitive deficits and possible anticholinergic-induced delirium are potential limiting side effects.

---

[5]AtypANs include bupropion, mirtazapine, and nefazodone.

Stress–diathesis model:

➤ MDD develops as a consequence of stressful life events or losses. Four of the most powerful stressors are:

✔ Death of a close relative.

✔ Being a victim of assault.

✔ Having serious marital problems.

✔ Dealing with separation or divorce.

➤ Genetics likely determine the vulnerability ("diathesis") to develop depression in response to a stressful event. However, after one or more depressive episodes, subsequent depressive episodes can occur without a stressful event (i.e., depression "takes on a life of its own"; becomes autonomous).

Neuroanatomic/neurotrophic model:

➤ Positron emission tomography (PET) and single photon emission computed tomography (SPECT) demonstrate anatomic and functional brain changes during depression:

✔ The limbic system ("visceral brain"; "mood center"):

■ Regulates mood.

■ Includes the hypothalamus, anterior nucleus of the thalamus, amygdala, limbic striatum, locus coeruleus, cingulate gyrus, septal nuclei, hippocampus, mammillary nuclei, and cingulate with projections to the prefrontal cortex. Limbic system dysregulation is prominent during depression and is reversed by treatment with antidepressants.

✔ The hippocampus:

■ Is involved in memory and learning. Hippocampal gray matter volume decreases during depression (as well as in schizophrenia). Antidepressants (SSRIs are the best studied) are purported to reverse the volume loss (i.e., neurogenic) when taken on an acute basis and to protect against further volume loss (i.e., neuroprotective) when taken on a maintenance basis.

✔ The hypothalamus:

■ Is involved with basic functions, such as sleep, appetite, and libido, among others. Poor appetite, sleep disturbances, and decreased libido are common findings during depression. Antidepressants improve these symptoms.

✔ The prefrontal cortex:

■ Regulates cognitive functioning and awareness. When depressed, gray matter volume decreases, resulting in impairments in the ability to concentrate, focus, and remember. Antidepressants (SSRIs are the best studied) are purported to reverse the volume loss (i.e., neurogenic) when taken on an acute basis and to protect from further volume loss (i.e., neuroprotective) when taken on a maintenance basis.

✔ The basal ganglia:

■ Is a subcortical area involved with movement. The findings of apathy, restricted affect, stooped posture, and motor slowing in depression are similar to symptoms seen in disorders of the basal ganglia. Depression commonly develops as a consequence of movement disorders originating from the subcortical region (e.g., Parkinson's disease, Huntington's chorea) and can be effectively treated with antidepressants.

Neuroendocrine models:

➤ Depression is linked to the hypothalamic-pituitary-adrenal (HPA) axis and cortisol production:

✔ Cortisol (endogenously produced or exogenously given as a glucocorticoid) can induce significant mood swings, including depression.

✔ Corticotropin-releasing factor (CRF) released from the hypothalamus is hypersecreted in depression, resulting in an increase in secretion of adrenocorticotropic hormone (ACTH), which then triggers the adrenal cortex to release excess cortisol.

✔ Unipolar and bipolar depression are often associated with elevated cortisol levels (that cannot be suppressed with dexamethasone). Ketoconazole lowers cortisol levels and can be helpful in some patients with unipolar or bipolar treatment-resistant depression.

➤ Depression is linked to the hypothalamic-pituitary-thyroid (HPT) axis and thyroid hormone production:

✔ Hypothyroidism is one of the most prevalent medical disorders associated with depression. Thyroid hormone augmentation can be helpful for treatment-resistant unipolar and treatment-resistant bipolar depression.

Sleep disturbance model:

➤ Insomnia or hypersomnia is usually associated with depression and is normalized with effective treatments.

➤ Sleep deprivation provides a transient antidepressant effect and may be predictive of an eventual positive response to somatic treatments.

➤ Characteristic changes in rapid eye movement (REM; dreaming phase) during depression involve an accentuation of REM sleep patterns, including:

✔ Reduced onset (shortened latency) to the first REM period.

✔ Increased length of the first REM period.

✔ Increased REM sleep during the first half of the night.

✔ Increased REM sleep density.

Infectious model:

➤ An infectious agent (e.g., Borna virus) is suspected as a possible cause of depression. The antiviral medication amantadine (Symmetrel) is helpful in some individuals to treat depression.

Psychological models:

➤ Psychodynamic models:

✔ Mood disorders result from fixation of development at the oral stage.

✔ Depression results from early childhood losses that lead to insecurity, difficulty in establishing attachments in adult life, dependency on others, low self-esteem, and vulnerability to losses.

✔ Mania results from "denial of depression."

➤ Behavioral model:

✔ Depression develops because of lack of social skills.

➤ Cognitive (Beck) model:

✔ Negative views lead to depression and can be corrected through cognitive therapy.

➤ Learned helplessness model:

✔ Past failures will continue unabated.

Novel considerations:

➤ Substance P (a neuropeptide) antagonists (SPAs) are showing promise as antidepressants with the potential benefit of a favorable side-effect profile. Their mechanism may involve facilitation of monoamine neurotransmission of the neurokinin 1 (NK1) receptor.

➤ There is increasing evidence that medications directed at altering glutamate neurotransmission may provide antidepressant effects.

➤ Brain-derived neurotrophic factor (BDNF) exerts antidepressant effects in animal models. Downregulation of BDNF can therefore result in depression and has been linked to decreased hippocampal volume. Medications that increase BDNF may have antidepressant effects. Increasing BDNF may also provide neurotrophic benefits to reverse hippocampal volume loss observed during depression. A BDNF gene has been implicated in the genesis of unipolar and bipolar depression.

MOOD DISORDERS DUE TO A GENERAL MEDICAL CONDITION AND SUBSTANCE-INDUCED MOOD DISORDERS

General Considerations

➤ Mood symptoms are frequent sequelae of physical illness, substances of abuse, and medication side effects but are often overlooked as causes of depressive symptoms. Always include these categories in your differential diagnosis for any patient presenting with mood symptoms. Be prepared to be asked to list a number of medical disorders and substances that can cause depressive symptoms. However, it may be very difficult to determine if the mood symptoms are due to the direct physiological effects of the medical condition or the substance or are due to factors associated with having a medical illness or using a substance (e.g., dysfunction from the medical illness, job loss from substance abuse).

➤ A number of symptoms routinely assumed by psychiatrists to be attributed to a primary depressive disorder may be due to the attributes of the physical illness itself (e.g., poor sleep, fatigue, poor appetite, decreased energy, generalized aches and pains). Pay particular attention to emotional/cognitive symptoms (e.g., depressed mood, tearfulness, hopelessness), which, if present, are more likely indicative of a comorbid depressive disorder.

➤ High rates of depression are found in outpatient primary care settings (5%–25% of patients), hospital settings of medically ill patients (20%–33% of patients), and nursing homes (up to 50% of patients).

➤ The mechanism(s) by which a physical illness can induce depression is not fully elucidated. A purported mechanism is suggestive that stress from physical illness leads to sustained increases in adrenal corticosteroids, thereby generating a depressive disorder.

Mood Disorders Due to a General Medical Condition

Clinical and diagnostic considerations:

➤ Mood disorders due to a general medical condition:

   ✔ Should always be listed as a potential cause of depression in your differential diagnosis.

   ✔ Are coded as to the name of the disorder and the phase of the mood. For example:

      ■ Hypothyroidism leading to depression would be coded as *mood disorder due to hypothyroidism, with depressive features.*

■ Cushing's disorder causing a manic episode would be coded as *mood disorder due to Cushing's disease, with manic features.*

Medical disorders associated with depression:

Hypothyroidism:

➤ Induces depression in up to 40% of affected individuals and, therefore, should always be considered in your differential as a cause of depression.

➤ Typically presents with vegetative symptoms of fatigue, lethargy, and weakness before cognitive or mood changes appear.

➤ Is diagnosed when thyroid-stimulating hormone (TSH) is elevated. For a more detailed description, refer to "Psychiatric Manifestations of Thyroid Disorders" section of Chapter 9 ("Miscellaneous Topics").

➤ Is effectively treated by adding thyroid hormone to correct the deficiency. This does not preclude concurrent treatment of the depression with antidepressants or psychotherapy. Thyroid hormone augmentation is also an effective strategy for patients who respond poorly to antidepressants, raising the possibility that some of these patients may have subclinical hypothyroidism.

➤ Is also a risk factor for bipolar depression and depression with postpartum onset.

➤ Is an excellent example of the diagnostic dilemma of assessing the cause of depression when physical illness is present. Given a patient with elevated TSH and depressive symptoms satisfying DSM-IV-TR for MDD, two possibilities are relevant:

✔ Depression is due to the intrinsic nature of the hypothyroidism (i.e., mood disorder due to hypothyroidism, with depressive features).

✔ The patient presents with MDD unrelated to the hypothyroidism.

Cushing's disease (hypercortisolism):

➤ Is one of the most likely medical illnesses to be associated with depression.

➤ Symptoms are nearly identical to those of a primary mood disorder (MDD).

➤ Is more frequent in women than men by a ratio of 5 to 1.

Diabetes:

➤ Purportedly increases the risk for unipolar and bipolar depression and possibly schizophrenia. In turn, depression purportedly increases the risk for diabetes.

➤ Depression may adversely affect adherence to prescribed therapies, possibly resulting in poorer glycemic control.

Autoimmune disorders:

➤ Systemic lupus erythematosus, rheumatoid arthritis, and multiple sclerosis are associated with depression. Treatment of the underlying disorder may not completely resolve the depression because of the chronic and debilitating nature of these illnesses.

Nutritional deficiencies:

➤ Deficiencies of B vitamins (especially vitamins B_9 [folic acid], B_6 [pyridoxine], and B_{12} (cyanocobalamin]) are implicated in causing depression. Furthermore, deficiencies of B_{12} and B_9 reduce the effectiveness of antidepressant treatment.

➤ Screening for B_9 and B_{12} vitamin deficiencies is recommended when assessing for the cause of depression in the elderly or in treatment-refractory depression.

Myocardial infarction and cardiovascular disease:

➤ Clinical issues:

✔ There is compelling evidence that depression (and perhaps anxiety) can increase the risk for cardiovascular disease (especially atherosclerosis) and dramatically worsen the outcome of persons who have suffered an MI.

✔ Approximately 15%–22% of persons who survive an MI become clinically depressed. Mortality (especially in the first 6 months after an MI) and morbidity are further increased if the depression remains undertreated or untreated.

✔ Beta-blockers and statins have previously been associated with causing depression, but these findings are not conclusive and further studies are needed.

➤ Treatment considerations:

✔ TCAs can cause serious and life-threatening cardiovascular side effects (e.g., orthostatic hypotension, exacerbation of congestive heart failure, quinidine-like antiarrhythmic effects, bundle branch block, QTc interval prolongation possibly leading to torsade de pointes), especially in the elderly and in persons with underlying cardiac disease. TCAs are contraindicated for 6 months following an MI and are a poor choice for patients with underlying cardiovascular disease.

✔ Cognitive-behavioral therapy (CBT) can be effective and may reduce or eliminate the need for somatic therapies.

✔ SSRIs, SNRIs, and AtypANs are the preferred somatic treatments. However:

■ SSRIs have mild anticoagulant effects that should be taken into account when utilizing anticoagulants.

■ Venlafaxine can adversely increase diastolic blood pressure, producing sustained hypertension at higher doses.

■ Mirtazapine can induce significant weight gain, thereby increasing the workload on the heart.

- Fluoxetine, paroxetine, and bupropion significantly inhibit cytochrome P450 (CYP) 2D6, which are involved with the metabolism of some antihypertensive medications (e.g., the beta-blockers metoprolol and betaxolol).

- Most antidepressants (except for venlafaxine, citalopram, and escitalopram) are highly protein bound and compete with and can displace cardiovascular medications that are also highly protein bound (e.g., digoxin, warfarin).

- Nefazodone is a potent inhibitor of CYP 3A4, which is responsible for the metabolism of many medications used to treat cardiovascular disease (e.g., calcium channel blockers).

- ECT can transiently increase the workload of the heart but is not contraindicated in patients with cardiovascular disease.

Cerebrovascular accident:

➤ Clinical issues:

  ✔ Depression:

    - May increase the risk for a first CVA.

    - Commonly develops after a CVA (incidence of 27%–40%) and increases poststroke morbidity and mortality.

    - May be more prevalent with left-hemisphere brain injury (controversial).

  ✔ Poststroke emotional lability (i.e., "emotional incontinence") with unprovoked episodes of crying and depressed mood is a common finding not always leading to clinically significant depression.

  ✔ Silent subcortical strokes (i.e., subcortical strokes without obvious physical manifestations) can be associated with depression. The organic etiology is easily missed and may only be evident with brain imaging.

➤ Treatment considerations:

  ✔ Antidepressants without appreciable cardiovascular or cognitive side effects (e.g., SSRIs, SNRIs, AtypANs) are preferred. However, TCAs and trazodone can also be effective, with recognition of their greater side-effect burden. Studies utilizing fluoxetine and nortriptyline demonstrated an increased survival rate for post-CVA patients with or without comorbid depression. A lower starting and target dosages and a slow upward titration is recommended.

  ✔ Stimulants (e.g., methylphenidate), ECT, and repetitive transcranial magnetic stimulation (rTMS) have been used with good results but are not as well studied as antidepressants.

Parkinson's disease:

➤ Clinical issues:

  ✔ Parkinson's disease:

    ■ Presents with physical symptoms of bradykinesia, rigidity, resting tremor (often the first symptom to develop), and postural instability secondary to loss of DA in the substantia nigra.

    ■ Presents with apathy and restricted affect due to loss of DA, making the assessment for depression more difficult.

    ■ Is highly associated with depression (~40% of patients), which speeds the progression of the physical and cognitive deficits of the disease.

➤ Treatment considerations:

  ✔ SSRIs are first-line treatments. Venlafaxine, mirtazapine, and bupropion have also been shown to be effective. TCAs are second-line treatments, and ECT can be beneficial for treatment-refractory depression.

    ■ Anticholinergic side effects of TCAs can improve motor symptoms but further impair cognition.

    ■ ECT can additionally reduce rigidity, tremors, and bradykinesia.

Cancer:

➤ Clinical issues:

  ✔ Depression:

    ■ Is often unrecognized, undertreated, or untreated in this group (i.e., "they have good reason to be depressed").

    ■ Develops in ~20%–30% of cancer patients, depending on the type of cancer and research methods used to assess for depression.

    ■ Is more likely to develop in cancer patients with a prior history of depression.

  ✔ Suicidal ideation, suicide attempts, and completed suicides are higher in cancer patients than in the general population. Suicide risk is greatest in cancer patients who have marked physical impairment, significant pain, and a poorer long-term prognosis.

  ✔ Pancreatic carcinoma is the most often cited cancer correlating with depression, but any cancer can be associated with depression. The intensity of depression seems to be proportional to the extensiveness of cancer involvement and may be greatest with metastatic disease.

  ✔ Chronic depression in older individuals may increase the risk of cancer. A proposed mechanism involves the negative impact of depression on immune system functioning, decreasing the body's innate ability to destroy developing cancer cells.

➤ Treatment considerations:

✔ Antidepressants with a lower side-effect burden (e.g., SSRIs, SNRIs, AtypANs) are preferred. However, some SSRIs may adversely increase blood levels of anticancer drugs through their impact on the CYP isoenzyme system.

✔ TCAs can induce adverse central and peripheral anticholinergic side effects, but their impact on increasing appetite can be beneficial.

HIV infection and AIDS:

➤ Clinical issues:

✔ Depressed mood and mood disorders are common in persons with HIV/AIDS. The depression may stem from the direct physiological effects of the virus on the brain, the psychological awareness of what having HIV means, or from medications used to treat the illness.

✔ The risk of depression is greatest in individuals with a prior history of depression.

✔ Depression is not generally correlated with the stage of the illness, T-helper cell count, or the use of medications to treat HIV.

➤ Treatment considerations:

✔ Antidepressants with a low propensity to cause side effects are preferred (e.g., SSRIs, SNRIs, AtypANs). TCAs are usually poorly tolerated, especially with regard to anticholinergic-induced side effects. Psychotherapy with or without somatic treatments can be very helpful.

✔ Stimulants can be effective for the treatment of fatigue, slowed thinking, and apathy associated with HIV infection.

Dementia:

➤ Clinical issues:

✔ The incidence of some form of depression in Alzheimer's disease is ~11%.

✔ Dementia with comorbid depression results in more severe cognitive deficits than either disorder alone.

✔ Long-standing depression may be a risk factor for the development of dementia.

✔ *Pseudodementia* (dementia of depression) refers to dementia-like symptoms (especially cognitive impairment) that are actually due to depression and are therefore correctable.

➤ Family issues:

✔ Fifty percent of caretakers eventually become depressed.

➤ Treatment considerations:

   ✔ Antidepressants with a low potential for side effects are preferred (e.g., SSRIs, SNRIs, AtypANs). TCAs with marked anticholinergic side effects and MAOIs should be avoided.

   ✔ Stimulants are usually well tolerated and can be effective either alone (controversial) or as adjunctive medications (preferred) for the treatment of depression in patients with dementia. Stimulants are most useful when psychomotor retardation is a prominent symptom.

Seizure disorders:

➤ Depression develops in 20%–60% of persons with a seizure disorder and is especially prominent in temporal lobe epilepsy and with left-sided seizure foci.

➤ SSRIs, SNRIs, and AtypANs (except bupropion) have less impact than TCAs on reducing seizure threshold and are therefore preferred.

Infections:

➤ Depression (especially during times of stress) can increase the release of corticosteroids and catecholamines, substances known to suppress the immune system, thereby increasing the risk of infections and possibly the development of certain cancers.

Hypogonadal states:

➤ Decreased levels of estrogen in women and testosterone in men purportedly can result in depression (controversial).

➤ Treatment possibilities include antidepressants and/or hormone replacement with recognition of the increased potential for breast and uterine cancer in women secondary to adding estrogen and for prostate cancer and aggression in men secondary to adding testosterone.

Pain syndromes:

➤ "Chronic pain syndromes" often lead to depression, particularly dysthymic disorder. The most frequently cited pain syndrome associated with depression is fibromyalgia.

➤ Treatment considerations:

   ✔ Antidepressants can be effective in treating both depression and pain.

   ✔ Proposed mechanisms for antidepressants to reduce or ameliorate pain include:

      ■ Adequate treatment of depression to break the "depression–pain–depression" cycle.

      ■ Antidepressants with both NE and 5-HT activity (e.g., amitriptyline, imipramine, duloxetine, higher-dose venlafaxine, mirtazapine) purportedly reduce pain through a direct effect on descending pain pathways, independent of their antidepressant effects.

Substance-Induced Mood Disorders

Clinical and diagnostic considerations:

➤ In most cases, it can be difficult, if not impossible, to determine whether the depression is attributable to the direct physiological consequences of taking the substance (i.e., substance-induced mood disorder) or is attributable to a comorbid MDD. Always include both possibilities in your differential.

➤ Substance-induced mood disorders:

✔ Are common causes of depression and are often overlooked or left untreated.

✔ Significantly increase the risk of suicide attempts and completed suicides.

✔ Interfere with the positive impact of psychotherapy and somatic treatments.

✔ Are coded by referencing the substance and the phase of the mood. For example:

■ Depression developing as a consequence of alcohol abuse is coded as *alcohol-induced mood disorder, with depressive features.*

■ Mania developing as a consequence of using the antidepressant amitriptyline is coded as *amitriptyline-induced mood disorder with manic features.* A switch to mania or hypomania caused by an antidepressant is classified as a substance-induced mood disorder.

Common substances associated with clinical depression:

Alcohol:

➤ Depression is a common consequence of excessive alcohol use and should resolve after detoxification and continued abstinence. In such cases, there is a clear indication of an alcohol-induced mood disorder.

➤ If depression predates the use of alcohol or persists after detoxification, antidepressants with a low propensity to cause side effects or to interact adversely with alcohol (e.g., SSRIs, SNRIs, AtypANs) are preferred. Importantly, TCAs plus alcohol can be lethal, and duloxetine is not recommended for those who are actively drinking.

Stimulants (cocaine, methamphetamine):

➤ Depression is common in persons who chronically abuse stimulants. Chronic stimulant abuse eventually depletes brain DA, NE, and 5-HT. Stopping the stimulant should eventually reverse the depression, although antidepressants can be helpful if the depression persists.

➤ There are no U.S. Food and Drug Administration (FDA)–approved medications for the treatment of stimulant abuse or dependence.

Opiates:

➤ Opioids have been utilized as antidepressants for years, although their abuse is likely to lead to depression:

✔ Buprenorphine (partial mu agonist and potent kappa antagonist) has been advocated (although not fully substantiated) for treatment-resistant depression.

✔ Oxycodone and oxymorphone were shown to provide significant antidepressant effects in treatment-resistant depression.

✔ If depression is secondary to a chronic pain syndrome, appropriate use of opioids can improve depression by reducing the pain-depression-pain cycle.

Marijuana:

➤ Marijuana can induce an "amotivational syndrome," but studies are inconclusive as to its role in causing depression. However, there is growing evidence that marijuana is used at times to self-treat dysphoric feelings.

Anabolic steroids ("roids"):

✔ Testosterone and testosterone derivatives (abused or prescribed) have been implicated in causing depression, anger, and violent outbursts ("roid rage"). These symptoms may persist for months after the anabolic steroid is stopped.

Nicotine:

➤ Cigarette smoking is associated with depression:

✔ Nicotine may provide mild antidepressant and anxiolytic effects. Thus, it is conceivable that some patients may smoke as a means of self-treatment of underlying depression and anxiety.

✔ The lifetime frequency of depression is higher in smokers than nonsmokers.

✔ Withdrawal from nicotine is frequently associated with dysphoric mood or depression, perhaps secondary to "unmasking" the depression formerly treated with nicotine.

Prescription medications (partial listing):

➤ Medications that purportedly can induce depression include:

✔ Cardiovascular and antihypertensive medications (e.g., reserpine, methyldopa, guanethidine, digitalis, some diuretics, clonidine). Beta-blockers and statins are not as clearly defined but are not thought to induce depression.

✔ Steroids (e.g., glucocorticoids, anabolic steroids, birth control pills with high levels of progesterone).

✔ Antimicrobials (e.g., sulfonamides, D-cycloserine).

✔ Anxiolytics and CNS depressants (e.g., benzodiazepines, barbiturates).

✔ Interferon and peginterferon (treatments for hepatitis C).

✔ Mefloquine (malaria prevention).

ASSESSMENT, WORKUP, AND TREATMENT OF A DEPRESSIVE DISORDER

Clinical Issues Related to Diagnosis

➤ Always assess for medical and substance-related causes of depression before attributing a depressive episode to MDD.

➤ With so many diagnostic possibilities, it is difficult, if not impossible, to accurately determine the type of depression after viewing or conducting a short interview. Additionally, comorbidities (e.g., Axis I + Axis II) can further complicate the picture. A broad differential diagnosis for a patient presenting with mood, cognitive, and/or neurovegetative symptoms of depression would commonly include:

✔ Mood disorders (e.g., MDD, depressive phase of bipolar I and II disorders, mixed bipolar episodes, cyclothymic disorder, dysthymic disorder, minor depressive disorder, depressive disorder not otherwise specified [NOS]). In addition, many of these disorders can be associated with specifiers (e.g., atypical features, catatonic features, postpartum onset, melancholic features, seasonal pattern), further complicating the assignment of an accurate diagnosis.

✔ Psychotic disorders other than mood disorders, which are often accompanied by or associated with mood symptoms (e.g., schizophrenia, schizoaffective disorder, brief psychotic disorder).

✔ Anxiety disorders with associated mood symptoms (e.g., obsessive-compulsive disorder, posttraumatic stress disorder [PTSD]).

✔ Dementias (Alzheimer's disease, Huntington's chorea).

✔ Personality disorders (e.g., borderline personality disorder).

✔ Mood disorder due to a general medical condition (e.g., hypothyroidism, B vitamin deficiency, Cushing's disease).

✔ Substance-induced mood disorder:

   ■ Substances of abuse (e.g., alcohol, cocaine, anabolic steroids).

   ■ Medications that can induce depression as a side effect (e.g., reserpine, corticosteroids, benzodiazepines, birth control pills with high progesterone–estrogen ratios).

Symptom Rating Scales and Screening Instruments

➤ Psychological testing, screening, and rating scales are useful to help establish or confirm the diagnosis and quantitate the degree of impairment:

✔ Minnesota Multiphasic Personality Inventory–II (see Chapter 1 ["Schizophrenia and Other Psychotic Disorders"]).

✔ Hamilton Rating Scale for Depression (HAM-D) (see Table 2–1 for scoring key).

■ Table 2–1   Scoring key for Hamilton Rating Scale for Depression

Score	Approximate level of depression
0–7	No depression
8–12	Mild depression
13–17	Less than major depression
18–29	Major depression
30+	Major depression with psychotic features

✔ Zung Depression Scale:

- Twenty-question self-rating scale. Higher scores are indicative of more severe depression.

✔ Primary Care Evaluation of Mental Disorders (PRIME-MD):

- Screens for mood, anxiety/panic, alcohol, eating, and somatoform disorders in primary care settings.

✔ Geriatric Depression Scale:

- Fifteen- (short form) or 30-item (long form) questionnaire to screen for depression in the elderly. Can be used for those with mild to moderate cognitive impairment.

✔ Beck Depression Inventory II (self-report questionnaire; see Table 2–2 for scoring key):

- Twenty-one questions provide a general (nondiagnostic) assessment of the severity of depression. Not as reliable when concomitant physical illness is present.

✔ Montgomery-Åsberg Depression Rating Scale (MADRS), Clinical Global Impressions—Severity Scale (CGI-S), Clinical Global Impressions—Improvement Scale (CGI-I), and a host of other clinical tests are used in clinical research studies to document the severity of and progression of improvement in depression.

■ Table 2–2   Scoring key for Beck Depression Inventory II

Score	General level of depression
<7–10	Nondepressed
10–14	Mildly depressed
15–22	Moderately depressed
23+	Severely depressed

Commonly Proposed Mechanisms of Action of Antidepressants

Theorized two-step process:

➤ Antidepressants improve depression presumably by a two-step process:

✔ First step—increase monoamine activity in the synaptic cleft or at the postsynaptic receptor through one or more of the following mechanisms:

- Blocking the reuptake into presynaptic vesicles of 5-HT, NE, and/or DA (TCAs, SSRIs, SNRIs, and AtypANs [except mirtazapine]) via interfering with monoamine transporter proteins (highly influenced by genetic factors).

- Blocking central presynaptic alpha$_2$-adrenergic inhibitory autoreceptors and heteroreceptors, resulting in an increased release of 5-HT and NE into the synaptic cleft (mirtazapine).

- Blocking the metabolism of 5-HT and NE (MAO-A inhibitors) or DA (MAO-B inhibitors).

- Blocking 5-HT$_{2A}$ and 5-HT$_{2C}$ postsynaptic receptors (nefazodone, trazodone), both principally increasing 5-HT activity.

✔ Second step—the 1- to 3-week delay (can be shorter or longer) before antidepressant effects become evident may be due to:

- Downregulation of 5-HT, NE, and DA postsynaptic receptors, which requires several weeks to re-equilibrate.

- Antidepressant regeneration of brain cells in the hippocampus and prefrontal cortex (neuroregenerative activity, possibly through an increase in BDNF).

- Antidepressant stimulation of cellular release of monoamines, which, via a negative feedback mechanism, requires several weeks to become desensitized. Despite immediate release of monoamines, the required "downstream" effects on neuronal pathways require time.

➤ Recent evidence brings into question that antidepressants require several weeks before they become clinically effective. Careful meta-analyses support an almost immediate response in antidepressant effect on mood and a 7- to 10-day lag for functional improvement.

Therapeutic effects and side effects of antidepressants:

Therapeutic effects based on neurotransmitter activity:

➤ Therapeutic effects of antidepressants attributable to:

- ✔ 5-HT include antidepressant effects, reduced anxiety, reduced panic, reduced obsessions and compulsions, reduced bulimic behavior, reduced symptoms of PTSD, reduced agitation/aggression, and reduced suicidal ideation/behavior.

- ✔ NE include antidepressant effects, increased alertness, improved concentration, increased energy, increased interest, and reduced fatigue.

- ✔ DA include antidepressant effects, increased motivation, improved reactivity to pleasurable experiences, decreased craving for substances, appetite suppression, and improved cognition.

Side effects based on neurotransmitter activity:

➤ Side effects of antidepressants attributable to:

   ✔ 5-HT include gastrointestinal upset, nausea, vomiting, diarrhea, headache, weight gain (5-HT$_{2C}$), and sexual dysfunction.

   ✔ NE include anxiety, irritability, tremors, sweating, increased heart rate, increased blood pressure, and blockade of antihypertensive effects of guanethidine.

   ✔ DA include psychomotor activation and increased potential for inducing or exacerbating psychosis.

Side effects secondary to postsynaptic receptor blockade:

➤ Side effects of antidepressants attributable to:

   ✔ Blockade of histaminic (H$_1$) postsynaptic receptors include sedation and weight gain. Ordering of side effects (from highest to lowest):

   ■ Mirtazapine > doxepin >> amitriptyline >> imipramine >> desipramine > SSRIs/venlafaxine/duloxetine/bupropion.

   ■ Blockade of cholinergic (muscarinic [M$_1$]) postsynaptic receptors include dry mouth, blurred vision, exacerbation of narrow-angle glaucoma, constipation, obstipation, urinary hesitancy/retention, sinus tachycardia, impaired cognition, and confusion. Ordering of side effects (from highest to lowest):

   ■ Amitriptyline > clomipramine > imipramine > desipramine > SSRIs/SNRIs/AtypANs.

   ✔ Blockade of alpha$_1$-adrenergic postsynaptic receptors include dizziness, postural hypotension, falls, and reflex tachycardia. Ordering of side effects (from highest to lowest):

   ■ Doxepin > amitriptyline/nefazodone > imipramine/desipramine > SSRIs/SNRIs/AtypANs.

Overview of Somatic Treatments for Major Depressive Disorder

➤ Table 2–3 presents a summary of somatic treatments for MDD.

Augmentation With Aripiprazole (Abilify)

➤ Aripiprazole, at dosages up to 15 mg/day, is FDA approved for adjunctive treatment of MDD when added to antidepressants.

➤ Refer to Chapter 1 of this volume, "Schizophrenia and Other Psychotic Disorders," for a more complete description of indications and side effects.

■ Table 2–3   Somatic treatments for major depressive disorder (MDD)

Medication or treatment	Recommended adult dosage, starting/ maximum, mg/day[a]	Neuro-transmitter producing therapeutic effect	Proposed mechanism of action	Blockade of histaminic, cholinergic, and alpha-adrenergic receptors	Potential for weight gain	Potential for early GI side effects	Potential for sexual side effects	Safety margin in overdose	Clinically relevant considerations
Selective serotonin reuptake inhibitors (SSRIs)									
Fluoxetine (generic, Prozac, Prozac Weekly)	20/80 (fluoxetine) 90 mg/week (fluoxetine weekly)	5-HT	5-HT reup-take inhibi-tion	Minimal	Low–medium	High	High	High	Significant inhibition of CYP 2D6 and mild to moderate inhibition of CYP 2C19 isoenzymes. Very long half-life (84 hours), with an active metabolite with an even longer half-life. Aggregate half-life is 10–16 days. Initial weight loss, long-term mild weight gain. Minimal withdrawal syndrome. Activating. Only antidepressant approved for persons < age18 years.
Paroxetine (generic, Paxil, Paxil CR)	20/50 (paroxetine) 25/50 (paroxetine CR)	5-HT	5-HT reup-take inhibi-tion	Minimal	Low–medium	High	High	High	Significant inhibition of CYP 2D6 isoenzyme system can cause clinically meaningful drug interactions. Dose-dependent anticholinergic side effects. Perhaps the most potent SSRI. Noradrenergic at higher doses. Potentially harsh withdrawal syndrome if stopped abruptly. Potentially significant weight gain, sedation, and sexual dysfunction. Wide range of FDA approvals.

■ Table 2–3 Somatic treatments for major depressive disorder (MDD) (continued)

Medication or treatment	Recommended adult dosage, starting/ maximum, mg/day[a]	Neurotransmitter producing therapeutic effect	Proposed mechanism of action	Blockade of histaminic, cholinergic, and alphaadrenergic receptors	Potential for weight gain	Potential for early GI side effects	Potential for sexual side effects	Safety margin in overdose	Clinically relevant considerations
Selective serotonin reuptake inhibitors (SSRIs) (continued)									
Sertraline (Zoloft)	50/200	5-HT	5-HT reuptake inhibition	Minimal	Low–medium	High	High	High	Significant inhibition of CYP 2D6 isoenzymes at high doses can cause clinically meaningful drug interactions. Can be activating. Mild to moderate withdrawal syndrome. Can cause weight loss. No dosage reduction in the elderly.
Fluvoxamine (Luvox, Luvox CR)	50/300	5-HT	5-HT reuptake inhibition	Minimal	Low–medium	High	High	High	Significant inhibition of CYP 2C19, 1A2, and 3A4 isoenzymes can cause clinically meaningful drug interactions (e.g., raise risperidone levels). Potentially harsh withdrawal syndrome. FDA approved for obsessivecompulsive disorder, but not for depression.

Table 2–3   Somatic treatments for major depressive disorder (MDD) *(continued)*

Medication or treatment	Recommended adult dosage, starting/maximum, mg/day[a]	Neuro-transmitter producing therapeutic effect	Proposed mechanism of action	Blockade of histaminic, cholinergic, and alpha-adrenergic receptors	Potential for weight gain	Potential for early GI side effects	Potential for sexual side effects	Safety margin in overdose	Clinically relevant considerations
Selective serotonin reuptake inhibitors (SSRIs) *(continued)*									
Citalopram (Celexa)	20/60	5-HT	5-HT reuptake inhibition	Minimal	Very low	High	Medium	High	Higher doses often more effective. Minimal inhibition of CYP isoenzymes. Contraindicated for use with pimozide (Orap). Mild to moderate withdrawal syndrome. H₁ blockade can cause sedation and weight gain.
Escitalopram (Lexapro)	10/20	5-HT	5-HT reuptake inhibition	Minimal	Very low	Medium	Medium	High	Most serotonin-selective of the SSRIs. Higher dosages often more effective. Minimal inhibition of CYP isoenzymes. Low protein binding. Contraindicated for use with pimozide (Orap). Mild to moderate withdrawal syndrome.

Table 2–3 Somatic treatments for major depressive disorder (MDD) (*continued*)

Medication or treatment	Recommended adult dosage, starting/maximum, mg/day[a]	Neuro-transmitter producing therapeutic effect	Proposed mechanism of action	Blockade of histaminic, cholinergic, and alpha-adrenergic receptors	Potential for weight gain	Potential for early GI side effects	Potential for sexual side effects	Safety margin in overdose	Clinically relevant considerations
Serotonin–norepinephrine reuptake inhibitors (SNRIs) and atypical antidepressants (AtypANs)									
Serotonin–norepinephrine reuptake inhibitors									
Venlafaxine (generic immediate release; Effexor XR)	37.5/375 (inpatient) 37.5/225 (outpatient)	5-HT (+ NE at higher doses)	5-HT and NE reuptake inhibitor	Minimal	Low	High	Medium	High	Pure 5-HT reuptake inhibitor until higher doses (~150–225 mg/day), when NE also becomes available. At even higher doses, DA may increase. Blood pressure increase possible with increasing dose (as NE becomes available). Nausea (minimized with long-acting preparations) is the principal side effect. Elevated cholesterol in 8% of users. Can be activating. Very low protein binding. Minimal inhibition of CYP isoenzymes. Potentially harsh withdrawal syndrome. May be especially effective for severe depression at higher doses.

Table 2–3   Somatic treatments for major depressive disorder (MDD) *(continued)*

Serotonin–norepinephrine reuptake inhibitors (SNRIs) and atypical antidepressants (AtypANs) *(continued)*

Serotonin–norepinephrine reuptake inhibitors (continued)

Medication or treatment	Recommended adult dosage, starting/maximum, mg/day[a]	Neuro-transmitter producing therapeutic effect	Proposed mechanism of action	Blockade of histaminic, cholinergic, and alpha-adrenergic receptors	Potential for weight gain	Potential for early GI side effects	Potential for sexual side effects	Safety margin in overdose	Clinically relevant considerations
Duloxetine (Cymbalta)	60/120 for all disorders	5-HT + NE	5-HT + NE reuptake inhibition	Low	Low	Low	Low	High	Early side effects include nausea, headache, and sedation (should resolve in 7–10 days). Start with 30 mg/day to reduce initial side effects. NE and 5-HT reuptake inhibition at all dosages. Mild to moderate CYP 2D6 inhibition. Approved for peripheral diabetic neuropathy. FDA approved for GAD and the maintenance phase of MDD. Do not use with active alcohol abuse.

Table 2–3 Somatic treatments for major depressive disorder (MDD) (continued)

Medication or treatment	Recommended adult dosage, starting/maximum, mg/day[a]	Neuro-transmitter producing therapeutic effect	Proposed mechanism of action	Blockade of histaminic, cholinergic, and alpha-adrenergic receptors	Potential for weight gain	Potential for early GI side effects	Potential for sexual side effects	Safety margin in overdose	Clinically relevant considerations
Serotonin–norepinephrine reuptake inhibitors (SNRIs) and atypical antidepressants (AtypANs) *(continued)*									
Serotonin antagonists and serotonin reuptake inhibitors									
Trazodone (generic, Desyrel)	150/600	5-HT >> NE	Potent blockade of $5\text{-}HT_{2A}$ and $5\text{-}HT_{2C}$ receptors Moderate 5-HT and NE reuptake inhibition (5-HT >> NE)	Minimal	High	Very low	Medium	Low (but better than TCAs)	Highly sedating; most often used for insomnia. Typically requires 200–400 mg/day for adequate antidepressant responsiveness, but poorly tolerated at these higher doses because of histamine blockade causing sedation. Priapism (very low incidence, but can lead to impotence) is a medical emergency. Principally a 5-HT agonist.
Nefazodone (generic)	200/600	5-HT >> NE	Potent blockade of post-synaptic $5\text{-}HT_{2A}$ and $5\text{-}HT_{2C}$ receptors Moderate 5-HT and NE reuptake inhibition (5-HT >> NE)	Minimal	Low	Medium	Low	High	Less weight gain and sedation than with trazodone. Significant inhibition of CYP 2D6 isoenzymes can cause clinically meaningful drug interactions. Twice-daily dosing. Higher doses often more effective. Can cause dizziness, blurred vision, and "vision trails." Idiopathic hepatic failure (black box warning). Mild to moderate elevation of liver function in ~4% of patients. Brand-name Serzone (but not generic) withdrawn from U.S. market. Principally a 5-HT agonist. Rarely used.

Table 2–3   Somatic treatments for major depressive disorder (MDD) (continued)

Serotonin–norepinephrine reuptake inhibitors (SNRIs) and atypical antidepressants (AtypANs) (continued)

Norepinephrine–dopamine reuptake inhibitor

Medication or treatment	Recommended adult dosage, starting/ maximum, mg/day[a]	Neuro-transmitter producing therapeutic effect	Proposed mechanism of action	Blockade of histaminic, cholinergic, and alpha-adrenergic receptors	Potential for weight gain	Potential for early GI side effects	Potential for sexual side effects	Safety margin in overdose	Clinically relevant considerations
Bupropion (generic immediate release [IR], generic sustained release [SR], Wellbutrin SR, Wellbutrin XL, Zyban)	100/400 (XR) 150/450 (XL) 100/400 (IR); use with caution	DA + NE	DA + NE reuptake inhibitor (due to hydroxy-bupropion)	Minimal	Low	Medium	Low	High (except for seizures)	Hydroxybupropion (metabolite) provides the major activity. Bupropion is thus a prodrug. Potential for seizures increases with increasing dose, with the immediate-release formulation, and in patients with a history of head injury, active alcohol withdrawal, or active bulimia. Seizures are most likely within several days of dosage increase and soon after administration of the dose. For the immediate-release formulation, do not exceed maximum daily dosage of 400 mg (seizure incidence is ~0.4% at 400 mg/day) and maximum single dose of 200 mg. Activating as opposed to sedating. Possibly anxiolytic. The XL formulation allows for once-daily dosing. May improve libido (but not erectile dysfunction), help with weight loss, and reduce craving for nicotine. Often added to an SSRI. Significant inhibition of CYP 2D6 isoenzymes.

Table 2–3 Somatic treatments for major depressive disorder (MDD) (continued)

Medication or treatment	Recommended adult dosage, starting/maximum, mg/day[a]	Neurotransmitter producing therapeutic effect	Proposed mechanism of action	Blockade of histaminic, cholinergic, and alpha-adrenergic receptors	Potential for weight gain	Potential for early GI side effects	Potential for sexual side effects	Safety margin in overdose	Clinically relevant considerations
Serotonin–norepinephrine reuptake inhibitors (SNRIs) and atypical antidepressants (AtypANs) *(continued)*									
Serotonin–norepinephrine receptor antagonist									
Mirtazapine (generic, Remeron SolTab)	15/45	5-HT + NE	Blockade of $5\text{-}HT_{2A}$ and $5\text{-}HT_3$ receptors; presynaptic $alpha_2$-adrenergic blockade	High (H_1)	Low	Very low	Low	High	Unique but complex mechanism of action (not a reuptake inhibitor) that increases 5-HT and NE in the synaptic cleft. Considered a second- or third-line agent because of significant potential for sedation, appetite increase, and weight gain. Agranulocytosis (0.1%) is the most serious side effect. Often combined with an SSRI (advantageous because of complementary mechanisms of action). Minimal inhibition of CYP isoenzymes. Low incidence of agitation, nausea, and anticholinergic and sexual side effects. Higher doses are less sedating.

■ **Table 2–3   Somatic treatments for major depressive disorder (MDD)** *(continued)*

Medication or treatment	Recommended adult dosage, starting/ maximum, mg/day^a	Neuro-transmitter producing therapeutic effect	Proposed mechanism of action	Blockade of histaminic, cholinergic, and alpha-adrenergic receptors	Potential for weight gain	Potential for early GI side effects	Potential for sexual side effects	Safety margin in overdose	Clinically relevant considerations
Heterocyclic antidepressants									
Tricyclic antidepressants (TCAs)									
Tertiary-amine TCAs (amitriptyline [Elavil], imipramine [Tofranil], doxepin [Sinequan], trimipramine [Surmontil], clomipramine [Anafranil])	75/up to 300	5-HT > NE	5-HT + NE reuptake inhibition	High	High	Very low	High	Low	Very effective agents but harsh side-effect profile at therapeutic doses. Very sedating. Dangerous when combined with alcohol. Minimal involvement with CYP isoenzyme system. Doxepin also approved for the treatment of anxiety and pruritis. Harsh side-effect profile, dangerous in overdose, and dangerous when combined with alcohol; limits usefulness. Clomipramine approved for OCD but not for depression.

■ Table 2–3   Somatic treatments for major depressive disorder (MDD) (continued)

Medication or treatment	Recommended adult dosage, starting/maximum, mg/day[a]	Neurotransmitter producing therapeutic effect	Proposed mechanism of action	Blockade of histaminic, cholinergic, and alpha-adrenergic receptors	Potential for weight gain	Potential for early GI side effects	Potential for sexual side effects	Safety margin in overdose	Clinically relevant considerations
Heterocyclic antidepressants (continued)									
Tricyclic antidepressants (TCAs) (continued)									
Secondary-amine TCAs (nortriptyline [Pamelor], desipramine [Norpramin], protriptyline [Vivactil, Aventyl])	Nortriptyline: 50/150 Desipramine: 100/300 Protriptyline: 10/60	NE > 5-HT	5-HT + NE reuptake inhibition	High	High	Very low	Medium	Low	Very effective agents, but moderate to harsh side-effect profile at therapeutic doses. Less sedating than the tertiary-amine TCAs. Desipramine is a virtually pure NE reuptake inhibitor. Dangerous when combined with alcohol. Minimal involvement with CYP isoenzyme system. Protriptyline is considered activating.
Tricyclic antidepressant with D_2 blockade									
Amoxapine (Asendin)	100/400	5-HT + NE	5-HT + NE reuptake inhibition of parent compound and active metabolites; metabolite blocks postsynaptic D_2 receptors	Low	High	Very low	High	Low	TCA with antipsychotic benefit for depression with psychotic features. Lethality in overdose similar to that of other TCAs. Possible EPS and TD. Use only when psychotic features are present.

■ Table 2–3   Somatic treatments for major depressive disorder (MDD) *(continued)*

Medication or treatment	Recommended adult dosage, starting/ maximum, mg/day[a]	Neuro-transmitter producing therapeutic effect	Proposed mechanism of action	Blockade of histaminic, cholinergic, and alpha-adrenergic receptors	Potential for weight gain	Potential for early GI side effects	Potential for sexual side effects	Safety margin in overdose	Clinically relevant considerations
Heterocyclic antidepressants (continued)									
Tetracyclic antidepressant									
Maprotiline (Ludiomil)	75/150	NE	NE reuptake inhibitor	Potent H_1 blockade; minimal alpha$_1$-adrenergic blockade	Moderate	Moderate	Variable	Low	Tetracyclic antidepressant with significant morbidity secondary to the potential for seizures at therapeutic doses. Overdose particularly dangerous. Weight gain and sedation secondary to H_1 receptor blockade.
Monoamine oxidase inhibitors (MAOIs)									
Selegiline transdermal (EmSam)	6/12	5-HT + NE + DA	Inhibition of MAO A and B, but not gastrointestinal MAO	None	Medium	Very low	Medium	High at 6 mg/day, low at 12 mg/day (because of drug and food interactions)	Likely a first choice when an MAOI is desired. Hypertensive crisis only at 12 mg/day dosage. Usual precautions to prevent serotonin syndrome (e.g., do not use with SSRIs, meperidine).
Phenelzine (Nardil)	45/90	5-HT + NE	Inhibition of MAO	None	Medium	Very low	Medium	Low (because of drug and food interactions)	Because of dangerous drug and food interactions, use with extreme caution. Multiple daily doses required. Sedating.
Tranylcypromine (Parnate)	20/60	5-HT + NE	Inhibition of MAO	None	Medium	Very low	Medium	Low (because of drug and food interactions)	Because of dangerous drug and food interactions, use with extreme caution. Multiple daily doses required. Activating.

■ Table 2–3 Somatic treatments for major depressive disorder (MDD) *(continued)*

Medication or treatment	Recommended adult dosage, starting/maximum, mg/day[a]	Neuro-transmitter producing therapeutic effect	Proposed mechanism of action	Blockade of histaminic, cholinergic, and alpha-adrenergic receptors	Potential for weight gain	Potential for early GI side effects	Potential for sexual side effects	Safety margin in overdose	Clinically relevant considerations
Monoamine oxidase inhibitors (MAOIs) *(continued)*									
Isocarboxazid (Marplan)	30/30	5-HT + NE	Inhibition of MAO	None	Medium	Very low	Medium	Low (because of drug and food interactions)	Because of dangerous drug and food interactions, use with extreme caution. Activating.
Other medications									
Stimulants (indirect agonists)	Various, depending on specific medication	DA (principally) + NE + 5-HT	Release DA + NE; block reuptake of DA + NE; inhibit MAO-A	None	None	Medium	Low	Medium, because of pressor effects and potential for dependence	Highly activating. Can induce weight loss. Not approved for treatment of depression. Potentially significant cardiovascular and CNS stimulation. Potential for drug dependency.
Nonmedication treatments									
ECT	NA	?	?	None	None	None	None	NA	Most effective of all treatments for MDD. Anterograde and/or retrograde amnesia widely publicized.
Phototherapy	NA	NA	?	None	None	None	None	NA	Excellent for treatment of SAD. Safe with proper light source. Can be used with antidepressants.
Newer, less well validated, and alternative treatments									
Repetitive TMS (rTMS)	NA	?	?	None	None	None	None	NA	Investigational use with great promise.
Vagus nerve stimulation (VNS)	NA	?	?	None	None	None	None	NA	FDA approved for treatment-resistant depression.

■ Table 2–3   Somatic treatments for major depressive disorder (MDD) *(continued)*

Medication or treatment	Recommended adult dosage, starting/ maximum, mg/day[a]	Neuro- transmitter producing therapeutic effect	Proposed mechanism of action	Blockade of histaminic, cholinergic, and alpha- adrenergic receptors	Potential for weight gain	Potential for early GI side effects	Potential for sexual side effects	Safety margin in overdose	Clinically relevant considerations
Newer, less well validated, and alternative treatments *(continued)*									
Deep brain stimulation	NA	?	?	None	None	None	None	NA	Investigational use with promise.
Sleep deprivation	NA	?	?	None	None	None	None	NA	
Exercise	NA	Possibly beta-endorphins	Release with exercise	None	None	None	None	NA	Excellent homeopathic treatment for depression and weight loss. Can improve maintenance benefits. Requires initial and follow-up checks for physical status.
St. John's wort	300 mg tid (oral)	Possibly 5-HT + NE + DA	Possible inhibition of MAO	Minimal	?	?	?	?	Potentially effective for mild to moderate levels of depression. May possess properties of MAOIs and/or SSRIs. Photosensitization. CYP isoenzyme induction. Switch to mania in bipolar depression. Dose standardization can be problematic. Can be purchased without prescription.
SAM-e	200/1,600	?	?	Minimal	?	?	?	?	Likely effective for depression. Can be purchased without a prescription.

Note.   5-HT = 5-hydroxytryptamine (serotonin); CNS = central nervous system; CR = controlled release; CYP = cytochrome P450; DA = dopamine; ECT = electroconvulsive therapy; EPS = extrapyramidal side effects; FDA = U.S. Food and Drug Administration; GAD = generalized anxiety disorder; GI = gastrointestinal; MAO = monoamine oxidase; MAOI = monoamine oxidase inhibitor; NA = not applicable; NE = norepinephrine; SAD = seasonal affective disorder; SAM-e = S-adenosylmethionine; SGMMA = second-generation mixed-mechanism antidepressant; SR = sustained release; SSRI = selective serotonin reuptake inhibitor; TCA = tricyclic antidepressant; TD = tardive dyskinesia; ? = unknown; TMS = transcranial magnetic stimulation.
aExcept fluoxetine weekly.

Antidepressant Medications

Selective serotonin reuptake inhibitors (SSRIs), serotonin-norepinephrine reuptake inhibitors (SNRIs), and atypical antidepressants (AtypANs):

General considerations:

➤ Available since 1987 with the introduction of fluoxetine, followed by bupropion (1989), sertraline (1992), paroxetine (1993), venlafaxine (1994), nefazodone (1995), mirtazapine (1996), citalopram (1998), escitalopram (2002), and duloxetine (2004).

➤ Neurotransmitter considerations:

✔ Sertraline at doses of 200 mg/day is purported to also increase DA in addition to increasing 5-HT.

✔ Paroxetine at doses of 50 mg/day is purported to also increase NE in addition to increasing 5-HT.

✔ Venlafaxine at doses greater than 200 mg/day is purported to also increase NE in addition to increasing 5-HT.

✔ Bupropion increases both NE and DA secondary to reuptake blockade by its principal active metabolite, hydroxybupropion. However, it has no effect on 5-HT.

✔ Fluoxetine and its active (but slowly metabolized) metabolite, norfluoxetine, are both effective SSRIs.

✔ Duloxetine increases both 5-HT and NE at all dosage levels.

➤ SSRIs, venlafaxine, duloxetine, and nefazodone produce minimal blockade of alpha$_1$-adrenergic, cholinergic (M$_1$), and H$_1$ receptors. They have a low potential to cause cardiovascular side effects, a low potential to induce seizures, a low potential to induce orthostatic hypotension, an initially low potential for appetite increase (although weight gain after long-term use is recognized as a side effect of SSRIs), a high margin of safety in overdose, and a high margin of safety when used with alcohol. Similar properties hold for mirtazapine, with the exception of significant H$_1$ blockade leading to appetite increase and sedation; for bupropion, with the exception of an increased potential for seizures at higher doses of the immediate-release formulation or in patients with bulimic behaviors or a prior history of a seizure disorder; for venlafaxine, with the exception of dose-dependent increases of diastolic blood pressure and the possibility of developing sustained hypertension; and for duloxetine, with the exception of a contraindication for concomitant use with active alcohol abuse.

➤ Bupropion, desipramine, escitalopram, and protriptyline are more often activating than sedating.

➤ The adage "start low, go slow" regarding the use of the first-generation antidepressants (e.g., TCAs, MAOIs) can be modified for SSRIs/SNRIs/AtypANs as "start low, go slow, but go up." Greater caution regarding raising doses is always advised in elderly, substance-abusing, and medically ill patients.

➤ There is growing recognition of the *possible* impact of SSRIs in *lowering* DA levels, possibly secondary to presynaptic inhibition by 5-HT receptors on DA release (somewhat controversial). This concept has been proposed to explain the "poop-out" phenomenon (possibly a DA deficit syndrome) often reported after long-term SSRI use and the inordinate popularity of adding bupropion (an NE and DA reuptake inhibitor) to SSRIs to restore DA activity. Poop-out may also be associated with decreased libido, increased appetite and weight, and increased cigarette smoking.

➤ SSRI blood levels can be useful for monitoring compliance but not clinical effectiveness. Blood levels vary greatly in responders and nonresponders. Concentrations in the CNS, not the blood, confer activity.

Therapeutic considerations:

➤ The major benefits of the SSRIs/SNRIs/AtypANs over first-generation antidepressants are greater tolerability due to fewer and less-intense side effects, greater safety in medically ill patients, greater safety in overdose, and greater safety with concurrent use of other medications, alcohol (except for duloxetine), or illicit drugs. The consideration that first-generation antidepressants are purportedly more effective in severe depression remains unresolved.

➤ SSRIs can also improve psychological anxiety (e.g., worry, fear) associated with low 5-HT levels, and reduce the intensity and frequency of panic attacks, usually at somewhat higher doses than used for the treatment of depression. Bupropion can increase psychological anxiety, and neither bupropion nor trazodone is effective for the treatment of panic disorder. For patients with significant comorbid anxiety, begin with half the normal starting dose if possible, and slowly titrate upward.

Side-effect considerations:

➤ Many of the side effects of this group of medications develop early in the course of treatment; are secondary to increases in 5-HT, NE, and/or DA; are typically dose dependent; and may decrease or resolve over time. If side effects are very problematic or are persistent, reducing the dose, administering adjunctive medications (e.g., benzodiazepines for sleep), or switching medications can be helpful.

➤ The impact of this group of medications on cardiovascular function (except for venlafaxine, which can cause dose-dependent increases in diastolic blood pressure, and mirtazapine, which can cause an increased workload on the heart due to weight gain) is minimal. On average, SSRIs reduce heart rate by 3–4 beats per minute.

➤ Sudden discontinuation of short-half-life antidepressants (e.g., paroxetine, venlafaxine) can generate a harsh discontinuation syndrome, possibly within hours after the dose is missed.

➤ Dropout rates correlate with the frequency and intensity of antidepressant side effects (TCAs/MAOIs > SSRIs/SNRIs/AtypANs):

✔ TCAs with strong anticholinergic and sedating properties have the highest dropout rates, and bupropion and escitalopram (few side effects) have the lowest dropout rates.

✔ Discontinuing antidepressants prior to achieving recovery greatly increases the risk of relapse.

✔ Antidepressant dropout rates are astoundingly high, with only 50% of patients continuing treatment past 3–6 months.

➤ Nefazodone, a 5-HT agonist, can cause idiosyncratic liver failure. Although the brand-name product (Serzone) is no longer marketed, generic formulations are available.

➤ Duloxetine should not be used in the presence of active alcohol abuse/ dependence.

➤ SSRIs/SNRIs/AtypANs are much less likely than TCAs/MAOIs to be lethal in overdose, although rarely deaths have been reported.

➤ Insomnia develops in about 15%–20% of patients taking SSRIs. Switching the time of dosing (e.g., morning to night) or providing a hypnotic for a short time can be beneficial.

➤ All antidepressants have the potential to induce a switch to mania or hypomania in patients with bipolar depression. Bupropion, paroxetine, and sertraline may have a lower risk, although recent studies suggest that all antidepressants likely have equal propensity to induce the switch.

➤ All antidepressants are regarded by the FDA as having an increased potential to increase suicidal ideation in adolescents and young adults (black box warning).

Sexual side effects:

➤ Are dose dependent, may or may not improve or resolve with time, and have a prevalence ranging from 20% to 80% (depending on the study).

➤ Are not clearly defined mechanistically as to etiology. Sexual dysfunction is possibly caused by increased 5-HT and/or decreased DA, although other mechanisms have been proposed. Serotonin receptors 5-HT_2 and 5-HT_3 are purportedly involved.

➤ Can negatively impact on all phases of sexual response (e.g., decreased libido, erectile dysfunction, ejaculatory delay, anorgasmia).

➤ Are potentially amenable by:

✔ Waiting 4–6 weeks to see if symptoms resolve (may compromise compliance).

✔ Reducing the dose (may compromise antidepressant effectiveness).

✔ Providing a "drug holiday" (may induce withdrawal symptoms and possibly compromise therapeutic outcome).

✔ Switching to another antidepressant with an inherently lower potential for inducing sexual dysfunction (bupropion, nefazodone, mirtazapine).

✔ Adding an "antidote," such as:

■ Phosphodiesterase (PDE-5) inhibitors:

● Can significantly improve SSRI-induced erectile dysfunction but do not improve libido. Purportedly helpful in females as well.

● Include sildenafil (Viagra; dosage range: 25–100 mg), vardenafil (Levitra; dosage range: 2.5–20 mg), and tadalafil (Cialis; dosage range: 5–20 mg).

● Caution for unusual side effects (e.g., color discrimination [blue/green], sudden loss of vision, optic neuropathy, cardiac risks associated with increased sexual activity).

● Contraindicated in patients taking nitrates.

■ Dopaminergic agents (e.g., bupropion, amantadine, bromocriptine, ropinirole [Requip], pramipexole [Mirapex]).

■ Other purportedly useful agents include trazodone, CNS stimulants, loratadine (Claritin; an H_1 receptor antagonist), Buspar (a serotonergic agonist), cyproheptadine (Periactin; a serotonergic antagonist), yohimbine, bethanechol, and granisetron (5-HT_3 receptor antagonist).

Weight gain:

➤ Recognized as side effect of SSRIs: Occurs more often than previously reported.

✔ Weight gain with SSRIs/SNRIs/AtypANs is not usually associated with carbohydrate craving (except mirtazapine) and is more likely to occur after several months of use.

✔ A wellness approach (i.e., behavioral modification), to include reduced caloric intake and greater caloric expenditure (exercise), can produce dramatic results.

Suicidal thinking and suicidal behavior:

➤ Although a direct correlation between the use of antidepressants and suicidal ideation/behaviors has not been firmly established, the FDA recommends careful observation for suicidal thinking and suicidal behavior in adolescents and adults. Only fluoxetine is approved for treatment in persons younger than age 18 years.

➤ A definitive correlation between the use of antidepressants and suicidal ideation/behavior has not been firmly established.

➤ The risk–benefit ratio must be assessed individually for each patient.

Serotonin syndrome:

➤ See Monoamine Oxidase Inhibitors section later in this chapter.

Metabolism issues:

➤ The ideal antidepressant would have a 24-hour half-life, permitting once-daily dosing; no active metabolites; no interaction with the CYP isoenzyme system; minimal or no side effects; no impact on protein binding; no adverse effects when used with alcohol; no variability of effects or side effects based on genetic influences; no requirement for dosage reduction in the elderly; no requirement for dosage reduction in patients with hepatic or renal impairment; and no discontinuation syndrome.

➤ Antidepressant drug interactions involving the CYP isoenzyme system can be complex, with clinical implications not always predictable. For example:

✔ Inhibition of the CYP 2D6 enzyme pathway by fluoxetine, paroxetine, and bupropion can inhibit the metabolism of TCAs, raising TCA blood levels to potentially toxic levels. Increases in TCA-induced cardiotoxicity (e.g., QTc), orthostasis, seizures, and central/peripheral anticholinergic side effects can then become significant.

✔ TCAs have minimal impact on the metabolism of other antidepressants.

✔ Fluoxetine and paroxetine can inhibit their own metabolism through the CYP 2D6 enzyme pathway.

✔ Genetic influence on CYP isoenzyme activity can be dramatic. Rapid metabolizers can possibly be translated as "treatment resistant," and slow metabolizers can experience serious side effects as drug levels rise higher than would be expected. Further, a very slow or nonmetabolizer of a prodrug (e.g., bupropion) may result in a totally nonresponsive individual.

Discontinuation (withdrawal) syndrome:

➤ Commonly starts within 6–48 hours after abruptly (or at times slowly) stopping the shorter-half-life SSRIs (e.g., paroxetine, sertraline) or venlafaxine.

➤ Presents with flu-like symptoms, paresthesias (e.g., electric shock–like sensations), and variable mental status changes (e.g., vivid dreams, agitation).

➤ Can be minimized by gradually discontinuing the antidepressant over several weeks or months (not more than a 25% reduction each week).

Use during pregnancy and lactation:

➤ Untreated depression during pregnancy can lead to a lower infant birth weight, preeclampsia, preterm delivery, and an increased risk of miscarriage.

➤ Fluoxetine is the best studied and appears to be the "safest" SSRI to use during pregnancy, but it is excreted into breast milk to a greater extent than are other SSRIs.

➤ Paroxetine has been associated with a two- to threefold increase in congenital and cardiac anomalies when administered in the first trimester and persistent pulmonary hypertension in the newborn when administered in the third trimester.

➤ Withdrawal symptoms in the newborn (e.g., tremors, sleep problems, transient hypoglycemia) have been reported. Paroxetine can have a prominent withdrawal syndrome in the neonate.

➤ Psychotherapy may reduce or eliminate the need for antidepressants during pregnancy.

➤ In order of greater-to-lower transfer into breast milk: fluoxetine > citalopram > paroxetine. SSRIs are deemed "compatible with breast feeding," although the risk–benefit ratio must be assessed on an individual basis.

Heterocyclic antidepressants (tricyclic and tetracyclic antidepressants):

General considerations:

➤ Heterocyclic antidepressants are highly effective but also carry a relatively high side-effect profile.

➤ Amitriptyline (a tertiary amine) is metabolized to nortriptyline (a secondary amine), whereas imipramine (a tertiary amine) is metabolized to desipramine (a secondary amine). Amitriptyline and imipramine have a dual mode of action, blocking the reuptake of both 5-HT and NE (with a predominance toward 5-HT), whereas desipramine and nortriptyline preferentially block the reuptake of NE.

➤ Amoxapine is a TCA with antipsychotic properties secondary to D_2 receptor blockade.

➤ Maprotiline is a tetracyclic antidepressant with principally NE reuptake inhibition.

➤ Trazodone was considered the first "safe" antidepressant. Although trazodone is less toxic than the TCAs, overdose deaths have been reported.

Therapeutic effects:

➤ Heterocyclic antidepressants may be more effective than SSRIs/SNRIs/AtypANs for severe depression.

Side effects:

➤ Often dramatically compromise compliance.

➤ Are due mostly to postsynaptic alpha$_1$-adrenergic, cholinergic (M_1), and H_1 receptor blockade and can have a dramatic negative impact on compliance. The tertiary-amine TCAs are more side-effect prone, more dangerous in overdose, and more dangerous in combination with alcohol than the second-ary-amine TCAs. In turn, the extent and impact of these side effects for the secondary-amine TCAs are generally still greater than for the SSRIs/SNRIs/AtypANs (except for mirtazapine's H_1 receptor blockade). Nortriptyline is the least anticholinergic TCA. Consequences of postsynaptic receptor blockade are summarized in Table 2–4.

■ **Table 2–4   Consequences of postsynaptic receptor blockade**

Postsynaptic blockade of	Possible side effects	Possible interventions
Central cholinergic (M_1) receptors	Hyperthermia Cognitive impairment Confusion Delirium	Lower the dosage. Switch to desipramine. Switch to SSRIs/SNRIs/AtypANs. Add intravenous physostig-mine for acute emergency.
Peripheral cholinergic (M_1) receptors	Dry mouth Constipation Urinary hesitancy or retention Tachycardia (sustained 11 beats per minute) Blurred vision Precipitation or worsening of narrow-angle glaucoma	Wait for tolerance to develop. Lower the dose. Add bethanechol 25–50 mg bid. Use sugarless gum for dry mouth. Switch to desipramine. Switch to SSRIs/SNRIs/AtypANs.
Histaminic H_1 receptors	Sedation (less often insomnia) Appetite increase with carbohydrate craving Weight gain	Wait for tolerance to develop. Lower the dose. Switch to SSRIs/SNRIs/AtypANs.
Alpha$_1$-adrenergic receptors	Postural hypotension (falls) Reflex tachycardia	Wait for tolerance to develop. Lower the dose. Switch to SSRIs/SNRIs/AtypANs.

Note. AtypAN = atypical antidepressant (bupropion, mirtazapine, nefazadone); SNRI = serotonin-norepinephrine reuptake inhibitor; SSRI = selective serotonin reuptake inhibitor.

➤ Also include:

✔ A switch to mania or hypomania or induction of rapid cycling in bipolar depressed patients.

✔ Reduction of the seizure threshold.

✔ Potentially dangerous cardiovascular side effects:

   ■ Quinidine-like cardiac effects (type IA antiarrhythmic effects), which can alter conduction rhythms (i.e., slow cardiac conduction), rendering TCAs especially dangerous in patients with preexisting cardiac disease.

   ■ QRS widening, which serves as an indicator of the degree of TCA cardiovascular toxicity in emergency settings.

   ■ An increase in heart rate of approximately 11 beats per minute, further increasing the cardiac workload in patients with congestive heart failure or heart disease.

   ■ Induction of heart block in patients with preexisting bundle branch block.

   ■ QTc interval prolongation (may be a cause of death in overdose).

   ■ Orthostatic hypotension, with an increased potential for dizziness and falls.

   ■ Toxicity in patients with a recent MI. TCAs are contraindicated for the treatment of depression until 6 months after an MI.

✔ Sexual dysfunction (e.g., arousal, erectile, and orgasmic difficulties) in both sexes.

✔ Sedation (e.g., amitriptyline, imipramine, nortriptyline, doxepin) or activation (e.g., desipramine, protriptyline):

   ■ Sedation can be helpful for patients with insomnia.

   ■ Activation can be helpful for patients with anergia.

✔ Weight gain (often significant, usually with carbohydrate cravings).

Safety considerations:

➤ TCAs have a low margin of safety and should be used with extreme caution (if at all) in patients who are:

✔ Physically ill (particularly with cardiovascular, pulmonary, cognitive, or seizure disorders).

✔ Impulsive or suicidal.

✔ Abusing substances or have a potential to abuse substances, especially alcohol or benzodiazepines.

✔ Advancing in age (the elderly are more sensitive to anticholinergic and orthostatic effects).

Dosing considerations:

➤ Typically, "start low, and go slow," especially in the elderly.

➤ Nortriptyline, imipramine, and desipramine have an advantage of recommended therapeutic plasma-level ranges (therapeutic windows). Refer to Table 2–5.

■ Table 2–5 Recommended therapeutic plasma-level ranges for selected tricyclic antidepressants (TCAs)

TCA	Recommended therapeutic trough-level ranges, ng/mL, 10–14 hours after the last dose
Nortriptyline (Pamelor)	50–150
Imipramine (Tofranil)	200–250 (imipramine + desipramine)
Desipramine (Norpramin)	125–200

Contraindications:

➤ Absolute contraindications:

   ✔ MI (until 6 months after the MI).

   ✔ Narrow-angle glaucoma.

➤ Relative contraindications:

   ✔ Cardiac disease (a baseline ECG is recommended).

   ✔ Prostatic hypertrophy or other obstructive uropathy (secondary to anticholinergic side effects).

Drug interactions:

➤ TCAs have minimal effects on CYP isoenzymes, but their own metabolism is greatly affected by the CYP 1A2, 2C19, 2D6, and 3A4 isoenzyme pathways.

➤ TCAs combined with MAOIs can produce serotonin syndrome.

➤ TCA anticholinergic side effects are additive when TCAs are combined with other agents with anticholinergic activity (e.g., diphenhydramine, benztropine mesylate).

➤ Table 2–6 summarizes common TCA–drug interactions.

■ Table 2–6 Common TCA–drug interactions

Combining TCAs and	Potential result
Barbiturates, carbamazepine, cigarette smoking	Metabolism of TCA is increased, lowering TCA plasma levels and possibly reducing therapeutic effectiveness.
Fluoxetine/paroxetine/bupropion	Metabolism of TCA is decreased, raising TCA plasma levels and possibly inducing TCA toxicity.
MAOIs	Serotonin syndrome.
Other anticholinergic agents	Increased central and peripheral anticholinergic side effects.

Note. MAOI = monoamine oxidase inhibitor; TCA = tricyclic antidepressant.

TCA overdose:

➤ TCAs have a very narrow margin of safety, with therapeutic levels approximately 50% of toxic levels. Ingestion of 1–2 g (less if taken with alcohol) can be fatal.

➤ Cardiovascular side effects of TCAs cause the greatest morbidity and mortality secondary to hypotension and conduction disturbances (especially QRS widening and QTc prolongation). Neurological side effects (e.g., delirium), pulmonary side effects (e.g., aspiration pneumonia, pulmonary edema), and complications from anticholinergic overload (e.g., urinary retention, obstipation) are common findings.

➤ There is a resurgence of use of TCAs for disorders other than depression (e.g., chronic pain syndromes, peripheral neuropathy, migraine prophylaxis, panic and phobic disorders, obsessive-compulsive disorder). Seventy percent of TCA overdose deaths occur before the patient reaches the hospital.

➤ TCA overdose is treated with gastric lavage, cooling blankets for hyperthermia, sodium bicarbonate for cardiac arrythmias, ECG monitoring, and benzodiazepine for seizures.

Discontinuation (withdrawal) syndrome:

➤ Abruptly (or at times slowly) stopping a TCA can produce a withdrawal syndrome. Symptoms include gastrointestinal disturbances, anxiety, withdrawal dyskinesia (amoxapine), and paradoxical behavioral activation (e.g., hypomanic- or manic-type symptoms).

➤ As with SSRIs/SNRIs/AtypANs, a slow taper is recommended.

Use during pregnancy and lactation:

➤ Like SSRIs, TCAs appear to have a relatively low potential for teratogenicity.

➤ Nortriptyline appears to be the safest TCA for use during pregnancy.

➤ Strongly anticholinergic TCAs (e.g., tertiary-amine TCAs) can produce fetal tachyarrhythmia, urinary retention, and intestinal obstruction in the neonate.

➤ Trazodone has been reported to have a greater propensity for birth defects than other first-generation antidepressants.

➤ Less is known about the consequences of TCA excretion into breast milk.

Monoamine oxidase inhibitors:

General considerations:

➤ MAOIs:

✔ Exert their antidepressant effects by raising monoamine (5-HT, NE, and/or DA) levels in the synaptic cleft by blocking monoamine metabolism through deactivation of the enzyme monoamine oxidase (MAO). Inhibition of at least 70%–85% platelet monoamine oxidase is needed to confer antidepressant effectiveness.

✔ Are only FDA approved for MDD and are especially effective for MDD with atypical features and for treatment-resistant depression.

✔ Are rarely used, but may see a resurgence with the recent FDA approval for transdermal selegiline (EmSam) with purportedly less danger of hypertensive crisis at the 6-mg/day dosage.

Therapeutic considerations, side effects, drug and food interactions, and toxicity:

➤ Clinical response typically requires 2–6 weeks, as with many antidepressants.

➤ Side effects include orthostatic hypotension, weight gain, sexual dysfunction, insomnia, daytime sedation, and urinary hesitancy. MAOIs can be lethal in overdose.

➤ Drug-drug and food-drug interactions can be dangerous and can limit the usefulness of these highly effective agents:

✔ Serotonin syndrome (hyperpyrexic crisis):

■ Has been reported when an MAOI is combined with another 5-HT agonist (e.g., SSRIs), some opioids (e.g., meperidine, tramadol), over-the-counter cough preparations containing dextromethorphan, 5-HT_1 agonists (e.g., triptans), stimulants (e.g., cocaine, methamphetamine, MDMA), and dopamine agonists (e.g., buspirone, bromocriptine, amantadine). Rarely reported with a single 5-HT agonist.

■ Symptom development can be dramatic and consists of the triad of altered mental status (e.g., confusion, hallucinations), neuromuscular changes (e.g., hyperreflexia, rigidity, rhabdomyolysis with associated renal failure), and autonomic dysfunction (e.g., hyperpyrexia, tachycardia, unstable blood pressure).

■ Is treated with supportive care (e.g., fluids, protected airway) in an intensive care unit. Chlorpromazine and cyproheptadine (Periactin) can be helpful.

■ Can be avoided by observing the recommended waiting periods when switching from an SSRI to an MAOI (2 weeks, except for fluoxetine [5 weeks]) or from an MAOI to an SSRI (2 weeks).

✔ Noradrenergic syndrome (hypertensive crisis, "cheese reaction"):

■ MAOI + other agents with NE agonist qualities (e.g., dextromethorphan, ephedrine, TCAs) or tyramine from foods (e.g., ripe bananas, fava beans, aged cheeses) can cause autonomic instability, altered mental status, and physical changes (e.g., severe occipital headache, cerebrovascular accident).

■ Treatment is supportive. Nifedipine (Procardia) 10 mg sublingually or chlorpromazine 50 mg orally can abort an impending noradrenergic crisis.

Other Medications Used in the Treatment of Depression

Stimulants:

➤ Include:

  ✔ Amphetamine (Dexedrine), amphetamine salts (Adderall), and methylphenidate (Ritalin).

  ✔ Modafinil (Provigil)—carries an increased risk for serious rash and Stevens-Johnson syndrome.

➤ Are especially beneficial when:

  ✔ Added adjunctively to an antidepressant when psychomotor retardation is prominent.

  ✔ Used at the initiation of traditional antidepressant therapy to speed the onset of antidepressant response (i.e., to provide a "jump start").

  ✔ Used as a marker for predicting the eventual response to antidepressants (a positive response to a stimulant may be indicative of an eventual positive response to an antidepressant).

Nonmedication Treatments for Depressive Disorders

Electroconvulsive therapy:

Principal uses:

➤ MDD (especially effective for MDD with psychotic, melancholic, or catatonic features and for treatment-resistant depression). Effectiveness can approach 70%–90%.

➤ Maintenance therapy for MDD (especially for patients successfully treated with ECT).

➤ Bipolar disorder (with a risk of induction of mania in depressed patients).

➤ Schizophrenia (especially for the catatonic type when combined with a high-potency antipsychotic medication).

➤ Additional uses (not as well studied and less well validated):

  ✔ Parkinson's disease (to reduce rigidity and treat depression).

  ✔ Tardive dyskinesia (to reduce dyskinetic movements).

  ✔ Neuroleptic malignant syndrome (to reduce rigidity).

  ✔ Treatment-resistant obsessive-compulsive disorder (OCD).

  ✔ Chronic pain syndromes (to reduce pain).

  ✔ Catatonia of varying etiologies (can be very effective).

Pretreatment workup:

➤ History, physical examination, complete blood count (CBC), routine chemistries, thyroid panel, chest X ray, urinalysis, and ECG.

➤ Additional testing is warranted if there are concerns for a spinal compression fracture, brain lesion, or brain mass (e.g., spine/skull X rays, computed tomography [CT]/magnetic resonance imaging [MRI], electroencephalogram [EEG]).

Usual procedure (in order):

➤ Administer atropine to decrease secretions and block bradycardia.

➤ Administer general anesthesia with a rapid-onset/brief-duration anesthetic (e.g., methohexital sodium [Brevital Sodium]).

➤ Administer succinylcholine for muscle relaxation and paralysis. Look for fasciculations as evidence of distribution in the body.

➤ Administer oxygen throughout the procedure and during the recovery phase.

➤ Place electrodes:

  ✔ Nondominant unilateral electrode placement results in less memory loss and fewer side effects than bilateral placement but is generally considered less effective than bilateral electrode placement.

➤ Provide brief pulsed current to induce a seizure for at least 25 seconds:

  ✔ Seizure duration can be assessed by electroencephalography, by visualizing the induced tremor (by tightening a blood pressure cuff on a leg prior to administering succinylcholine), or by monitoring changes in blood pressure and pulse.

  ✔ If a seizure cannot be induced, provide hyperventilation, use less anesthesia, reduce or eliminate medications that raise the seizure threshold, or add a stimulant (e.g., caffeine, theophylline).

  ✔ If a seizure cannot be terminated (status epilepticus), add more anesthetic or administer diazepam.

  ✔ If seizures are too short, pretreat with theophylline or caffeine.

Potential side effects:

➤ Headache (common).

➤ Postictal delirium, lasting 1–2 days (more likely in neurologically compromised patients and patients treated with bilateral electrode placement).

➤ Memory loss:

  ✔ Is well recognized and can consist of postictal confusion, anterograde amnesia, and/or retrograde amnesia.

  ✔ Is more likely with bilateral electrode placement, higher electrical dosages, and an increased number of treatments.

Contraindications:

➤ Absolute contraindications:
  ✔ None.

➤ Relative contraindications include recent CVA, brain tumor, hypertension, seizure disorder, recent myocardial infarct, compression fractures of the spine, and severe osteoporosis or osteoarthritis.

Clinical issues:

➤ Spontaneous seizure activity was recognized in the eighteenth century to improve mood, and there are reports of seizure induction by administering camphor as far back as the sixteenth century.

➤ ECT is the most effective treatment for depression.

➤ Concurrent use of ECT and lithium can produce a short-term encephalopathy, resulting in confusion or delirium.

➤ Informed consent is required. If the patient is unable to provide informed consent, a court order or approval by a guardian may be needed. A concerned family member not court authorized may not legally be able to provide consent, despite the gravity of the circumstances.

➤ The risk of dying from ECT is equivalent to the risk of dying from general anesthesia.

➤ The number of treatments varies with the indication:

✔ MDD or bipolar depression typically requires 3–12 treatments, usually administered three times per week.

✔ Bipolar mania or treatment-refractory depression may require 10–20 treatments.

✔ Catatonia may require 1–4 treatments.

➤ Maintenance therapy (e.g., once monthly ECT, antidepressants, antidepressants + lithium, or liothyronine [T3; Cytomel]) is usually required after the acute illness resolves due to a high rate of relapse for patients who previously did not significantly improve with antidepressants.

Light therapy (phototherapy):

➤ Especially effective for MDD with seasonal pattern, jet lag, and some forms of insomnia.

➤ The patient self-administers 2,500–10,000 lux of bright light for 30 minutes to 2 hours daily utilizing a light box containing a full-spectrum, non-ultraviolet (UV) light source.

➤ Properly administered light does not cause retinal or eye damage. Side effects can include fatigue, sunburn, and short-term hypomania.

Newer, Less Well Validated, and Alternative Treatments

Repetitive transcranial magnetic stimulation (rTMS):

➤ Utilizes an electromagnet placed on the scalp to generate low-frequency magnetic field pulses nearly equal to the strength of an MRI scan. The magnetic pulses induce electrical currents (but not a seizure) in the underlying cerebral cortex. High-frequency left prefrontal rTMS has antidepressant properties.

➤ Mechanism of action is unknown but may involve the release of DA, which has an impact on the limbic system.

➤ Is a noninvasive procedure. The most significant side effects are headache and the unlikely possibility of inducing a seizure.

➤ A recent application for FDA approval for treatment-resistant depression was denied because of lack of robust effectiveness although safety was judged to be quite good.

Magnetic seizure therapy:

➤ A strong magnetic field induces a seizure like that of ECT while the patient is under general anesthesia. However, the seizures are more localized and of shorter duration than with ECT, such that antidepressant effectiveness is maintained while side effects (e.g., confusion, amnesia) are minimized. Not FDA approved for the treatment of depression.

Deep brain stimulation:

➤ Involves the placement of a stimulator ("brain pacemaker") in the subgenual cingulate region of the brain.

➤ Is FDA approved for the treatment of Parkinson's disease, dystonia, and essential tremor, but not for depression.

➤ Is a surgically invasive procedure (unlike ECT, rTMS, and magnetic seizure therapy) with accompanying risks.

Vagus nerve stimulation:

➤ FDA approved for treatment-resistant depression that has not improved after use of at least four other treatments (e.g., antidepressants, ECT).

➤ Involves the intermittent electrical stimulation of the 10th cranial nerve on the left side of the neck by implanting a stimulating device (pulse generator) in the chest. Signals from the stimulating device are sent to the vagus nerve approximately every 3–5 minutes for about 30 seconds.

➤ Minimal side effects (e.g., hoarseness, mild neck pain, cough). Memory loss is not problematic.

Sleep deprivation:

➤ Can be effective when used the entire night or during the second half of the night. Sleep deprivation during REM sleep appears to provide the most robust response.

➤ Produces temporary improvement, which may be predictive of an eventual positive response to antidepressants. Can be repeated every 4–5 days.

Exercise:

➤ Can be an effective treatment for mild to moderate depression. Validated as an effective treatment for depression for up to 6 months; longer-term effectiveness remains in question.

➤ Effectiveness for treating depression seems to increase with increasing frequency and intensity of exercise. The "recommended dosage" of exercise is 30–60 minutes of moderate-intensity physical activity per day.

➤ Performed on a regular basis may reduce the potential for relapse or recurrence of depression (i.e., exercise may constitute maintenance therapy).

➤ Is recommended as an augmentation strategy when "added" to an antidepressant/psychotherapy to improve overall effectiveness.

➤ Effectiveness appears to be at least in part related to:

✔ The release of beta-endorphins and neuropeptides that bind to opioid receptors in the brain producing a feeling of well-being.

✔ Increased brain levels of 5-HT, NE, and DA.

St. John's wort:

➤ Is marketed over-the-counter as a dietary supplement, is derived from the plant *Hypericum perforatum,* and purportedly has properties of an MAOI and SSRI.

➤ Effectiveness is not fully established. Although small studies are supportive as effective for mild depression, larger studies are not.

➤ The recommended dosage is 300 mg tid. However, there is great variability in the percentage of active ingredients from brand to brand and from batch to batch.

➤ Can be beneficial for smoking cessation.

➤ Has important drug interactions:

✔ Induces CYP 3A4 isoenzymes.

✔ Inhibits the metabolism of the protease inhibitor indinavir (used for the treatment of HIV infection).

➤ Reported side effects include photosensitization with sunburn, sinus tachycardia, gastrointestinal upset, fatigue, and (at high doses) difficulty with urination.

➤ Should not be used during pregnancy and can induce mania/hypomania in depressed bipolar individuals.

S-adenosylmethionine (SAM-e):

➤ Is a naturally occurring compound, marketed as a dietary supplement, and administered at a dosage of 800 mg/day in two divided doses for the treatment of depression. Recommendations are to take supplemental folic acid and vitamin B_{12} along with SAM-e.

➤ Purportedly increases 5-HT, NE, and DA in the synaptic cleft as well as being involved with vitamin B_{12} and folate metabolism.

➤ Effectiveness claims are based on small, at times poorly undertaken, clinical studies. However, some of these studies have shown a robust response for the treatment of depression.

Omega-3 fatty acids:

➤ Are products of fatty fishes, with active ingredients of eicosapentaenoic acid (EPA) and docosahexaenoic acid (DHA). A high ratio of EPA to DHA is preferred.

➤ May be helpful as an adjunctive treatment when added to:

✔ Mood stabilizers for the treatment of bipolar disorder.

✔ Antidepressants for the treatment of MDD.

✔ Antipsychotic medications for the treatment of schizophrenia.

➤ Are usually dosed at 1–2 g/day, but "megadoses" (up to 12 g/day) have also been advocated.

Placebo effect:

➤ Although the actual mechanism remains unknown, a placebo dosage form can provide up to a 30% benefit for the treatment of depression, at least on a short-term basis. A proposed mechanism is that the "therapeutic environment" has changed for the better, with the patient now hopeful for improvement secondary to the intervention.

Ultimate Treatment Goal

➤ The ultimate goal of treatment is recovery (rather than just a response). The presence of residual symptoms (i.e., incomplete recovery) greatly increases the risk for relapse and, potentially, the development of a chronic depression.

Phase-Specific Goals for Treatment of Major Depressive Disorder

Acute phase (0–16 weeks):

➤ The goal is to generate a robust response.

➤ The plan is to start an antidepressant medication:

✔ Although a positive response may occur within the first week, 12 weeks or more at a therapeutic dosage may be needed to generate a robust response.

✔ Improvements in appetite, anxiety, and sleep typically occur before improvement in mood.

➤ Predictors of a robust positive response to a first trial of an antidepressant (expected in ~30–50% of patients) include:

✔ Acute onset of depression and rapid intervention after onset.

✔ Depression with melancholic features or predominance of vegetative symptoms.

✔ Prior positive response to an antidepressant medication.

✔ Family history of a mood disorder (implies genetic underpinnings).

✔ Good family functioning and strong social supports.

➤ Predictors of a poorer response to a first trial of an antidepressant include:

✔ A long duration of depression prior to initiating treatment.

✔ Comorbid anxiety, panic attacks, and/or agitation.

✔ Comorbid substance abuse.

✔ Psychotic symptoms, especially if mood-incongruent.

➤ Results from the STAR-D study (see Chapter 9 of this volume, "Miscellaneous Topics") are strongly supportive of the importance of a robust response to the very first trial of an antidepressant. Improvement from switching to a different antidepressant diminishes as the number of switches increases.

Continuation phase (begins after the acute phase and lasts an additional 6–9 months):

➤ The goal is to continue the improvements already achieved and to prevent a relapse.

➤ The plan is to continue the antidepressant at the same dosage that was effective for the acute phase aiming for full recovery (absence of significant depressive symptoms for at least 2 months).

Maintenance phase (begins after recovery):

➤ The goal is to prevent a recurrence of depression (i.e., a new depressive episode).

➤ The plan is to continue the antidepressant for a period of time based on the patient's risk factors for a recurrence. In some cases, indefinite treatment will be needed. Usually, "the dose that gets you well keeps you well." Maintenance treatment is usually recommended if any of the following apply:

✔ The patient has experienced incomplete remission of a prior MDD.

✔ The patient is 50 years of age or older at onset of MDD.

✔ The patient has MDD, chronic.

✔ The patient has experienced three or more MDEs at any age.

✔ The patient has experienced two MDEs and any of the following:

- Family history of bipolar disorder.

- Family history of recurrent depression.

- Recurrence of MDD within 1 year after a previously effective medication was discontinued.

- First MDE before age 20 years.

- Both MDEs were severe (e.g., melancholic features, psychotic features, suicidal behavior), had a rapid onset, and occurred within the previous 3 years.

General Guidelines for Antidepressant Pharmacotherapy

Diagnostic considerations:

➤ Accurate diagnosis of depression can be especially difficult in:

✔ Men, who may deny depressed mood but complain of anxiety or anger management problems.

✔ Women, who may deny depressed mood but complain of physical symptoms that lack an organic basis (i.e., somatization).

✔ Elderly individuals, who may:

- Have significant comorbid physical disorders that often take precedence with primary care physicians leaving depression overlooked and untreated.

- Have undiagnosed alcohol abuse or dependence that contributes to or causes depression.

- Present predominantly physical complaints as the major presentation of depression.

✔ Persons belonging to minority groups, who may feel a negative stigma in asking for mental health help and may have higher rates of somatization.

✔ Individuals with comorbid physical illness, who may complain of pain, fatigue, and anergia that are inappropriately attributed solely to the medical illness rather than to depression.

✔ Individuals with more than one psychiatric disorder, who may receive attention for one disorder (e.g., PTSD, schizophrenia) but not for the comorbid depression.

Choice of antidepressant medication:

➤ When deciding which antidepressant to use, consider the following:

✔ Effectiveness and potential side effects (i.e., risk–benefit profile). Although it is generally recognized that all antidepressants are equally effective for the treatment of depression, clinicians choose antidepressants on the basis of varying criteria (e.g., personal experience, type of depressive symptoms, type of associated symptoms, side-effect profile).

✔ The patient's prior positive response to or preference for a particular antidepressant, if applicable (improves the likelihood of a positive response to that antidepressant).

✔ A prior positive response to a particular antidepressant in a close family member, if applicable (improves the likelihood of a positive response to that antidepressant).

✔ The age and medical status of the patient (increasing age and significant physical impairments correlate with a poorer response to antidepressant medications).

✔ Active substance abuse. Antidepressants are unlikely to be effective when substance abuse is active and in some cases can be dangerous or lethal (e.g., alcohol + TCA, MAOI + meperidine).

Bases for selection of an antidepressant medication:

American Psychiatric Association practice guidelines:

➤ Psychiatric management includes:

✔ Performing a diagnostic evaluation.

✔ Evaluating for safety of patient and others.

✔ Evaluating and addressing functional impairments.

✔ Determining the treatment setting (e.g., oupatient, day treatment, inpatient).

✔ Establishing and maintaining a therapeutic alliance.

✔ Monitoring psychiatric status and safety.

✔ Providing education to the patient and, when appropriate, to his or her family.

✔ Enhancing medication adherence (educational aspects of delay in feeling better, need to continue medications even when feeling better).

✔ Addressing early signs of relapse.

General treatment guidelines recognized by most treatment providers (to include psychotherapy):

➤ Based on the type of depression:

✔ Depression with atypical features: SSRIs and MAOIs preferred, avoid TCAs.

✔ Depression with seasonal features: light therapy alone or with antidepressants.

✔ Depression with postpartum onset: usual somatic therapies; adding estrogen can enhance response.

✔ Depression with psychotic features: antipsychotic medication added to an antidepressant; ECT; amoxapine.

➤ Based on the severity of depression (Ham-D scores):

✔ Mild: antidepressants or psychotherapy alone.

✔ Moderate to severe: antidepressants are preferred unless ECT is considered as a first intervention:

■ SSRIs/SSNIs/AtypANs are a good first choice. TCAs may have greater efficacy. MAOIs or ECT for treatment resistance.

➤ Based on gender: TCAs appear to be more effective in men and SSRIs appear to be more effective in women. However, decisions based on gender may not be clinically warranted.

➤ Based on race/ethnicity: genetic influence will, in time, be accessible such that predicting response and side effects of an antidepressant can be assessed prior to initiating treatment.

➤ Based on pain management considerations:

✔ The somatic symptoms accompanying depression (e.g., generalized aches and pains, irritable bowel) improve as depression improves, regardless of the treatment used.

✔ Antidepressants with both 5-HT and NE activity (e.g., higher-dose venlafaxine, duloxetine, amitriptyline, imipramine) provide pain relief (e.g., migraine headaches, peripheral diabetic neuropathy) in addition to antidepressant effects.

➤ Based on advancing age (late-life depression):

✔ SSRIs/SNRIs/AtypANs are clearly preferred over TCAs and MAOIs because of their reduced side effect burden:

■ SSRIs (2D6 metabolism inhibition with fluoxetine and paroxetine), bupropion (2D6 metabolism issues), mirtazapine (weight gain, sedation), nefazodone (3A4 inhibition of metabolism), nortriptyline (TCA side-effect profile, lethal in overdose), and venlafaxine (sustained hypertension) have been extensively studied in the elderly and are effective treatments.

➤ Based on treatment resistance. Some options include:

✔ Switching strategies:

■ From one SSRI to another SSRI (can result in significant improvement in up to 50% of patients).

■ From one TCA to another TCA (can result in significant improvement in up to 30% of patients).

■ From one antidepressant class to another antidepressant class (e.g., from an SSRI to a TCA or to an MAOI) or from an antidepressant to ECT (the improvement in response from switching to ECT can be as high as 70%).

✔ Augmentation strategies:

- ■ Adding lithium, liothyronine (T_3), or an atypical antipsychotic medication (especially aripiprazole) to an antidepressant can dramatically improve response.

✔ Combination strategies (examples):

- ■ Bupropion + SSRI (the most common augmentation strategy).
- ■ SSRI+TCA (particularly with the predominantly noradrenergic desipramine). Watch for serotonin syndrome.
- ■ SSRI + mirtazapine (mechanistically different).
- ■ ECT + atypical antipsychotic medication.

✔ Novel approaches (all off label):

- ■ High-dose (up to 90 mg/day) buspirone (a 5-HT agonist).
- ■ Amantadine (a DA agonist).
- ■ Buprenorphine (a partial mu opioid agonist).
- ■ Ketoconazole (may be beneficial in "hypercortisolemic depression").

Algorithm for the treatment of MDD:

➤ First (and always) rule out medical and substance-related causes of depression before assuming a diagnosis of MDD. Follow the American Medical Association guidelines (pp. 170–172) to work up the patient.

➤ Strongly consider starting with an SSRI, SNRI, or AtypAN because of the low side effect burden promoting compliance. A TCA may be appropriate under certain circumstances (e.g., prior robust response, robust response in a close family member, patient preference, severe depression).

➤ Expectations are for a positive response within 1–4 weeks after starting the medication. Antidepressants requiring titration to achieve a therapeutic dose may require a longer waiting period.

➤ If the desired level of response is not seen, implement the OACS (Optimize, Augment, Combine, Switch) strategy:

✔ First, *optimize* the dosage by:

- ■ Increasing the dosage:
  - ● For most SSRIs, SNRIs, and AtypANs, upward titration usually improves response (e.g., escitalopram, sertraline) although the degree of expected improvement may plateau at higher doses (e.g., paroxetine, fluoxetine).
- ■ For TCAs, start low and go slow. A baseline ECG may also be warranted (e.g., for the elderly, for medically ill patients). Titrate upward, perhaps utilizing serum levels as a guide (e.g., imipramine, desipramine, nortriptyline).

- Decreasing the dosage:
  - Usual dosages of antidepressants can lead to too-high antidepressant serum levels when:
    - ▸ Antidepressant metabolism is slowed (e.g., CYP drug interaction, genetic predisposition to slower metabolism, hepatic/renal impairment).
    - ▸ The antidepressant is displaced from protein binding sites by another drug that is highly protein bound.
    - ▸ The patient is elderly or is medically compromised.
- ✔ If optimization fails to achieve an adequate response, consider *augmentation, combining,* or *switching* strategies (order of choice based on clinical findings and physician preference):
  - Augmentation strategies (those strongly supported in the literature are noted with an asterisk [*]):
    - Add lithium* to achieve a serum level of at least 0.4–0.6 mEq/L. Lithium augmentation can take 2–4 weeks to become optimally effective.
    - Add liothyronine* (T_3; Cytomel) 25–50 µg/day. Liothyronine augmentation can be effective in both euthyroid and subclinically hypothyroid patients.
    - Add an atypical antipsychotic* (aripiprazole [Abilify] is FDA approved).
    - Add a stimulant* (e.g., methylphenidate 5–10 mg/day).
    - Add buspirone* 5–10 mg tid.
    - Add estrogen in postpartum, perimenopausal, and postmenopausal women.
    - Add testosterone in hypogonadal men.
    - Add pindolol (Visken) 2.5–5.0 mg bid–tid.
    - Add yohimbine (Yocon) 5.4 mg tid.
  - Combination strategies:
    - Combine an SSRI (5-HT activity) with desipramine (NE activity).
    - Combine bupropion (NE and DA activity) with an SSRI (5-HT activity).
    - Combine an SSRI and an MAOI (very controversial due to the strong potential for serotonin syndrome). Caution is strongly advised.
    - Combining two antidepressants from the same class (e.g., fluoxetine and escitalopram) is not clinically prudent.
  - Switching strategies (many options are possible, only a few of which are listed here):

- Switch from one antidepressant class to another class (e.g., SSRI to SNRI, SNRI to AtypAN), SSRI to TCA or MAOI).
- Switch from any antidepressant to ECT.
- If treatment fails after four therapeutic treatment trials consider vagus nerve stimulation.

Prognostic considerations:

➤ With a first trial of an antidepressant:

✔ Thirty percent to 50% of patients respond with complete or near-complete remission of symptoms (not the 75%–80% usually reported).

■ Remission: 30%–50% of patients.

■ Partial response: ~25% of patients.

■ Little to no response: ~20% of patients.

➤ Failure to achieve remission increases the risk for recurrent, chronic, or treatment-resistant depression.

➤ If remission is achieved, maintenance treatment is appropriate when there is a high risk for a recurrence of depression. Typically, maintenance dosages are the same as those used to effectively treat the depression. Fluoxetine, citalopram, escitalopram, sertraline, paroxetine, and venlafaxine are proven effective for preventing a recurrence of depression.

➤ When assessing expectations from drug therapy, apply the following axiom: *Expect a positive response when the **right drug** is used at the **right dosage**, for the **right duration**, for the **right diagnosis**.* Failure to adequately respond to an antidepressant may be due to:

✔ An inherently ineffective antidepressant (e.g., a 5-HT–based depression is treated with desipramine or bupropion).

✔ An antidepressant serum level outside (i.e., too low or too high) the therapeutic range (i.e., lack of optimization). Factors such as gender, weight, age, genetics, drug interactions, displacement from protein binding sites, and renal/hepatic functioning will greatly influence the ultimate dosage.

✔ An inadequate trial duration.

✔ Poor compliance due to denial of illness, medication side effects, inadequate financial resources, too-frequent dosage requirements, poor motivation for recovery, secondary gain, or lack of understanding as to how medications work or can be helpful.

✔ Inaccurate diagnosis (e.g., depression is secondary to bipolar disorder, substance of abuse, prescribed medication, medical illness).

➤ There is no clear consensus on how to proceed if optimization fails. Consider:

✔ Augmentation or combining strategies if the patient has a partial response to optimization.

✔ Switching strategies if there is little or no response to optimization.

➤ When tapering an antidepressant, a slow taper over several months is advisable because this approach:

✔ Avoids withdrawal symptoms, which can mimic signs of returning depressive symptoms.

✔ Tests the hypothesis that the timing is right to stop the antidepressant. If depressive symptoms return during the slow taper, the dosage can be increased and a taper can be reattempted at a later date if appropriate.

Major depressive disorder and suicide:

➤ The lifetime risk of suicide is 2%–6% (~7% in males and ~1% in females). Higher rates (~15%) are often reported in the literature and may be accurate for previously hospitalized patients.

➤ Approximately 60%–80% of persons who commit suicide are depressed.

➤ Females attempt suicide much more frequently than do males.

➤ Males complete suicide more frequently than do females.

➤ The peak incidence of suicide is in May, with a second peak in October.

➤ Suicide rates are particularly high for adolescents and the elderly. An added concern is the possibility that antidepressants may increase the risk for suicide in children and adolescents.

➤ Significant risk factors (nonexhaustive list) for completed suicide in persons with MDD include:

✔ Advancing age (often overlooked as a risk factor).

✔ Feelings of hopelessness (a powerful risk factor).

✔ Severe or chronic depression.

✔ Prior suicide attempt(s).

✔ Presence of psychotic symptoms (especially if mood-incongruent).

✔ Comorbid medical illness, especially if it is chronic, is painful, or is appreciated to result in death within a relatively short period of time. **Note.** The risk for suicide in this patient group is higher than in the general population even if the patient is not depressed.

✔ Agitation (can lead to impulsive suicide attempts).

✔ Active substance abuse.

Psychotherapeutic Treatment of Major Depressive Disorder

➤ Common psychotherapies used for the treatment of depression include:

✔ Cognitive-behavioral therapy (CBT):

■ Is time-limited and directed at examining why maladaptive thinking can cause depression, with behavioral changes to be forthcoming.

✔ Interpersonal therapy:

 ■ Is directed at improving disturbed interpersonal relationships that may have contributed to the development of depression.

 ■ Is limited in duration, often once weekly for 3–4 months.

 ■ Identifies "here and now" concerns rather than childhood or developmental issues. Some examples are dealing with grieving, loss of an important relationship, and transition to motherhood.

✔ Marital therapy:

 ■ Is especially valuable when marital discord is the stressor precipitating depression or is a consequence of the depression.

✔ Group therapy:

 ■ Can be very effective when patients with similar problematic issues join to discuss problems and provide mutual support.

✔ Psychodynamic and psychoanalytic psychotherapy:

 ■ Examines defenses, with a goal of personality changes through the understanding of past conflicts, defenses, ego distortions, and super-ego deficits.

➤ There is ongoing debate as to whether psychotherapy or antidepressant medication provides better results. In general, it is well accepted that:

 ✔ For mild depression, psychotherapy and antidepressant medications can be equally effective.

 ✔ For moderate to severe depression, antidepressant medication (or ECT) will likely be needed.

 ✔ For mild, moderate, and severe depression, a combination of an antidepressant and psychotherapy is better than either alone.

DYSTHYMIC DISORDER

DSM-IV-TR Diagnostic Criteria (Summary)

➤ Depressed mood for most of the day, for more days than not, for at least 2 years (Criterion A) and two or more of the following symptoms while depressed (Criterion B):

 ✔ Poor appetite or overeating.

 ✔ Insomnia or hypersomnia.

 ✔ Low energy or fatigue.

 ✔ Low self-esteem.

 ✔ Poor concentration or difficulty making decisions.

 ✔ Feelings of hopelessness.

➤ During the 2-year period, the person has never been without the symptoms in Criteria A and B for more than 2 months at a time.

➤ No MDE has been present during the first 2 years of the disturbance.

➤ There has never been a manic episode, a mixed episode, or a hypomanic episode, and criteria have never been met for cyclothymic disorder.

➤ The disturbance does not occur exclusively during the course of a chronic psychotic disorder, such as schizophrenia or delusional disorder.

➤ Symptoms are not caused by a medication, substance of abuse, or medical condition.

➤ The disturbance causes clinically significant distress or impairment.

Clinical Issues

➤ Dysthymic disorder:

✔ Is distinguished from MDD by:

■ The steady presence of depressive symptoms (as opposed to discrete episodes of depression). Usually, the intensity of the depression is less than in MDD.

■ The requirement for depressed mood as opposed to the requirement of *either* depressed mood *or* anhedonia in MDD.

✔ Is often described as a "chronic low-grade depression" or a "pervasive, lingering depressive disorder." Symptoms often include decreased energy, sleep and/or appetite disturbance, and low self-esteem.

✔ Was described in older literature as "neurotic depression." Some authorities feel that dysthymic disorder is more consistent with a personality disorder than with a mood disorder.

✔ Often presents with patients:

■ Noting or complaining that "I've been depressed as long as I can remember" or "I've been depressed all my life."

■ Presenting as being sarcastic, rigid, nihilistic, brooding, demanding, and habitually gloomy. Negative countertransference may develop.

■ Having substance abuse and/or social problems (e.g., divorce, unemployment).

✔ Is described by:

■ Akiskal as "habitually gloomy, introverted, broody, overconscientious, discouraged, pessimistic."

■ Eysenck with a description nearly the same as Akiskal's, but with the addition of anxious and depressed mood, worrying, and psychosomatic discomfort or distress.

✔ Can be comorbid with MDD if the major depressive episode develops 2 years after the established diagnosis of dysthymic disorder. This combination is described as "double depression." In this case, it is appropriate to code for both disorders.

✔ Can be comorbid with many other psychiatric and medical disorders (e.g., psychotic disorders, anxiety disorders, substance use disorders, eating disorders, personality disorders).

✔ Is associated with an increased risk of suicide and the eventual development of MDD or bipolar II disorder.

Epidemiology

➤ Lifetime prevalence is ~3%–5%. The disorder is more frequent in females (2:1).

Etiology

➤ The etiology of dysthymic disorder is poorly understood. Proposed risk factors include:

✔ Deficits in personality development.

✔ A family history of mood disorders, especially bipolar disorder.

Treatment Guidelines

➤ Aggressive treatment is warranted because of the considerable morbidity associated with the disorder.

➤ Dysthymic disorder has not been studied to the same degree as MDD:

✔ Classically, long-term psychotherapy (e.g., psychodynamic, insight-oriented) was considered the treatment of choice.

✔ More recent recommendations are for a combination of psychotherapy and long-term use of antidepressants.

MANIC, HYPOMANIC, AND MIXED EPISODES

Manic Episode

DSM-IV-TR diagnostic criteria (summary):

➤ A distinct period of abnormally and persistently elevated, expansive, or irritable mood, lasting at least 1 week (or any duration if hospitalization is necessary).

➤ During the period of mood disturbance, three (or more) of the following symptoms have persisted (four if the mood is only irritable) and have been present to a significant degree:

✔ Inflated self-esteem or grandiosity (may reach delusional proportions).

✔ Decreased need for sleep.

✔ More talkative than usual or pressure to keep talking.

✔ Flight of ideas or subjective experience that thoughts are racing.

✔ Distractibility.

✔ Increase in goal-directed activity or psychomotor agitation.

✔ Excessive involvement in pleasurable activities that have a high potential for painful consequences (e.g., engaging in unrestrained buying sprees, sexual indiscretions, or foolish business investments).

➤ The symptoms do not meet the criteria for a mixed episode.

➤ The mood disturbance is sufficiently severe to cause marked impairment in occupational functioning or in usual social activities or relationships with others, or to necessitate hospitalization to prevent harm to self or others, or there are psychotic features.

➤ The symptoms are not due to the direct physiological effects of a substance (e.g., a drug of abuse, a medication, or other treatment) or a general medical condition (e.g., hyperthyroidism).

Clinical issues:

➤ Mood and affect are typically euphoric or expansive but can quickly become labile, irritable, or angry. The potential for a sudden onset of threatening or assaultive behavior during a manic episode is high, and caution is always advised.

➤ Although not required to make the diagnosis:

✔ Depressive episodes may follow manic episodes. Although it may seem obvious, a manic episode is required for the diagnosis. Therefore, if the first few mood episodes are depressed, a diagnosis of MDD is appropriate until the first manic episode occurs, at which time the diagnosis is changed to and remains bipolar disorder. Therefore, the statement that the majority of bipolar patients are "misdiagnosed" for 7–10 years is not correct if a manic episode has never occurred. Actually, they are "delayed" in the assessment of their correct diagnosis of bipolar disorder.

✔ Psychotic features (e.g., delusions, hallucinations, disorganization) are present in 75% of individuals during a manic episode. Delusional themes usually include having great wealth, abilities, or powers.

➤ Speech is often loud, rapid, difficult to interpret, and difficult to interrupt, possibly with jokes, puns, or a play on words. The person may become theatrical, with singing or clang associations, resulting in an entertaining quality to the interview (while assaultive potential continues). In grossly psychotic states, speech can be incoherent.

➤ Thought content includes themes of self-confidence, possibly leading to tangentiality, flight of ideas, or looseness of associations (disorganization). Flight of ideas is the characteristic classic presentation of a manic episode but is not specific to bipolar disorder.

➤ Occupational and social dysfunction are often marked.

➤ Activity level is dramatically increased. Findings include diminished need for sleep, heightened arousal, impulsivity, impaired judgment (e.g., sexual indiscretions, stealing, increased spending), poor reliability, and lying/deceitfulness.

➤ The person often does not recognize or acknowledge that he or she is experiencing a manic episode (i.e., poor insight). Denial of illness is a common characteristic of the disorder and an important clinical manifestation of a manic episode.

➤ Hospitalization is often necessary for stabilization of a manic episode.

➤ A manic episode occurring as a consequence of a somatic treatment for depression (e.g., antidepressants, light therapy, ECT), the use of an illicit substance, or a medical illness does not lead to a diagnosis of bipolar disorder. The correct diagnosis may be either substance-induced mood disorder with manic features or mood disorder due to a general medical condition with manic features.

➤ The DSM-IV-TR definition of a manic episode is representative of "classic euphoric mania" but not of a mixed episode or a manic episode with rapid cycling.

Hypomanic Episode

DSM-IV-TR diagnostic criteria (summary):

➤ A distinct period of persistently elevated, expansive, or irritable mood, lasting throughout at least 4 days, that is clearly different from the usual nondepressed mood.

➤ During the period of the mood disturbance, three (or more) of the following symptoms have persisted:

✔ Inflated self-esteem or grandiosity.

✔ Decreased need for sleep (e.g., feels rested after only 3 hours of sleep).

✔ More talkative than usual or pressure to keep talking.

✔ Flight of ideas or subjective experience that thoughts are racing, distractibility (i.e., attention too easily drawn to unimportant or irrelevant external stimuli).

✔ Increase in goal-directed activity (either socially, at work or school, or sexually) or psychomotor agitation.

✔ Excessive involvement in pleasurable activities that have a high potential for painful consequences (e.g., engaging in unrestrained buying sprees, sexual indiscretions, or foolish business investments).

➤ The episode is associated with an unequivocal change in functioning that is uncharacteristic of the person when not symptomatic.

➤ The disturbance in mood and the change in functioning are observable by others.

➤ The episode is not severe enough to cause marked impairment in social or occupational functioning or to necessitate hospitalization, and there are no psychotic features.

➤ The symptoms are not due to the direct physiological effects of a substance (e.g., a drug of abuse, a medication, or other treatment) or a general medical condition (e.g., hyperthyroidism).

Clinical issues:

➤ A hypomanic episode:

✔ Presents with less-intense highs than does a manic episode.

✔ Is not associated with psychotic symptoms or a need for hospitalization.

✔ Is not diagnosed if the hypomania is secondary to the direct physiological effects of a medical illness or the use of a substance.

✔ May not be overly impairing in terms of level of functioning. Hypomania differs from most other psychiatric disorders in that functional impairment is not a requirement.

Mixed Episode

DSM-IV-TR diagnostic criteria (summary):

➤ The criteria are met for both a manic episode and an MDE (except for duration) nearly every day during at least a 1-week period.

➤ The mood disturbance is sufficiently severe to cause marked impairment in occupational functioning or in usual social activities or relationships with others, or to necessitate hospitalization to prevent harm to self or others, or there are psychotic symptoms.

➤ The symptoms are not due to the direct physiological effects of a substance (e.g., a drug of abuse, a medication, or other treatment) or a general medical condition (e.g., hyperthyroidism).

Clinical issues:

➤ Mixed episodes involve relatively rapid shifts between mania and depression experienced daily for at least 1 week. Although not clearly defined by

DSM-IV-TR, mania and depression can occur together ("depressive symptoms in the midst of mania").

➤ Mixed episodes are typically severe, impairing, and more treatment resistant than classic euphoric mania. Psychotic features and suicidal ideation are common, often necessitating hospitalization.

➤ Forty percent of manic episodes present with mixed features and are often followed by a depressive episode.

BIPOLAR I DISORDER, BIPOLAR II DISORDER, AND CYCLOTHYMIC DISORDER

Bipolar I Disorder

Diagnostic considerations:

➤ Basic diagnostic requirements are for the presence of at least one manic or mixed episode not accounted for by the effects of a substance or a medical illness:

✔ Depressive episodes commonly occur but are not required for the diagnosis.

✔ If only a single manic or mixed episode has developed, the diagnosis is *bipolar disorder, single manic (or mixed) episode.*

✔ If this episode is a recurrence of a manic (or mixed) episode, the diagnosis is *bipolar disorder, most recent episode manic (or mixed).*

Clinical issues:

➤ A history of a single manic (or mixed) episode distinguishes bipolar disorder from MDD, bipolar II disorder, and cyclothymic disorder.

➤ Historically, a classic distinction between schizophrenia and bipolar disorder was that interepisode functioning is "normal" in bipolar disorder but downwardly dysfunctional in schizophrenia. However, most bipolar patients have a depressive interepisode course with poor functioning rather than a euthymic interepisode course with good functioning.

➤ Bipolar I disorder is an episodic, incurable illness with a variable course and variable outcome. Even with treatment, outcomes can be poor, with high rates of relapse, persistence of residual symptoms after an acute manic or depressive episode, increased potential for cognitive loss, marked functional and psychosocial impairment, and high rates of suicide.

➤ Considerations:

  ✔ Substance abuse is very common (as high as 70%).

  ✔ With increasing age, the frequency and intensity of episodes tend to increase while the length of an episode tends to stay relatively constant.

  ✔ Although somewhat variable, depressive episodes are more common in the spring and fall, and manic episodes are more common in the summer.

  ✔ Interepisode moods are more likely depressed than euthymic by a ratio of 3:1.

  ✔ Manic, mixed, or depressive episodes can follow a seasonal pattern.

  ✔ There is a strong genetic component to the transmission of the disorder. The risk of developing bipolar I disorder is highly associated with the presence of a mood disorder in one or both parents (27% chance with one afflicted parent, 50%–75% chance with two afflicted parents).

➤ Children and adolescents with ADHD, adjustment disorder, oppositional defiant disorder, or conduct disorder and adults with antisocial or borderline personality traits or disorder may actually be showing signs of bipolar disorder.

➤ An earlier age of onset of the first bipolar episode correlates with increased chronicity and overall greater functional impairment.

➤ Onset of a manic episode is typically rapid (hours or days). Untreated, a manic episode typically lasts 3–4 months and a bipolar depressive episode typically lasts 6–9 months.

➤ Untreated, the average length of time between the first and second bipolar episodes is 5 years. After four or more episodes, the symptom-free interval is about 1 year.

➤ Sleep and mood charting can be extremely helpful in detecting an impending bipolar episode. A pattern of decreased need for sleep is highly predictive of an impending manic episode.

➤ Some physicians look for the "rule of 3" to help uncover bipolar disorder. Some examples include 3 marriages before 30 years of age, failure of 3 different antidepressants, 3 different careers by age 30 years, 3 first-degree relatives with a mood disorder, and 3 consecutive generations with a mood disorder.

➤ Prognosis is poorer for persons with:

  ✔ A rapid-cycling pattern or mixed episodes.

  ✔ A severe index episode.

  ✔ Active substance abuse.

  ✔ Psychotic symptoms during the manic episode or severe depressive episodes.

  ✔ Male gender.

✔ A younger age at initial onset.

✔ Increasing frequency of bipolar episodes.

✔ Low occupational status.

➤ Suicide attempts and completed suicides are a prominent risk, typically being greatest during a depressive period, especially if accompanied by psychotic symptoms.

➤ Always rule out secondary causes of mania before making a diagnosis of bipolar disorder. Some examples include:

✔ Medications (e.g., corticosteroids, methylphenidate, thyroid medications).

✔ Drugs (e.g., methamphetamine, cocaine).

✔ Endocrine disorders (e.g., hyperthyroidism, Cushing's disease).

✔ Neurological disorders (e.g., head injury, neoplasms, cerebral vascular accident).

✔ Infections (e.g., meningitis, HIV/AIDS, neurosyphilis).

Bipolar II Disorder

Diagnostic considerations:

➤ Basic diagnostic requirements are for the presence of at least one hypomanic episode, but without a history of a manic or mixed episode, and the presence of one or more MDEs. Mood episodes cannot be secondary to another psychiatric illness, a medical illness, a medication, or a substance of abuse. The symptoms must cause clinically significant distress or impairment in social, occupational, or other important areas of functioning.

Clinical issues:

➤ The presence or history of a single manic or mixed episode precludes the diagnosis of bipolar II disorder.

➤ Unlike bipolar I disorder, bipolar II disorder requires at least one depressive episode.

➤ Onset is usually in the late teens or early 20s.

➤ Psychotic symptoms during depressive episodes are less common than in bipolar I disorder.

➤ Marked changes in sleep–wake cycles (e.g., east-to-west travel across multiple time zones, sleep deprivation) can precipitate hypomanic or depressive episodes.

➤ Reverse vegetative symptoms (e.g., excessive sleeping and eating) are often characteristic of depression associated with bipolar II disorder.

➤ Individuals with bipolar II disorder:

✔ Often benefit from the hypomania, with achievements and artistic accomplishments.

✔ Are much more often depressed than hypomanic (by a ratio of 37 to 1).

✔ Likely have a genetic predisposition toward developing the disorder.

✔ Have significant morbidity associated with the disorder (most often during depressive episodes).

✔ Commonly abuse substances.

✔ Often have significant symptom overlap with narcissistic, histrionic, and borderline personality disorders. It may be difficult to determine whether bipolar II or a personality disorder is the correct diagnosis.

✔ Are as likely to commit suicide as are those with bipolar I disorder.

➤ By DSM-IV-TR criteria, a hypomanic episode does not cause significant functional impairment, whereas bipolar II disorder does cause significant functional impairment.

➤ Treatment guidelines are not clearly defined. Guidelines for use of mood stabilizers and augmenting, combining, and switching strategies are often empirically derived and based on the treatment strategies of bipolar I disorder.

Cyclothymic Disorder

Diagnostic considerations:

➤ Basic diagnostic requirements are for numerous periods of hypomanic symptoms (but never a manic or a mixed episode) and depressive symptoms (but never an MDE) over a 2-year period. Mood episodes cannot be secondary to another psychiatric illness, a medical illness, a medication, or a substance of abuse. The symptoms must cause clinically significant distress or impairment in social, occupational, or other important areas of functioning.

Clinical issues:

➤ Cyclothymic disorder is often characterized by alternating cycles of subsyndromal depression and subsyndromal hypomania.

➤ Almost all persons with cyclothymic disorder also have periods of mixed symptoms (i.e., both subsyndromal hypomanic and subsyndromal depressed symptoms concurrently) with irritability, moodiness, or negativism. However, about 50% of persons have depressive symptoms as the major presentation. Individuals are often unproductive, with quick mood shifts, often within hours. Patients often feel that their moods are out of their control.

➤ Patients are more often depressed than hypomanic (as with bipolar I and bipolar II disorders).

➤ By definition, the disorder must cause significant functional impairment.

➤ Substance abuse is a common feature.

➤ It may be especially difficult to distinguish between cyclothymic disorder and narcissistic, histrionic, and borderline personality disorders because of symptom overlap.

➤ There is an increased risk for progression to bipolar disorder.

➤ Treatment guidelines are not clearly defined and are empirically derived utilizing the treatment guideline formulated for bipolar disorders:

✔ Mood stabilizers (e.g., lithium, divalproex) can be effective.

✔ Antidepressants are usually avoided secondary to concerns about an inadvertent switch to a hypomanic or manic episode.

✔ Psychotherapy (individual, group) and self-help groups can be beneficial.

Epidemiology of Bipolar I, Bipolar II, and Cyclothymic Disorders

Lifetime prevalence:

➤ Bipolar spectrum disorders (see section later in this chapter): found in about 2%–7% of the general population.

➤ Bipolar I disorder—found in ~1% of the general population; equally prominent in males and females.

➤ Bipolar II disorder—found in ~0.3%–2.0% of the general population, more prominent in females than males by a ratio of 3 to 1.

➤ Cyclothymic disorder—0.4%–1% of the population; equally prominent in males and females.

Age:

➤ Bipolar disorder is observed in children and adolescents but may be misdiagnosed as (or comorbid with) ADHD, oppositional defiant disorder, conduct disorder, or developing antisocial personality disorder.

➤ The first episode of bipolar I disorder typically occurs between 20 and 25 years of age, although mood symptoms may have been present for years.

➤ An earlier age at onset is associated with more frequent psychotic events (possibly leading to an inaccurate diagnosis of schizophrenia).

➤ Typically, an individual with bipolar disorder will have seen three or four physicians over 8–10 years before bipolar disorder is recognized.

Patterns:

➤ "Classic euphoria": found in about 15% of persons with bipolar I disorder; equally prominent in females and males.

➤ Mixed episodes: found in about 40% of persons with bipolar I disorder; more frequent in females.

➤ Rapid cycling: found in approximately 15%–20% of persons with bipolar I disorder. More frequent in bipolar II disorder and in females.

➤ Ultra-rapid cycling: rapid mood shifts, perhaps daily or several times daily.

Etiology and Risk Factors for Bipolar I, Bipolar II, and Cyclothymic Disorders

➤ There is strong evidence for genetic transmission of bipolar disorder:

✔ Preliminary findings are suggestive of a "susceptibility" bipolar gene located on or near chromosomes 1, 6, 10, 18, and 21.

✔ The risk of developing bipolar disorder increases with closer genetic ties to relatives with a history of a mood disorder (e.g., there is a 70% concordance of bipolar disorder in monozygotic twins).

➤ Alcohol dependence has been associated with an increased risk of manic episodes.

➤ Bipolar disorder is likely a manifestation of monoamine neurotransmitter (i.e., 5-HT, NE, DA) and/or glutamate dysregulation.

➤ The postpartum period (especially in mothers with a history of bipolar disorder) is a risk factor for a manic or a bipolar depressive episode.

➤ ADHD is a risk factor for bipolar disorder and is often comorbid with bipolar disorder. Classically, ADHD can be differentiated from bipolar disorder in that ADHD does not have a mood component and is not associated with psychosis.

➤ There is increasing evidence for neuroanatomic and functional brain changes in bipolar disorder:

✔ MRI demonstrates subtle neuroanatomic changes (e.g., increased subcortical white matter hyperintensities, increased lateral ventricle size, decreased cellebellar size, amygdalar changes).

✔ PET and functional magnetic resonance imaging (fMRI) demonstrate functional changes (e.g., prefrontal cortex abnormalities).

Psychiatric Disorders Commonly Comorbid With Bipolar I, Bipolar II, and Cyclothymic Disorders

Substance use disorders:

➤ The extent of substance abuse in all types of bipolar disorder is extremely high:

✔ Comorbidity with substance abuse is ~50%–70%, and abuse of more than one substance is common. Substance abuse is highest in bipolar I disorder, followed by bipolar II disorder and then cyclothymic disorder.

✔ Comorbid substance abuse is associated with an increased risk of suicide and an overall poorer prognosis.

Personality disorders:

➤ Personality disorders (especially antisocial, histrionic, and borderline) are frequently comorbid with or misidentified as bipolar II disorder.

Rating Scales for Bipolar I, Bipolar II, and Cyclothymic Disorders

➤ There are a multitude of rating scales, ranging from use for research purposes to self-rating scales. Some of the more popular scales are:

✔ Young Mania Rating Scale (YMRS)—11 questions with higher scores indicative of greater illness severity; widely used in research settings.

✔ Bipolar Spectrum Diagnostic Scale (BSDS)—A self-rating scale in which a story is assessed as to how closely it represents the individual.

✔ Mood Disorder Questionnaire (MDQ)—Yes/No questions to uncover a history of manic episodes.

✔ Mood/sleep charts—Patients chart their moods/sleep patterns over time to uncover trends.

BIPOLAR DEPRESSION AND RAPID CYCLING

Bipolar Depression

Diagnostic considerations:

➤ DSM-IV-TR does not provide a separate categorization or specific definition for bipolar depression, but rather classifies bipolar depressive episodes using the same diagnostic criteria as for MDD (i.e., unipolar depression). However:

✔ Bipolar depressive episodes are likely genetically distinct from unipolar depressive episodes. Therefore, the treatment of bipolar depression is not simply an extension of the usual treatments for unipolar depression.

✔ Depression, when part of bipolar disorder, should be considered as a phase of a lifelong, chronic illness.

✔ Distinguishing between unipolar and bipolar depression when there is a question of a history of manic, mixed, or hypomanic episode(s) is truly a diagnostic challenge, even for experienced clinicians. No single symptom distinguishes bipolar depression from unipolar depression. In comparison with individuals with unipolar depression, individuals with bipolar depression are more likely to:

■ Present with a greater severity of depressive symptoms (described as "rock bottom depression").

■ Have greater functional impairment.

- Have a more rapid onset of symptoms.
- Have a greater likelihood of presenting with psychotic features.
- Initially present with depression at an earlier age.
- Develop an MDE without an obvious stressor.
- Switch to an agitated hypomanic or manic state when treated with an antidepressant or ECT, or fail to respond to multiple trials of antidepressants.
- Present with comorbid substance abuse disorders.
- Have more frequent depressive episodes.
- Present with melancholic features (found in approximately 67% of bipolar depressed patients).
- Have reverse vegetative symptoms (bipolar II disorder).
- Make more frequent suicide attempts and have higher rates of completed suicide:
  - The suicide rate in bipolar disorder is ~15 times greater than in the general population.
  - Suicide occurs most often during depressive episodes (approximately 60%–90% of completed suicides).

Clinical issues:

➤ Persons with bipolar disorder can experience multiple recurrent depressive episodes before experiencing the first manic, mixed, or hypomanic episode. Because mania and hypomania are unlikely to be recalled by the patient as problematic, a screening tool (e.g., Mood Disorder Questionnaire) can be extremely useful to uncover bipolar disorder in patients with a reportable history of recurrent depressions but without a reportable history of manic, mixed, or hypomanic episodes.

➤ Patients are much less likely to seek or accept treatment for manic or hypomanic episodes than for episodes of bipolar depression.

➤ Interepisode periods are often punctuated with depression and poor functioning rather than euthymia.

➤ Overall, about 75% of individuals initially present with a bipolar depressive episode. A diagnosis of bipolar disorder cannot be made until there is a manic, mixed, or hypomanic episode.

Rapid Cycling ("Cycle Acceleration")

Diagnostic considerations:

➤ Rapid cycling requires at least four mood episodes over the previous 12 months. Episodes can be all of one polarity or shifts between polarities. The pattern is rarely consistent or predictable and is most often seen in bipolar II disorder (where the predominant mood is depressed).

➤ Clinically, mood shifts can be very frequent, at times occurring several times daily.

➤ Rapid cycling presents with more frequent depressive than manic episodes, more frequent time spent in an acute mood episode, and a greater likelihood of suicide.

➤ Risk factors for rapid cycling include prolonged use of antidepressants without concurrent treatment with a mood stabilizer (controversial), female gender, and clinical or subclinical hypothyroidism.

➤ Rapid cycling is a specifier applicable to bipolar I and II disorders, not a separate disorder (e.g., *bipolar I disorder with a rapid-cycling pattern*).

ASSESSMENT, WORKUP, AND TREATMENT OF BIPOLAR DISORDER

Evaluation and Assessment

➤ Medication management, either as an outpatient or an inpatient, is the cornerstone for the effective management of bipolar disorder.

➤ Consider hospitalization for:

✔ Diagnostic evaluation, especially if the patient is experiencing a first manic or psychotic episode. Assess for medical and substance-induced causes of mania or depression.

✔ Mood stabilization (either manic or depressed), especially when accompanied by dangerousness, poor self-care, complicated physical or psychiatric problems, or concomitant substance abuse.

➤ Obtain appropriate chemistries, depending on the clinical findings and situation (e.g., drug screen, digoxin level, thyroid panel, liver function tests, head CT/MRI).

Overview of Medications Used to Treat Bipolar Disorder

➤ Technically, a mood stabilizer effectively treats manic, mixed, and depressive bipolar episodes and protects against their recurrence (i.e., provides maintenance treatment; prophylaxis). Under this strict definition, no single FDA-approved medication meets all of these criteria, although lithium, olanzapine, and quetiapine come closest to satisfying this definition.

➤ Mood-stabilizing agents (as opposed to antidepressant medications or psychotherapy) are the treatment of choice for all phases of bipolar disorder.

➤ *Maintenance treatment* implies continual and indefinite treatment.

➤ FDA-approved mood-stabilizing agents are lithium, divalproex (Depakote), valproic acid (Depakene), carbamazepine extended release (Equetro), olanzapine (Zyprexa), olanzapine + fluoxetine (Symbyax), risperidone (Risperdal), quetiapine (Seroquel), aripiprazole (Abilify), ziprasidone (Geodon), and lamotrigine (Lamictal).

➤ Antiepileptic medications (AEDs), as a class effect, appear to increase the risk of suicidal ideation and suicidal behavior. Advisory warnings by the FDA may be forthcoming. AEDs are widely used as mood-stabilizing agents.

➤ Many other medications are commonly used off-label, including many that have generally *failed* to consistently demonstrate efficacy in clinical trials (designated with an asterisk [*]):

✔ Antiseizure medications:

■ Carbamazepine immediate release (Tegretol).

■ Oxcarbazepine (Trileptal; a keto-congener of carbamazepine).

■ Tiagabine* (Gabitril).

■ Topiramate* (Topamax).

■ Gabapentin* (Neurontin).

■ Levetiracetam (Keppra).

✔ Second-generation antipsychotic medications (SGAs) other than those that are FDA approved:

■ Clozapine (Clozaril).

✔ Anxiolytics (benzodiazepines)—provide short-term calming effects, but do not have proven antimanic properties for long-term usage.

✔ Antidepressants:

■ Despite warnings to the contrary, antidepressants are at times used without a mood stabilizer to treat the depressive and maintenance phases of bipolar disorder.

➤ Table 2–7 lists medications used in the treatment of bipolar disorder.

Mood-Stabilizing Medications

Lithium (carbonate immediate release; citrate immediate release; carbonate sustained release):

General considerations:

➤ Clinically available since 1970, lithium is considered "the standard therapy for euphoric mania" and "the gold standard for the treatment of bipolar disorder."

➤ Lithium is considered less effective for mixed states ("dysphoric mania") and for rapid cycling than for classic euphoric mania.

➤ Lithium has proven antisuicidal properties, yet in overdose can be lethal.

■ **Table 2–7   FDA-approved medication for the treatment of bipolar disorder**

	Approved for acute mania	Approved for mixed states	Approved for bipolar depression	Approved for the maintenance phase of bipolar disorder
Lithium	Yes	No	No	Yes
Divalproex (Depakote)	Yes	Yes	No	No
Valproic acid (Depakene)	Yes	Yes	No	No
Olanzapine (Zyprexa)	Yes	Yes	No	Yes
Risperidone (Risperdal)	Yes	Yes	No	No
Quetiapine (Seroquel)	Yes	No	Yes	No
Ziprasidone (Geodon)	Yes	Yes	No	No
Aripiprazole (Abilify)	Yes	Yes	No	Yes
Chlorpromazine (Thorazine)	Yes	No	No	No
Carbamazepine extended release (Equetro)	Yes	Yes	No	No
Lamotrigine (Lamictal)	No	No	No	Yes
Olanzapine + fluoxetine (Symbyax)	No	No	Yes	No
Topiramate (Topamax), carbamazepine (Tegretol), oxcarbazepine (Trileptal), gabapentin (Neurontin), tiagabine (Gabitril), verapamil (Calan), omega-3 fatty acids	None	None	None	None

Note.   FDA = U.S. Food and Drug Administration.

➤ Compliance is generally poor due to a broad range of adverse side effects, including mental sluggishness, tremor, polyuria, polydipsia, nausea/vomiting/diarrhea, acne, edema, metallic taste to foods, and weight gain. Tolerability may be improved by:

✔ Initiating treatment at a lower dose (if clinically appropriate), with gradual dosage increases.

✔ Using a sustained-release or liquid formulation.

✔ Using a single nighttime dose decreases polyuria, but may have an adverse long-term impact on renal functioning.

Proposed mechanism(s) of action:

➤ Lithium inhibits the enzyme glycogen synthase kinase-3 (GSK-3). This pathway is perhaps the most studied and is felt to be responsible for the neuroprotective features of lithium.

➤ Lithium lowers the elevated excitatory neurotransmitter glutamate level at the synapse in bipolar mania and raises the lowered glutamate level at the synapse in bipolar depression.

➤ Lithium increases NE and 5-HT activity, which may help explain its antidepressant effects.

➤ Lithium regulates the protein kinase C signaling cascade by inhibiting recycling of inositol.

FDA-approved indications (indicated with an asterisk [*])
and purported non-FDA-approved uses:

➤ Acute bipolar mania*:

✔ Lithium is most effective for patients presenting with:

■ Classic euphoric mania (absence of mixed episodes, absence of rapid cycling).

■ Fewer than three previous bipolar episodes. Effectiveness decreases as the number of mood episodes increases.

■ Prior positive response to lithium.

■ Good interepisode functioning and euthymia between episodes.

■ Absence of neurological impairment, psychotic symptoms, and active substance abuse.

■ Sustained higher plasma lithium levels.

✔ Under these ideal conditions, lithium is effective in ~80% of patients.

✔ Lithium is slow working, requiring 10–14 days to stabilize a manic episode. An antipsychotic medication and/or a benzodiazepine can be helpful until lithium becomes effective.

✔ Augmentation of lithium with another mood stabilizer, a benzodiazepine, or an antipsychotic medication can be an effective strategy. There is a general consensus that antidepressants are not an appropriate choice.

✔ Olanzapine + lithium, risperidone + lithium, and quetiapine + lithium are FDA approved for the treatment of manic episodes associated with bipolar disorder. Cotherapy appears to be more effective than lithium monotherapy but additive side effects may compromise compliance.

➤ Maintenance treatment of bipolar disorder*:

✔ Lithium has proven efficacy for preventing relapses into mania or bipolar depression.

➤ Bipolar depression:

✔ Lithium is effective as a monotherapy in 60%–70% of depressed bipolar patients, although:

■ It is not FDA approved for this indication.

■ Six to 8 weeks may be required for lithium to become optimally effective.

■ Higher lithium levels than used to treat mania may be needed.

■ Combining lithium with lamotrigine, olanzapine, or quetiapine would seem to be logical choices for combining mood stabilizers that also have proven effectiveness for bipolar depression.

■ Augmentation of lithium with liothyronine (T_3) can improve effectiveness.

➤ MDD:

✔ Lithium has limited usefulness as a monotherapy for the acute management of MDD.

✔ The chief indications for lithium in MDD are to augment antidepressants for treatment-resistant depression and (new finding) for maintenance treatment of MDD.

➤ Schizophrenia and schizoaffective disorder: lithium can be helpful when combined with an antipsychotic medication, but is not effective as a monotherapy.

➤ Bipolar II disorder and cyclothymic disorder (one of the few antimanic medications studied for this disorder).

➤ Mania due to physical disorders or substances: Lithium is less likely to be effective than carbamazepine ER, divalproex, olanzapine, risperidone, quetiapine, aripiprazole, or ziprasidone.

➤ Borderline personality disorder and other "emotionally unstable" personality disorders (short-term use for exacerbations).

➤ Impulse-control disorders: Lithium can help reduce aggressiveness. Other useful agents include carbamazepine, divalproex, antipsychotic medications, and beta-blockers.

➤ Premenstrual syndrome when associated with cyclic periods of depression.

Treatment considerations:

➤ A workup prior to initiating lithium therapy should include medical/psychiatric history, physical examination, routine blood and urine chemistries, CBC with differential, ECG if the patient is older than 40 years or has a history of heart disease, thyroid panel with TSH, blood urea nitrogen, serum creatinine, and a pregnancy test (if applicable).

➤ Lithium:

✔ Can adversely affect the brain (neurotoxic in overdose), kidney (impaired concentration ability, potentially nephrotoxic), thyroid (hypothyroidism, goiter), hematopoietic system (benign increases in leukocyte production), and heart (impairs sinus node functioning, potentially leading to heart block).

✔ When discontinued or used in a stop-and-start fashion can lead to high relapse rates. Each bipolar episode further increases the risk for relapse and the potential for decreasing effectiveness of lithium.

Pharmacokinetics and dosing:

➤ Pharmacokinetics:

✔ Plasma level peaks 0.5–4.0 hours after dosing with the immediate-release formulation, possibly with transient gastrointestinal upset, fine hand tremor, and lethargy.

✔ Lithium does not bind to serum proteins.

✔ Elimination is principally by renal excretion of unchanged lithium. Changes in hydration or renal excretion of sodium and potassium can have a marked impact on lithium plasma levels:

■ Dehydration, sodium depletion, coadministration with non-potassium-sparing diuretics (e.g., thiazides, furosemide), renal insufficiency (e.g., caution for use in the elderly), and the puerperium (time period immediately after birth) can result in elevated and possibly toxic lithium levels.

■ Excessive dietary sodium and pregnancy can result in significantly reduced and possibly subtherapeutic lithium levels (due to increased renal clearance).

✔ The elimination half-life of lithium averages 20–24 hours, with plasma level equilibration in 5–7 days. Check the plasma level within 3–7 days of initiating or changing the dose. The plasma level is taken 12 hours after the last dose but before the next dose is due.

✔ Therapeutic plasma level range is 0.6–1.2 mEq/L for acute mania and 0.7–1.0 mEq/L for maintenance therapy. A general consensus is that higher lithium levels are more protective against relapses at the expense of greater side effects.

➤ Considerations for use:

✔ Initiate dosing of the immediate or sustained release formulations with 300 mg tid or 450 mg bid, and titrate upward utilizing lithium plasma levels as a guide.

✔ Sustained release preparations provide for a more constant lithium plasma level than the immediate release formulation but may actually increase the potential for polyuria.

✔ Lithium can be combined with other mood stabilizers, antidepressants (e.g., for refractory MDD), antipsychotic medications, thyroid medications, and benzodiazepines.

Side-effect and safety considerations:

➤ General considerations:

✔ Lithium has the narrowest ratios of toxic-to-therapeutic plasma levels of all psychotropic medications (TCAs are next in line).

➤ Frequently cited side effects:

✔ Thyroid:

■ Hypothyroidism occurs in 5%–35% of lithium users, is more frequent in women, typically develops 6–18 months after starting lithium, can be diagnosed by an elevated TSH level, and is reversible by stopping lithium. Treatments include changing medications or adding a thyroid medication.

■ Diffuse nontoxic goiter with or without hypothyroidism (reversible by stopping lithium).

✔ Renal:

■ Renal insufficiency:

● Most often develops in patients on long-term lithium therapy. Changes include interstitial fibrosis, tubular atrophy, and glomerular sclerosis, possibly reflected by increased serum creatinine.

■ Decreased urine-concentrating ability, resulting in:

● Polyuria (excessive urination) with accompanying polydipsia (excessive thirst), secondary to the antagonism of antidiuretic hormone. Can be especially problematic at night.

● Nephrogenic diabetes insipidus (i.e., "severe polyuria").

✔ Neurological (hand or finger fine tremor, often worsening with higher lithium levels). Switching from the immediate-release to the slow-release formulation can help. A coarse hand tremor is more likely indicative of lithium toxicity.

✔ Cardiac:

   ■ Benign electrocardiographic conduction changes resemble hypokale-mia, with T-wave flattening or inversion.

   ■ Arrhythmias and, rarely, sudden death have been reported in patients with preexisting cardiac disease.

   ■ Impaired sinus node function with potential heart block. Lithium should not be used in patients with sick sinus syndrome.

✔ Weight gain:

   ■ Altered carbohydrate metabolism leading to weight gain and fluid retention (peripheral edema). Weight gain can be substantial, is greater for patients with preexisting weight problems, and can be dif-ficult to manage even with exercise and diet control.

✔ Gastrointestinal:

   ■ Dyspepsia, nausea, vomiting, or diarrhea. These findings could be benign side effects of lithium or an early sign of lithium toxicity. Check the lithium level.

   ■ If symptoms are due to a lithium side effect and not to lithium toxicity, treat by giving lithium more often but at a lower dose, administering lithium with food, changing the lithium formulation, or switching to another mood stabilizer.

✔ Cognitive dulling (patients frequently complain of decreased creativity while taking lithium), impaired memory, lethargy, and sedation.

✔ Dermatological (acne, psoriatic skin changes, allergic skin rash, alope-cia).

✔ Metallic taste to foods.

✔ Benign leukocytosis.

➤ General strategies to reduce adverse side effects of lithium:

   ✔ Decrease the dosage (helps with many side effects but may decrease effectiveness).

   ✔ Administer the daily dose in smaller increments at more frequent inter-vals.

   ✔ Administer the entire daily dose at bedtime to reduce polyuria (contro-versial).

   ✔ Use a sustained-release preparation (decreases upper gastrointestinal cramping and nausea). However, lower–gastrointestinal system side effects (e.g., diarrhea) may then become problematic.

   ✔ Use lithium citrate liquid formulation (may reduce skin rash and gas-trointestinal side effects).

✔ Combine or augment lithium with another mood-stabilizing agent to allow for a reduction in the lithium dosage.

✔ Switch to another mood stabilizer.

Lithium toxicity:

➤ General considerations:

✔ Lithium and haloperidol can usually be safely used together. However, cases of an encephalopathic syndrome (characterized by symptoms similar to neuroleptic malignant syndrome) have rarely been reported and a warning about this risk appears in the product literature.

✔ Lithium has a very narrow therapeutic window, requiring careful detail to the emergence of side effects that may easily progress to toxicity.

✔ Lithium levels greater than 1.5 mEq/L are in the toxic range, and toxicity increases with increasing serum lithium levels. Lithium levels in the 2- to 3-mEq/L range can be lethal.

✔ If a dose of lithium is missed, doubling the next dose is *not* appropriate.

✔ Dehydration and lack of adequate sodium chloride are the most common causes for unintended rises in the lithium level.

➤ Signs and symptoms of lithium toxicity (nonexhaustive listing):

✔ Early signs can include nausea, vomiting, diarrhea (i.e., flulike symptoms), and a fine hand tremor. However, a fine hand tremor may also be evident at therapeutic serum levels.

✔ As serum levels increase, neurological findings can include a coarse hand tremor, nystagmus, increased deep tendon reflexes, ataxia, altered mental status, lethargy, blurred vision, and confusion. Cardiac arrhythmias, seizures, and coma can follow, and permanent neurological damage or death may result.

✔ Significant toxicity can result in death in 10%–15% of patients. Those who survive may have permanent neurological and/or renal damage.

✔ Treatment of toxicity may require management in a medical intensive care unit. Administration of polyethylene glycol (GoLYTELY) with gastric lavage/aspiration is recommended to reduce further lithium absorption. Hemodialysis, cardiac monitoring, treatment of arrhythmias, reduction of further lithium absorption, maintenance of hydration, and treatment of electrolyte imbalances are vital considerations.

Use in the elderly:

➤ The elderly are more sensitive to the side effects of lithium.

➤ A natural decrease in renal clearance with advancing age promotes higher blood levels in elderly than in younger individuals when both groups are administered the same dosage.

➤ Dehydration (more likely in the elderly) will promote higher lithium levels.

➤ The elderly are more likely to be on non-potassium-sparing diuretics, which can further increase the lithium level.

Use during pregnancy and lactation:

➤ Lithium is potentially teratogenic (pregnancy risk category D):

✔ The potential for teratogenicity is greatest during the first trimester of pregnancy but is present throughout pregnancy. Ebstein's anomaly (a severe and sometimes fatal malformation of the tricuspid valve that enters the right ventricle) is the most common finding. Recent studies give an incidence of 1 per 1,000, whereas older studies gave an incidence of 3%. A fetal echocardiogram between 16 and 18 weeks of gestation will normally demonstrate Ebstein's anomaly.

✔ The risk of relapse from stopping lithium must be weighed against the potential for teratogenicity. This issue must be discussed with the patient, who, if competent, should help decide on the course of treatment with the clinical information (risk–benefit considerations) provided by the psychiatrist. A consultation with a psychiatrist or treatment center with expertise in the use of medications in pregnancy is strongly recommended.

✔ Consider using antipsychotic medications (which appear to have a lower potential for teratogenic effects) or ECT during the first trimester of pregnancy as an alternative to lithium. Valproic acid and carbamazepine also carry significant risks to the developing fetus.

➤ Renal clearance of lithium increases during pregnancy, with a resulting decline in lithium levels. At birth, there is a rapid and precipitous rise in the maternal lithium level due to massive fluid loss. To avoid patient and neonatal toxicity, reduce the lithium dosage by 50% prior to delivery.

➤ Lithium toxicity in the newborn may cause flaccidity (e.g., floppy baby syndrome), lethargy, and decreased sucking reflex.

➤ Lithium is secreted in sufficient amounts into breast milk that patients taking lithium should not breast-feed (American Academy of Pediatrics). Newborns exposed to lithium during breast-feeding can develop lethargy, poor muscle tone, and electrocardiographic changes.

Valproic acid, sodium valproate, divalproex extended release, and divalproex sodium:

General considerations:

➤ Valproic acid and valproate salts are marketed for the treatment of mania as:

✔ A free acid—valproic acid (Depakene).

✔ A sodium salt—sodium valproate (Depakene syrup).

✔ A 1:1 mixture of the free acid and sodium salt—divalproex sodium (Depakote; also available as a "sprinkle" capsule and an extended release formulation [Depakote ER]).

➤ When referring to divalproex sodium ("divalproex"), equivalent therapeutic considerations are implied for valproic acid and sodium valproate. However, divalproex sodium has a lower propensity to cause the gastrointestinal side effects typically found with valproic acid (e.g., anorexia, nausea, vomiting, dyspepsia).

FDA-approved indications and off-label uses:

➤ Divalproex:

   ✔ Is FDA approved for the treatment of acute mania (effective for classic euphoric mania, mixed episodes, and rapid cycling), alone or in combination with olanzapine, risperidone, or quetiapine:

   ■ Depakote ER (extended release) is not FDA approved for the treatment of manic episodes of bipolar disorder.

   ■ Additional FDA approvals are for prophylaxis for migraine headaches and the treatment of simple and complex absence seizures.

   ✔ Is more effective than lithium for mixed episodes and for rapid cycling.

   ✔ Is also used (although not FDA approved) for the treatment of:

   ■ Maintenance phase of bipolar disorder (as effective as lithium).

   ■ Agitation, aggression, and behavioral dyscontrol.

   ■ Neuropathic pain syndromes.

   ■ Alcohol and benzodiazepine withdrawal syndromes.

   ■ PTSD.

   ■ Borderline personality disorder.

   ■ Schizophrenia (improves response when added to an antipsychotic medication; minimal value as a monotherapy).

   ■ MDD (maintenance phase).

   ■ MDD (augmenting agent to SSRIs).

Pharmacokinetics and dosing considerations:

➤ Divalproex:

   ✔ Acts more rapidly than lithium (3–5 days rather than 10–14 days).

   ✔ Achieves therapeutic effectiveness with serum levels between 50–120 µg/mL (as measured 12 hours after the last dose but before the next dose).

   ✔ Has a wider margin of safety than lithium although the effective serum level range is fairly narrow.

   ✔ Has no significant effects on renal or thyroid functioning.

Proposed mechanisms of action:

➤ The precise mechanism of action is not known; however, divalproex purportedly imparts its antimanic activity by one or more of the following mechanisms:

✔ Enhances 5-HT functioning.

✔ Augments the inhibitory effect of gamma-aminobutyric acid (GABA), thereby promoting GABAergic activity.

✔ Decreases the activity of glutamate on the N-methyl-D-aspartate (NMDA) receptor.

✔ Regulates protein kinase C signaling cascade (as with lithium).

✔ Blocks voltage-dependent sodium channels thereby inhibiting neuronal activity.

✔ Inhibits high-frequency repetitive action potentials.

Pretreatment workup:

➤ Workup should include a medical/psychiatric history, physical examination, routine chemistries, CBC with differential, platelet count, liver function tests, renal function tests, serum amylase, and pregnancy test (if applicable).

Dosage and monitoring:

➤ Initiate dosing of divalproex with 250 mg at 4 P.M. and 500 mg at bedtime, increasing the dose by 250–500 mg every 2–3 days, with the objective of attaining a therapeutic serum level of 50–120 µg/mL.

➤ Divalproex can also be dosed on a mg/kg basis. Usually start with 15 mg/kg/day administered bid, with a maximum dosage of 60 mg/kg/day.

➤ For inpatients, divalproex loading may be suitable, providing a rapid therapeutic onset comparable to olanzapine. A rough rule of thumb is to take the patient's weight in pounds and multiply by 10. This represents the approximate initial daily loading dose in mg. Alternatively, an initial loading dose of 20 mg/kg/day for 3 days can achieve a stable therapeutic serum level. Provide frequent plasma level checks (e.g., every 1–3 days) and careful dosage titration.

Side-effect and safety considerations:

➤ Common side effects:

✔ Gastrointestinal upset, sedation, increased appetite with significant weight gain, tremor, skin rash, cognitive dulling, hair brittleness, alopecia (try B-complex vitamins, zinc, or selenium), and benign leukopenia/thrombocytopenia.

➤ Serious or life-threatening side effects:

✔ Black box warnings for hepatic toxicity (possibly fatal), hemorrhagic pancreatitis, and teratogenicity. The risk of hepatic toxicity is greatest during the first 6 months of treatment and in children younger than 2 years of age.

✔ Platelet dysfunction, dose-related thrombocytopenia, and coagulopathies (prominent warning in the product monograph).

✔ Stevens-Johnson syndrome, toxic epidermal necrolysis, or erythema multiforme (both are life-threatening skin reactions).

✔ Agranulocytosis (prominent warning in the product monograph).

✔ Polycystic ovarian syndrome (PCOS) in patients with epilepsy (somewhat controversial). Divalproex may increase testosterone levels in teenage girls, which can lead to PCOS after long-term use. Symptoms include hirsutism, acne and alopecia, and irregular or absent menses. However, bipolar disorder may itself confer an increased risk of PCOS.

✔ Possibly fatal in overdose.

Combination and augmentation strategies:

➤ Divalproex can be combined with antidepressants, lithium, antipsychotic medications, and benzodiazepines. Divalproex is FDA approved for the treatment of manic episodes when combined with olanzapine, risperidone, and quetiapine.

Common drug interactions:

➤ The metabolism of divalproex is approximately 25% by CYP isoenzyme metabolism and approximately 75% by phase II metabolism (glucuronidation). Therefore, drug interactions involving the CYP isoenzyme systems have only a minor to moderate impact on overall divalproex metabolism:

✔ Phenobarbital, phenytoin, and carbamazepine can lower divalproex levels by CYP isoenzyme induction.

✔ Aspirin, fluoxetine, isoniazid, ibuprofen, erythromycin, and phenothiazines can raise divalproex levels by CYP isoenzyme inhibition.

➤ Divalproex is 90% protein bound and therefore can displace (and be displaced by) other strongly protein-bound medications (e.g., aspirin, carbamazepine, digoxin, warfarin), resulting in increased activity or toxicity of these displaced medications.

➤ Divalproex can significantly raise lamotrigine (Lamictal) levels secondary to enzyme inhibition. Reduce the lamotrigine dosage by approximately 50%.

Use during pregnancy and lactation:

➤ Divalproex is potentially teratogenic (pregnancy risk category D), with a 1%–2% incidence of neural tube defects (spina bifida). Craniofacial defects may also occur. The danger is greatest in the first trimester. Folic acid 0.4–1.0 mg/day can be protective. Serum alpha-fetoprotein levels and ultrasound can help detect spina bifida in utero.

➤ Divalproex is excreted in small but measurable amounts into breast milk. The benefits (protection from relapse in the mother) versus risks (e.g., potential for hepatic damage in the neonate) should be evaluated on an individual basis.

Lamotrigine (Lamictal):

➤ Lamotrigine is FDA approved for the maintenance phase of bipolar disorder and is effective, but not FDA approved, for bipolar depression. It is not considered to be as effective for manic or mixed episodes (somewhat controversial).

➤ Purported mechanisms of action are inhibition of glutamate at the NMDA receptor site and/or inhibition of voltage-sensitive sodium channels.

➤ The usual dosage range is 100–400 mg/day administered in two divided doses starting with 25 mg once or twice daily and titrating slowly upward (50 mg dosage change per week) as clinically warranted. Monotherapy dosages higher than 200 mg/day are not recommended.

➤ Blood level monitoring is not required, and maintenance therapy can often be accomplished with once-daily dosing.

➤ The elimination half-life is approximately 24 hours via hepatic glucuronidation. Unlike divalproex (inhibitor of CYP isoenzymes) or carbamazepine (inducer of CYP isoenzymes), lamotrigine has no effect on CYP isoenzymes.

➤ Side effects include headache (the most commonly reported side effect) and an early-onset prominent skin rash (approximately 10% of patients), which can be minimized by a slow titration schedule. Headaches, muscle aches, dizziness, blurred vision, back pain, dry mouth, nausea, vomiting, and sedation can occur. Cognitive dulling at dosages greater than 200 mg/day is fairly common. Weight gain is unusual (as with carbamazepine).

➤ The most dangerous complications are "serious rashes" (e.g., Stevens-Johnson syndrome, toxic epidermal necrolysis), occurring at a rate of 1:1,000, which can be life-threatening. These serious rashes occur most often within the first 8 weeks of treatment and can be minimized (but not entirely avoided) by initiating treatment at a low dosage and titrating upward slowly. Discontinue lamotrigine and, unless absolutely necessary, do not rechallenge. Polypharmacy with valproic acid may increase the propensity of developing a serious rash.

➤ Carbamazepine induces (potentially reducing effectiveness) and divalproex inhibits (potentially increasing the risk of side effects or toxicity) the metabolism of lamotrigine. Dosage adjustments are therefore necessary (e.g., one-half the normal lamotrigine dosage should be used when combined with divalproex). Birth control pills may reduce lamotrigine levels.

➤ Lamotrigine is pregnancy risk category C and is associated with an approximately twofold increase in major congenital malformations, including cleft palate. Breast feeding is not recommended.

Carbamazepine extended release (Equetro):

General considerations:

➤ FDA approved only as the extended-release formulation (Equetro) for the treatment of manic and mixed episodes of bipolar I disorder.

➤ Other purported uses include reducing aggression, treating alcohol withdrawal syndromes, providing maintenance treatment for bipolar disorder, and treating depressive episodes.

➤ Prior to the introduction of the sustained release formulation, carbamazepine was used much less often than other mood stabilizers because of erratic oral absorption, a complex drug interaction profile, and an unfavorable side-effect profile. The newly approved Equetro is designed to improve the oral absorption pattern and to reduce some of the troubling side effects.

➤ Significant weight gain is unusual (as with lamotrigine).

Combination and augmentation strategies and concerns:

➤ Carbamazepine can be combined with antidepressants, lithium (anecdotal reports of increased neurotoxicity), antipsychotic medications, and benzodiazepines.

➤ Carbamazepine is highly protein bound and can displace other medications from protein binding sites, potentially leading to their toxicity (e.g., digoxin, warfarin).

➤ Structurally, carbamazepine is related to the TCAs. At least theoretically, serotonin syndrome can occur when carbamazepine is combined with TCAs or MAOIs.

➤ With the addition of an oxygen atom, carbamazepine becomes oxcarbazepine (Trileptal). Although not widely studied for the treatment of bipolar disorder, oxcarbazepine does not have carbamazepine's potential for agranulocytosis.

Potential drug interactions:

➤ Carbamazepine is a potent inducer of CYP P450 1A2 and 3A4 isoenzymes. As a consequence, blood levels of a wide number of medications are reduced, including some antipsychotic medications, TCAs, benzodiazepines, antiseizure medications (including itself), and estrogen in birth control pills. Unplanned pregnancies and subsequent fetal exposure to the teratogenic effects of carbamazepine are then possible. Carbamazepine is one of several antiepileptic medications that induce CYP isoenzymes. Other enzyme-inducing antiseizure medications commonly used in psychiatry include oxcarbazepine and topiramate (the three T's: Tegretol, Trileptal, Topamax).

➤ Contraindicated for use with MAOIs (because of the close structural similarity of carbamazepine to TCAs).

Side-effect and safety considerations:

➤ Common side effects include:

✔ Dermatitis (common finding).

✔ Nausea, vomiting, and diarrhea (an especially common complaint that is markedly improved with the extended-release formulation).

✔ Dizziness, acute confusional states, ataxia, and diplopia (all dose-dependent).

✔ Mild anticholinergic side effects due to the tricyclic structure.

✔ CNS depression, sedation (common), and cognitive impairment.

✔ Mild nonprogressive decreases in blood indices.

➤ Potentially serious or life-threatening side effects:

✔ Stevens-Johnson syndrome and toxic epidermal necrolysis especially during the first 2–8 weeks of treatment (recent advisory warning by the FDA). The likelihood of developing these disorders is greater in patients with allele *HLA-B*1502,* which is more common in Asian populations.

✔ Hepatitis or hepatic failure.

✔ Agranulocytosis or aplastic anemia (1 in 20,000; black box warning).

✔ Syndrome of inappropriate antidiuretic hormone (SIADH) due to vasopressin release.

Pretreatment workup:

➤ Workup prior to initiating carbamazepine therapy should include a medical/psychiatric history, a physical examination, routine chemistries, a CBC with differential, a platelet count, liver function tests, renal function tests, and a pregnancy test (if applicable).

Dosage and monitoring (Equetro):

➤ Initiate at a dose of 200 mg bid, increasing the dose 200 mg at weekly intervals until a plasma level of 6–12 μg/mL is achieved (measured 12 hours after the last dose and before the next dose is due). The usual dosage range is 800–1,200 mg/day. A favorite protocol is to try to achieve a dosage of 1,200 mg/day, which is likely at the high end of the therapeutic plasma level.

➤ Routinely monitor carbamazepine level, CBC, platelet count, liver function, and renal function.

➤ Carbamazepine induces its own metabolism (i.e., autoinduction), gradually resulting in a decrease in the carbamazepine serum level without a change in the dose. Dosage increases may eventually be needed.

Use during pregnancy and lactation:

➤ Carbamazepine is potentially teratogenic (pregnancy risk category D), with a 0.5%–1% incidence of spina bifida. Craniofacial defects and developmental delay in the neonate have also been reported. The danger is greatest during the first trimester of pregnancy. Serum alpha-fetoprotein levels and ultrasound can help detect spina bifida. Folic acid 0.4–1.0 mg/day is recommended if carbamazepine is used during pregnancy.

➤ Carbamazepine is excreted in small but measurable amounts into breast milk. The benefits (protection from relapse in the mother) versus risks (e.g., potential for hepatic damage in the neonate) should be considered on an individual basis.

Gabapentin (Neurontin):

➤ Is a selective GABA reuptake inhibitor (i.e., a GABAergic agent).

➤ Is FDA approved for the treatment of seizure disorders and postherpetic neuralgia. It is widely used off label for bipolar disorder, neuropathic pain and prophylaxis of migraine headaches, and nystagmus. Ninety percent of prescriptions for gabapentin are for off-label uses.

➤ Is typically dosed at 900–3,000 mg/day in two to three divided doses. Blood levels are not required.

➤ Is eliminated principally by renal excretion and thus, like lithium, does not share the CYP-related drug interactions of divalproex (inhibitor) and carbamazepine (inducer). Half-life is 5–7 hours. May be especially useful in patients with impaired hepatic functioning.

➤ Is not FDA approved for the treatment of bipolar disorder.

➤ Is not considered effective for the treatment of bipolar disorder (based on large-scale studies) but is widely used in clinical practice. However, some physicians feel that gabapentin is a very effective augmenting medication for the treatment of bipolar disorder.

➤ Has potential side effects of sedation (prominent), dizziness, and ataxia.

➤ Has few, if any:

✔ Drug interactions and is relatively safe in overdose.

✔ Hematological or hepatic side effects (unlike divalproex and carbamazepine).

➤ Is pregnancy risk category C.

Topiramate (Topamax):

➤ Is FDA approved for the treatment of seizure disorders and prophylaxis of migraine headaches.

➤ Is likely not as useful for the treatment of the manic phase of bipolar disorder as once thought (controversial).

➤ Is potentially helpful for comorbid conditions associated with bipolar disorder (e.g., anxiety disorders, eating disorders, impulse control disorders, substance use disorders). Not FDA approved for the treatment of bipolar disorder (or any other psychiatric disorder).

➤ Is typically dosed at 100–400 mg/day, administered in two divided doses, starting with 25 mg bid and slowly titrating upward as warranted.

➤ Potential side effects include anorexia with accompanying weight loss, nephrolithiasis, acute myopia, secondary angle-closure glaucoma, decreased sweating with a potential for hyperthermia, and metabolic acidosis.

➤ Can induce metabolism of estrogen in birth control pills (i.e., an enzyme inducer), possibly leading to menstrual irregularities and unplanned pregnancies.

➤ Is pregnancy risk category C.

Atypical Antipsychotic Medications

➤ Olanzapine (Zyprexa), risperidone (Risperdal), and quetiapine (Seroquel) are FDA approved for the treatment of mania and mixed episodes associated with bipolar disorder, alone or in combination with lithium or divalproex sodium.

➤ Ziprasidone (Geodon) and aripiprazole (Abilify) are FDA approved for the treatment of mania and mixed episodes associated with bipolar disorder.

➤ Olanzapine is FDA approved for the maintenance treatment of bipolar disorder and, when combined with fluoxetine (Symbyax), for the treatment of depression associated with bipolar disorder. Quetiapine is FDA approved for the treatment of depression associated with bipolar disorder. Aripiprazole is FDA approved for the maintenance treatment of bipolar disorder.

➤ As a group, atypical antipsychotic medications are gaining recognition and acceptance as effective mood stabilizers independent of their antipsychotic properties.

➤ Side effects of the atypical antipsychotic medications are covered in detail in Chapter 1 ("Schizophrenia and Other Psychotic Disorders").

➤ All FDA-approved, second-generation atypical antipsychotics for the treatment of bipolar disorder are pregnancy risk category C.

➤ Clozapine (pregnancy risk category B) is an effective mood stabilizer for manic episodes of bipolar I disorder, but it is not FDA approved.

Benzodiazepines

Clonazepam (Klonopin), lorazepam (Ativan), and others:

➤ Are most often used to augment other mood stabilizers for the treatment of bipolar disorder, providing a calming effect and helping with sleep.

➤ Are potentially abusable medications. Caution is advised for use in patients with a history of substance abuse or who are suspected of abusing substances (as are a high proportion of bipolar patients).

➤ Are pregnancy risk category C or D.

Antidepressants

➤ Can be used to treat bipolar depression but may induce a switch to mania/hypomania or a rapid-cycling pattern.

✔ There is no absolute consensus as to which antidepressants are better or worse to induce a switch. TCAs and MAOIs are thought to be greater offenders, but this may not be accurate.

✔ Risk factors for a switch include a prior antidepressant-induced switch to mania/hypomania, comorbid substance abuse, younger age, and early illness onset.

➤ When used, should be combined with a mood stabilizer to help protect against a switch to mania/hypomania:

✔ Olanzapine + fluoxetine (Symbyax) is FDA approved for the treatment of bipolar depression (2004). Start with a combination of 3–6 mg of olanzapine and 25 mg of fluoxetine, with upward titration as warranted to a maximum of 12 mg of olanzapine and 50 mg of fluoxetine. The addition of fluoxetine does not protect from olanzapine-induced weight gain.

➤ Are gradually being replaced by lamotrigine (effective for bipolar depression without the risk of a switch to mania/hypomania).

Other Somatic Treatments for Bipolar Disorder

Electroconvulsive therapy:

➤ Is useful for the treatment of acute mania and bipolar depression.

➤ Should be considered for bipolar patients who are in need of immediate symptom control (e.g., patients who are suicidal, psychotic, or unable to care for themselves).

➤ Can cause a switch to mania or hypomania in bipolar depressed patients.

General Guidelines for Somatic Treatment of Bipolar Disorder

Pharmacotherapeutic considerations:

➤ The successful treatment of bipolar disorder is an art requiring considerable experience, expertise, and patience. There are no universally accepted algorithms (although there are a multitude to choose from). A review of the literature demonstrates that there are as many ways to treat bipolar disorder as there are prescribing physicians. "Creative" uses of combinations of mood stabilizers and augmentation of mood stabilizers with antipsychotic medications and/or benzodiazepines are becoming common treatment options for patients whose conditions are refractory to monotherapies.

➤ The difficulty arises because of the multiple variants of the disorder, the possibility that an intervention to stabilize one phase might inadvertently worsen another, the lack of availability of a "universal agent" that will effectively treat all phases of the disorder, the rather unfavorable side-effect profile of the majority of available antimanic medications, the adverse effects of concurrent substance abuse, the paucity of good clinical studies, the greater treatment resistance of rapid cycling and mixed states, and patient unwillingness to comply with treatment recommendations (often due to denial of illness, preference for a substance of abuse rather than medications to stabilize moods, and/or unwillingness to tolerate undesirable side effects of available treatments).

➤ Effective management of bipolar disorders is grounded in medication management. Psychotherapeutic treatments are becoming more effective in diminishing emotional lability and educating patients and families, but cannot replace somatic treatments. Mood stabilizers are indicated for all phases of bipolar disorder.

➤ FDA-approved medications for the various phases of bipolar disorder are as follows:

✔ Manic episodes—carbamazepine ER, lithium, divalproex, olanzapine, risperidone, quetiapine, ziprasidone, aripiprazole, and chlorpromazine.

✔ Mixed episodes—carbamazepine ER, divalproex, olanzapine, risperidone, ziprasidone, and aripiprazole (but not lithium, quetiapine, or chlorpromazine).

✔ Depressive phase—olanzapine + fluoxetine combination, quetiapine.

✔ Hypomania—none.

✔ Maintenance phase—lithium, olanzapine, aripiprazole, and lamotrigine.

➤ When possible, monotherapy is preferred. If symptom control cannot be achieved with monotherapy, the options for combining or switching medications are almost endless.

➤ When combining medications, consider the increased burden of additive side effects:

✔ Olanzapine, divalproex, risperidone, quetiapine, and lithium can cause significant weight gain.

✔ Olanzapine, divalproex, risperidone, carbamazepine, and quetiapine can cause sedation.

✔ Lithium and divalproex can cause a hand tremor.

✔ Lithium, carbamazepine, and divalproex can cause gastrointestinal distress.

✔ Carbamazepine, oxcarbazepine, and topiramate can increase the metabolism of estrogen in birth control pills.

✔ Carbamazepine and divalproex can reduce the white blood cell count.

➤ When switching mood stabilizers, it is extremely important to overlap medications rather than abruptly stopping one and starting another. Otherwise, there is a high risk that mood symptoms will worsen during the transition period.

➤ The time interval for assessing the serum level of the mood stabilizer and ancillary chemistries is individualized, ranging from days in patients in acute manic states to 3–6 months in medically healthy, well-stabilized patients. Elderly and medically ill individuals are more likely to have decreases in renal and hepatic functioning, necessitating lower dosages and more frequent serum level checks.

Treatment of a manic episode:

➤ Initiate treatment with an FDA-approved medication (lithium, divalproex, olanzapine, quetiapine, risperidone, aripiprazole, ziprasidone, carbamazepine ER). Carbamazepine ER may or may not be considered first-line; the high index of enzyme induction (including autometabolism) may limit first-line suitability.

➤ For additional symptom control, adding a second medication that works by a mechanism different from the initially implemented medication and does not share the same side-effect profile seems prudent (e.g., olanzapine [increased weight] + carbamazepine [weight neutral], lithium [weight gain] + aripiprazole [weight neutral]).

➤ Olanzapine, risperidone, quetiapine, aripiprazole, and ziprasidone are logical choices when significant agitation or psychosis is part of the presentation and an immediate response is desired.

➤ Clozapine is an effective medication for the treatment of bipolar disorder but is not FDA approved.

➤ Chlorpromazine (Thorazine) is FDA approved for the treatment of mania. Haloperidol can be effective to ameliorate manic symptoms while waiting for a response to a mood stabilizer. Rarely, an encephalopathy can occur when lithium is combined with haloperidol.

➤ ECT is an effective treatment for medication-refractory manic episodes or when a rapid response is needed.

➤ A benzodiazepine can be added to reduce anxiety and insomnia.

Treatment of rapid cycling:

➤ Rule out medical and substance-induced causes of frequent mood shifts.

➤ Correct or remove offending agents (e.g., discontinue antidepressants, re-establish regular sleep patterns, discontinue substances of abuse).

➤ Utilize mood stabilizers that have been demonstrated in clinical trials to be effective (e.g., divalproex, olanzapine, and perhaps quetiapine).

➤ If treatment-refractory, consider ECT.

➤ A special form of CBT adapted to bipolar disorder can reduce depressive symptoms.

Treatment of mixed episodes:

➤ Providing effective treatment can be a challenge. Polypharmacy is likely necessary, and outcomes may be suboptimal:

✔ Monotherapies with proven efficacy include divalproex, olanzapine, aripiprazole, ziprasidone, risperidone, and carbamazepine.

✔ Combination strategies (combining two mood stabilizers) can be effective.

✔ Antidepressants should be avoided.

✔ ECT can be effective for patients with treatment-refractory illness.

Treatment of the depressive phases of bipolar disorder:

➤ Olanzapine-fluoxetine combination and quetiapine are FDA approved and are appropriate first choices.

➤ Lamotrigine and lithium are also effective but are not FDA approved.

➤ Despite the finding that as many as 50% of bipolar depressed patients receive an antidepressant as part of their treatment, there is no compelling evidence that response rates improve with antidepressant use while, at the same time, the patient is at increased risk for a switch to mania/hypomania. Utilizing lamotrigine rather than an antidepressant seems a prudent choice.

➤ For treatment-refractory patients, the choices are more limited in that adequate clinical trials are not available. Small studies are suggestive of the following options:

✔ Pramipexole (Mirapex [a dopaminergic agent]).

✔ MAOIs (high rates of switching).

✔ Modafinil (Provigil) added to a mood stabilizer.

✔ Ziprasidone.

✔ Aripiprazole.

✔ Beta-blockers (e.g., high-dose propranolol).

✔ Omega-3 fatty acids (1–2 g/day) added to a mood stabilizer.

✔ Calcium-channel blockers (e.g., verapamil, diltiazem).

✔ High-dose thyroid hormone.

✔ ECT alone or in combination with low-dose clozapine.

✔ Psychotherapy, in addition to medications, can be helpful when the depression is in response to a stressor.

Treatment of cyclothymic disorder:

➤ Treatment guidelines are not clearly defined and are often empirically derived:

✔ Mood stabilizers (e.g., lithium, divalproex) can be provided on a continual basis or only when dysfunction is evident (no clear guidelines in the literature).

✔ Antidepressants are usually (but not always) avoided secondary to concerns for an inadvertent switch to a hypomanic or manic episode.

✔ Psychotherapy (individual, group) and self-help groups can be beneficial.

Treatment of hypomanic episodes as part of bipolar II disorder:

➤ There are no medications that are FDA approved for the treatment of hypomania, and DSM-IV-TR clearly indicates that hypomania does not necessarily impart a dysfunctional course. Therefore, careful assessment and clinician judgment must be exercised.

➤ The real danger is the potential reversal to clinical depression consistent with a diagnosis of bipolar II disorder. Therefore, many clinicians advocate treatment of hypomania on a long-term basis using the general guidelines advocated for bipolar I disorder:

✔ Patients with hypomania frequently refuse treatment for hypomanic episodes.

✔ Because the majority of dysfunction from bipolar II disorder is secondary to the depressive phase, aggressive treatment of depression is always mandated and usually readily accepted by the patient.

Treatment of the maintenance phase of bipolar disorder:

➤ The primary goal is to prevent a relapse to a manic, hypomanic, or bipolar depressive episode. The general consensus is that since bipolar disorder is a lifelong illness, treatment should be life-long as well.

➤ Lithium, lamotrigine, aripiprazole, and olanzapine are FDA approved for the maintenance phase of bipolar disorder.

➤ Other reportedly effective (but not FDA-approved) treatments include:

✔ Divalproex.

✔ Carbamazepine.

✔ Atypical antipsychotic medications, either alone or in combination with lithium or divalproex.

Treatment of bipolar disorder during pregnancy:

➤ Pregnancy is not necessarily protective of mood, especially if medications are discontinued prior to or during pregnancy to protect the fetus from potential teratogenic effects.

➤ Bipolar individuals are especially prone to postpartum depression and postpartum psychosis.

➤ Patients should be advised before becoming pregnant as to the:

   ✔ Benefits of stopping medications (protection from fetal damage).

   ✔ Benefits of staying on medications (protection from manic or bipolar depressive episodes).

   ✔ Risks of stopping medications (illness exacerbation).

   ✔ Risks of staying on medications (potential teratogenicity and potential subsequent impact on the child's developing neurological system).

➤ Patients should share in the responsibility of choosing a treatment option before, during, and after pregnancy.

➤ Lithium, divalproex, and carbamazepine are potentially teratogenic (approximate risks of teratogenicity are 0.1%, 2%–5%, and 1%–3%, respectively). Less is known about the other approved medications.

➤ ECT and antipsychotic medications appear safer than lithium, carbamazepine, and divalproex for the treatment of bipolar disorder during pregnancy.

➤ CBT may provide significant benefits, possibly allowing for a reduction or elimination of medications during pregnancy (controversial).

Treatment of bipolar disorder during lactation:

➤ Lithium is excreted into breast milk to a greater extent than divalproex and carbamazepine. Less is known about the other FDA-approved mood stabilizers. The benefits versus risks should be individually assessed for use of mood stabilizers during breast-feeding, with the recognition that safer alternatives (bottled milk) are readily available.

Outcome and Functional Issues in Bipolar Disorder

➤ Bipolar disorder is an illness that "benefits mankind at the expense of the individual" (Kay Redfield Jamison). This statement refers to the special creativity often exhibited by individuals with bipolar disorder, as evidenced by the many famous writers, painters, and poets diagnosed with this disorder. Typically, creative periods are evident during hypomanic episodes. Equally impressive are periods of extreme dysfunction during manic highs and depressive lows, significant interepisode depression, high rates of suicide, and a remarkably high prevalence of comorbid substance abuse.

➤ Bipolar I disorder carries the highest morbidity of the bipolar spectrum disorders, especially when accompanied by mixed episodes, a rapid-cycling pattern, and/or substance abuse.

➤ Functional impairment is very high in all forms of bipolar disorder. Interepisode depression or depressive symptoms are frequent and at times chronic (new findings contradict the older assumption of euthymic interepisode functioning). Divorce, impairment at work, and job loss are frequent consequences of bipolar disorder.

➤ In a patient whose condition is well stabilized on medications, a bipolar episode can be precipitated by:

✔ Discontinuation of stabilizing medications.

✔ Sleep or sleep-wake cycle changes.

✔ Initiation or exacerbation of substance abuse.

✔ Experiencing a significant stressor.

✔ Finally achieving a significant goal.

✔ Experiencing seasonal changes.

✔ Engaging in east-to-west travel.

✔ Nothing at all.

➤ Medication noncompliance is one of the best predictors of outcome. After recovery from a manic episode, there is a 60% chance of relapse within 1 year if mood-stabilizing medications are discontinued.

➤ The suicide-completion rate in patients with bipolar disorder is the highest of all psychiatric disorders:

✔ Although difficult to quantify, the suicide rate has been shown in some studies to be as high as 50% (untreated), with an overall range between 15% and 50%. The most-cited statistic is that suicide occurs in approximately 30% of bipolar patients.

✔ Suicide occurs most often (but not exclusively) during depressive or mixed episodes, especially when there is comorbid substance abuse and/or comorbid anxiety.

✔ An increased frequency of bipolar episodes is associated with higher suicide rates.

➤ Reducing the frequency and severity of bipolar episodes through adequate treatment can dramatically decrease morbidity and mortality and can regain 7–10 years of improved functioning that would otherwise be lost. Therefore, indefinite maintenance treatment to protect against future bipolar episodes is the recommended approach, as opposed to initiating medication treatment only when a bipolar episode develops.

Psychotherapeutic Approaches to Treatment of Bipolar Disorder

➤ The advisability and potential benefits of insight-oriented individual psychotherapy or CBT are a matter of much debate. Psychotherapy is effective to enhance overall treatment compliance through the development of a therapeutic alliance with the patient and, if possible or practical, the patient's family. CBT may be helpful to reduce the intensity of depressive symptoms. Therapeutic issues of discussion include:

✔ Education of the patient (and possibly the patient's family) regarding the impact of psychosocial stressors on precipitating relapses.

✔ Denial of illness and/or reluctance to give up manic or hypomanic highs.

✔ Long-term compliance with side effect–prone medications.

✔ The negative impact of substance abuse (or possibly even substance use) in destabilizing moods.

✔ Promotion of a structured routine, to include regular patterns of sleep and exercise. Changes in mood, hours of sleep, and activity patterns can be a signal of an impending bipolar episode. It is extremely valuable for patients to chart their moods (elevated, normal, or depressed), level of anxiety, level of irritability, and sleeping patterns.

✔ A pristine lifestyle with great regularity of activities provides the best nonsomatic treatment for stabilizing bipolar disorder.

BIPOLAR SPECTRUM DISORDERS

➤ Constitute a spectrum (i.e., heterogeneous group) of disorders characterized by manic episodes, mixed episodes, hypomanic episodes, rapid cycling, bipolar depressive episodes, and cyclothymic disorder.

➤ Represent a prolific area of research. Old presumptions are being challenged, improved understandings of etiologies are emerging, and new and promising treatments are rapidly evolving.

➤ Have a prevalence of 2%–7%, depending on the study.

➤ Can present broadly with five symptom clusters:

✔ Manic episodes, mixed episodes, hypomanic episodes, and hypomanic symptoms.

✔ Bipolar depressive episodes and depressive symptoms.

✔ Psychotic symptoms (delusions, hallucinations, disorganized thinking, disorganized behavior).

✔ Cognitive changes (e.g., easy distractibility, poor insight, poor judgment).

✔ Behavioral disturbances (e.g., impulsivity, aggressiveness, violent behavior).

MOOD DISORDER NOT OTHERWISE SPECIFIED

➤ The "Not Otherwise Specified" categorizations are used when the mood symptoms do not fully meet the diagnostic criteria for any specific mood disorder and it is difficult to choose between depressive disorder NOS and bipolar disorder NOS:

✔ Depressive disorder NOS:

- Depressive symptoms do not meet the full criteria for another Axis I depressive disorder (e.g., MDD, dysthymic disorder, adjustment disorder with depressed mood). Examples are:
  - Premenstrual dysphoric disorder (more severe than premenstrual syndrome in that symptoms cause marked interferences with usual activities, including work and school).
  - Minor depressive episode (2-week history of mood symptoms, but with fewer than the five items required to diagnose MDD).
  - A depressive disorder is present but it cannot be determined whether it is primary, due to a general medical condition, or substance induced.

✔ Bipolar disorder NOS:

- Bipolar symptoms do not meet the full criteria for a specific bipolar disorder. Examples are:
  - Rapid cycling that does not meet the minimum-duration criterion for a manic episode or an MDE.
  - Recurrent hypomanic episodes without intercurrent depressive symptoms.
  - A bipolar disorder is present but it cannot be determined whether it is primary, due to a general medical condition, or substance induced.

3

ANXIETY DISORDERS

Principal DSM-IV-TR Anxiety Disorders

Generalized anxiety disorder
Panic disorder with and without agoraphobia
Specific phobia
Social anxiety disorder (social phobia)
Obsessive-compulsive disorder
Posttraumatic stress disorder
Acute stress disorder
Anxiety disorder due to a general medical condition
Substance-induced anxiety disorder
Anxiety disorder not otherwise specified

GENERAL CLINICAL ISSUES

➤ *Worry, apprehension, uncertainty, helplessness, nervousness,* and *fear* are examples of lay terms for anxiety.

➤ Anxiety and/or panic attacks are the core symptoms of the anxiety disorders. Symptoms are uncontrollable, unpleasant (ego-dystonic), and impairing:

✔ Anxiety can involve both psychological ("psychic") and "somatic" (physical) attributes:

■ Psychological anxiety—includes worry and fear.

■ Somatic anxiety—includes restlessness, gastrointestinal complaints, headaches, muscle aches, and increased heart rate and respiration.

✔ In *generalized anxiety disorder* (GAD), anxiety develops insidiously, tends to be persistent, and is in excess of what is warranted.

✔ In *panic disorder,* discrete severe anxiety episodes (i.e., panic attacks) repeatedly recur, most often without a specific stimulus. Anticipatory anxiety and agoraphobia may develop as the disorder progresses.

✔ In specific phobia and social phobia, anxiety or panic attacks are prompted by contact with a stimulus that the individual knows can generate anxiety.

✔ In *obsessive-compulsive disorder* (OCD), anxiety symptoms occur when the individual tries to resist the obsession. The anxiety can be relieved (temporarily) with compensatory compulsions.

✔ In *posttraumatic stress disorder* (PTSD) and acute stress disorder, anxiety may develop when the trauma occurs and may recur with reexperiencing the trauma (e.g., flashbacks [while awake], nightmares [while asleep]). However, anxiety may NOT be a presenting or recurring symptom of PTSD.

✔ In *anxiety disorder due to a general medical condition* and *substance-induced anxiety disorder,* anxiety, panic attacks, obsessions, or compulsions develop as a consequence of the medical disorder or substance abuse, respectively. When the medical disorder or substance abuse is adequately treated or resolves, anxiety symptoms are expected to resolve.

➤ Anxiety disorders are:

✔ The most prevalent psychiatric disorders.

✔ More frequent in women (except possibly for OCD, where the prevalence is nearly equal in men and women).

✔ More likely to develop at an early age, although treatment may be delayed for years.

✔ Chronic, with symptom intensity waxing and waning over time. At times, symptoms may totally remit, only to return at a later date.

✔ Often disabling, with large numbers of individuals receiving disability benefits.

✔ Associated with high rates of somatization (the expression of feelings or emotions through physical symptoms or complaints).

✔ Most often treated by primary care physicians, usually without an accurate diagnosis or adequate treatment.

✔ Often induced by or comorbid with a large number of medical disorders and substances:

■ Considerations for medical causes of anxiety ALWAYS take precedence. The listing for medical disorders that can cause anxiety symptoms is prolific, and a number of life-threatening physical disorders (e.g., myocardial infarction, pulmonary embolism) can initially present with anxiety symptoms.

■ Substances (e.g., alcohol, illegal drugs, prescribed and over-the-counter medications) are often overlooked as potential causes of anxiety symptoms.

✔ Often comorbid with other psychiatric disorders (e.g., psychotic disorders, mood disorders, other anxiety disorders).

✔ Can be assessed by various rating scales:

■ Anxiety Disorder Interview Scale—Revised (ADIS-R).

■ Hamilton Anxiety Scale (HAM-A)—14 questions assessing psychological and physiological anxiety symptoms, measured on a 0–4 severity point scale.

■ Panic Attack Scale.

■ Self-rating scales (e.g., Beck Anxiety Scale, State-Trait Anxiety Inventory).

■ Yale-Brown Obsessive Compulsive Scale (Y-BOCS)—a 10-item checklist for measuring severity of OCD.

➤ Etiological formulations of anxiety symptoms (nonexhaustive listing):

✔ Neurological formulations:

■ The limbic system and locus coeruleus are implicated in the manifestations of GAD, PTSD, and panic disorder. The amygdala coordinates fear behaviors and responses, and the locus coeruleus releases norepinephrine. Overall, the limbic system "scans" the environment for danger ("limbic alert").

■ Brain imaging in persons with GAD and panic disorder may demonstrate organic pathology (e.g., lesions in the hippocampus, lesions in the frontal or temporal lobes) or functional pathology (e.g., dysregulation of cerebral blood flow).

■ The hippocampus tends to be smaller in individuals with PTSD.

■ Persons with OCD may have reduced amounts of white matter and overactivity of cingulum bundles in the prefrontal cortex. Symptoms can be reduced dramatically with a cingulotomy.

✔ Biochemical formulations:

■ Gamma-aminobutyric acid (GABA) is a natural inhibitory neurotransmitter that reduces anxiety by binding to $GABA_A$ receptor sites. When GABA binds to $GABA_A$ receptor sites, chloride ion channels open, resulting in reduced firing of neurons, producing a calming effect. Benzodiazepines (BDZs) potentiate the effectiveness of GABA by binding to specific sites on the $GABA_A$ receptor complex (different from where GABA binds). By binding to $GABA_A$:

● Chloride ion channels remain open longer, accentuating the effects of GABA.

● GABA activity at the $GABA_A$ receptor increases, further enhancing anxiolytic effects.

- Serotonin (5-hydroxytryptamine [5-HT]) and norepinephrine (NE) are important neurotransmitters in the pathophysiology of anxiety disorders. Epinephrine is released in the "fight or flight" response. Caffeine, intravenous lactate, yohimbine, and carbon dioxide can stimulate the release of NE, resulting in a panic attack in persons with panic disorder. Buspirone (a 5-HT$_{1A}$ agonist), selective serotonin reuptake inhibitors (SSRIs), and SNRIs (serotonin norepinephrine reuptake inhibitors; venlafaxine, duloxetine) are effective anxiolytic agents.

- Dysregulation of corticotropin-releasing factor [CRF] from the hypothalamus and adrenocorticotropic hormone [ACTH]) from the pituitary are implicated in the development of anxiety disorders as part of the hypothalamic-pituitary-adrenal (HPA) axis. In turn, excessive secretion of cortisol ("stress hormone") from the adrenal glands in response to ACTH can increase anxiety symptoms.

✔ Infectious etiologies:

- Streptococcal bacterial infection in susceptible individuals may lead to the development of obsessions and compulsions and possibly OCD.

✔ Genetic formulations:

- Individuals with close relatives with an anxiety disorder are at increased risk of developing anxiety disorders.

✔ Psychoanalytic formulations:

- Anxiety is related to unresolved unconscious conflicts or separation from a love object.

- Panic disorder represents an unsuccessful attempt to defend against anxiety-producing impulses.

✔ Psychosocial formulations:

- Panic disorder represents a learned response of classical conditioning from repeated exposure to anxiety-provoking situations.

➤ Disorders that can present with anxiety symptoms (partial listing):

✔ Physical disorders (especially those that result in decreased availability of oxygen or glucose to the brain):

- Cardiovascular disorders (e.g., myocardial infarction, angina, mitral valve prolapse [controversial], congestive heart failure, arrhythmias, labile hypertension).

- Pulmonary disorders (e.g., pulmonary embolus, hyperventilation, asthma, chronic obstructive lung disease).

- Infectious diseases (e.g., streptococcal infection, influenza, hepatitis, encephalitis, pneumonia).

- Endocrine disorders (e.g., hypoglycemia, hyperthyroidism, Cushing's disease, carcinoid syndrome, pheochromocytoma).

- Neurological disorders (e.g., transient ischemic attack, cerebrovascular accident, intracranial tumor, head trauma, migraine headaches, seizure disorders, Parkinson's disease, akathisia, peripheral neuropathy, vestibular dysfunction).
- Gastrointestinal disorders (e.g., irritable bowel syndrome and other nonspecific gastrointestinal complaints, gastrointestinal bleeding, porphyria).

✔ Psychiatric disorders (partial listing):

- Anxiety disorders (e.g., GAD, panic disorder, PTSD, phobic disorders, OCD).
- Mood disorders (especially high comorbidity with mood disorders).
- Psychotic disorders (e.g., schizophrenia, schizoaffective disorder, brief psychotic disorder).
- Adjustment disorder with anxiety.
- Personality disorders (e.g., dependent, histrionic, borderline).
- Somatoform disorder.
- Eating disorders.
- Cognitive disorders (dementia, delirium).

✔ Substance use disorders:

- Substance abuse and substance dependence.
- Substance intoxication (e.g., amphetamine, cocaine, marijuana, hallucinogens, anabolic steroids, anticholinergic agents, excess caffeine).
- Substance withdrawal (e.g., alcohol, sedatives/hypnotics).
- Side effects of medications (e.g., caffeine, theophylline and herbal remedies (e.g., ma huang [ephedrine]).

➤ Medications useful for the treatment of anxiety disorders (Tables 3–1 and 3–2):

✔ BDZs:

- General considerations:
  - Short-half-life BDZs (e.g., alprazolam, oxazepam, lorazepam) have the advantage of a lower risk of sedation, psychomotor impairment, and amnestic effects than the longer-half-life agents (e.g., clonazepam, diazepam, chlordiazepoxide).
  - The longer-half-life agents are less likely than the shorter-half-life agents to produce a discontinuation syndrome (i.e., rebound anxiety, nervousness, depression, insomnia).
  - BDZs can be grouped by their indications, duration of action, and dosage range. Longer-half-life medications require less frequent dosing but tend to accumulate. All are GABAergic agents and therefore are cross-tolerant with each other and with alcohol (Table 3–3).

■ **Table 3–1** **Somatic treatments of anxiety disorders classified by disorder**

Anxiety disorder	FDA-approved medications	Additional effective medications
Generalized anxiety disorder	Escitalopram Paroxetine Venlafaxine Duloxetine Alprazolam Other benzodiazepines ("anxiety disorders") Buspirone	TCAs Beta-blockers MAOIs Alpha-adrenergic agonists
Panic disorder	Fluoxetine Paroxetine Sertraline Alprazolam Venlafaxine Clonazepam	TCAs Beta-blockers MAOIs Alpha-adrenergic agonists (clonidine)
Specific phobia	None	Benzodiazepines on as-needed basis
Social phobia	Paroxetine Sertraline Venlafaxine Fluvoxamine CR	TCAs Beta-blockers MAOIs Benzodiazepines
Obsessive-compulsive disorder	Fluoxetine Paroxetine Sertraline Fluvoxamine Clomipramine Fluvoxamine CR	MAOIs Augmentation (e.g., atypical antipsychotic medications, clonazepam, buspirone, pindolol, opiates, gabapentin)
Posttraumatic stress disorder (PTSD)	Sertraline Paroxetine	TCAs MAOIs Antiseizure medications (topiramate, lamotrigine) Prazosin Carbamazepine
Acute stress disorder	None	As in PTSD

Note. CBT = cognitive-behavioral therapy; FDA = U.S. Food and Drug Administration; MAOI = monoamine oxidase inhibitor; TCA = tricyclic antidepressant.

■ **Table 3–2.** **Somatic treatments of anxiety disorders classified by medication**

Medication	FDA approval	Indication(s) or target symptoms
Clonazepam	Yes	Panic disorder
Alprazolam	Yes	GAD, panic disorder
Diazepam, chlordiazepoxide, lorazepam, oxazepam	Yes	"Anxiety disorders"
Fluoxetine	Yes	OCD, panic disorder
Paroxetine	Yes	Panic disorder, GAD, OCD, PTSD, SAD
Sertraline	Yes	PTSD, OCD, SAD
Fluvoxamine	Yes	OCD
Escitalopram	Yes	GAD
Venlafaxine XR	Yes	Panic disorder, GAD, SAD
Duloxetine	Yes	GAD
Doxepin	Yes	"Anxiety disorders"
Clomipramine	Yes	OCD
Other SSRIs, other TCAs, MAOIs, mirtazapine, trazodone	No	Various anxiety disorders
Adrenergic-inhibiting agent (e.g., propranolol, prazosin, clonidine)	No	PTSD, performance anxiety, SAD
Antiseizure medications (e.g., lamotrigine, divalproex)	No	PTSD
Antipsychotic medications (preferably SGAs)	No	Augmentation

Note. FDA = U.S. Food and Drug Administration; GAD = generalized anxiety disorder; MAOI = monoamine oxidase inhibitor; OCD = obsessive-compulsive disorder; PTSD = posttraumatic stress disorder; SAD = social anxiety disorder; SGA = second-generation antipsychotic; SSRI = selective serotonin reuptake inhibitor; TCA = tricyclic antidepressant.

■ **Table 3–3   Commonly used benzodiazepines and benzodiazepine-like medications**

Benzodiazepine/ benzodiazepine-like medication	FDA-approved psychiatric indication(s)	Duration of action	Active metabolite	Recommended usual dosage range, mg/day
Lorazepam (Ativan)	Anxiety	Medium	No	1–4
Oxazepam (Serax)	Anxiety, alcohol withdrawal	Short–medium	No	30–120
Alprazolam (Xanax)	Anxiety, panic disorder	Short	No	1–4
Clonazepam (Klonopin)[a]	Panic disorder	Long	No	1–4
Chlordiazepoxide (Librium)[b]	Anxiety, alcohol withdrawal	Long	Yes	10–100
Diazepam (Valium)[b]	Anxiety, alcohol withdrawal	Long	Yes	2–40
Clorazepate (Tranxene)[b]	Anxiety, alcohol withdrawal	Long	Yes	7.5–60
Triazolam (Halcion)	Insomnia	Short	No	0.125–0.25
Temazepam (Restoril)	Insomnia	Medium–long	No	15–30
Flurazepam (Dalmane)[b]	Insomnia	Long	Yes	15–30
Estazolam (Prosom)	Insomnia	Short	No	1–2
Zaleplon (Sonata)[c]	Insomnia	Short	No	5–20
Zolpidem (Ambien)[c]	Insomnia	Short	No	5–10
Zolpidem CR (Ambien CR)[c]	Insomnia	Medium	No	6.25–12.5

Note.   FDA = U.S. Food and Drug Administration.
[a] A long duration of action without an active metabolite.
[b] Prodrugs (not active themselves), each metabolized to an active metabolite(s).
[c] A nonbenzodiazepine.

■ Clinical indications:

- Anxiety (more effective for somatic anxiety than psychological anxiety).

- Insomnia (i.e., a hypnotic; a sedative).

- Augmentation of antidepressants, mood stabilizers, and antipsychotic medications to reduce anxiety until the primary medication becomes effective.

- Alcohol, BDZ, and hypnotic/sedative withdrawal.

- Seizure disorders (e.g., diazepam).

- Muscle strain (e.g., diazepam).

■ Advantages:

- Rapid onset of action.

- Proven efficacy in relieving anxiety symptoms.

- Intermittent use can provide transient relief of anxiety symptoms.

- High patient acceptability and favorable side-effect profile.

- Shorter-half-life agents without active metabolites (e.g., lorazepam, oxazepam) are less impairing, especially if used in the elderly.

- Longer-half-life agents (e.g., diazepam, chlordiazepoxide) are often used for alcohol, BDZ, and barbiturate withdrawal.

■ Disadvantages (the "seven D's"):

- Depression of central nervous system function (e.g., drowsiness, depressed mood, depressed mechanical performance).

- Dependence (physical and psychological).

- Disinhibition resulting in agitation and possibly behavioral dyscontrol.

- Deficits in memory (e.g., anterograde amnesia).

- Dizziness (ataxia).

- Drug inhibition of the metabolism of other sedating medications resulting in additive or synergistic sedative effects.

- Dangerous when combined with other agents that also depress pulmonary function (e.g., alcohol, opioids, barbiturates).

■ Considerations and cautions:

- Because of the potential for dependence, recommendations are for short-term rather than long-term use. However, many patients do well with long-term use without developing abuse or dependence, typically when the dosage is kept low.

- BDZs should not be used in patients with active substance abuse.

- BDZ use can be associated with poor mechanical and cognitive performance, poor judgment, and an increased potential for impulsivity secondary to disinhibition. These effects can be exacerbated by alcohol, which can add a considerable measure of morbidity and mortality when combined with BDZs.

- Overdosage is safer than with the barbiturates but can be lethal (respiratory failure) if combined with alcohol or other cross-tolerant agents (e.g., barbiturates).

- Cognitive impairment can be problematic, especially in the elderly.

- Malingering as a way of gaining access to BDZs should always be assessed.

- When discontinuing BDZs, reduce the dosage slowly (particularly for the shorter-half-life agents) to minimize the potential for withdrawal symptoms (e.g., elevated vital signs, rebound anxiety more intense than the original anxiety, insomnia, headaches, muscle aches, nausea, anorexia, hyperarousal, withdrawal seizures, paranoia).

- The potential for a withdrawal syndrome increases with higher doses given for longer periods of time. The withdrawal syndrome for alprazolam is possibly the most intense and problematic of the BDZs, and a very slow taper (e.g., ~10% every 3–5 days) is recommended.

- Nonbenzodiazepine medications helpful for sleep include ramelteon (Rozerem), diphenhydramine, hydroxyzine, and TCAs.

- Especially concerning for medical-legal considerations when:
  - Medical causes are overlooked as causative factors of anxiety.
  - BDZs are prescribed for patients with active comorbid alcohol or drug abuse/dependence.
  - Patients who are abusing BDZs are not recognized as malingering.
  - Cognitive impairment is not recognized when BDZs are prescribed.

- In regard to use during pregnancy and lactation, BDZs:
  - Are potentially teratogenic, with diazepam the most widely reported offending agent (e.g., cleft lip/palate, cardiac defects, pyloric stenosis, dysmorphic features, mental retardation). However, the absolute risk to induce teratogenic effects is not clearly established.
  - Can induce "floppy baby syndrome" (e.g., feeding difficulties, lower Apgar scores, irritability, hyperreflexia) in newborns when used during the third trimester of pregnancy.
  - Can potentially induce prominent and life-threatening withdrawal symptoms in the newborn at birth.

- Most are pregnancy risk category D and a few of the hypnotics are category X (temazepam, triazolam, flurazepam).
- Diphenhydramine and zolpidem are category B and may be safer alternatives.
- Are excreted in breast milk to a low but measurable extent and can cause fatigue in the neonate.

✔ Buspirone (BuSpar):

■ General considerations:

- Buspirone (chemically an azaspirone with an active metabolite) is a serotonergic agonist (a "serotonergic anxiolytic") that acts at the 5-HT$_{1A}$ receptor and is also a mixed agonist/antagonist at postsynaptic dopamine receptors.
- Most effective for psychological anxiety (e.g., worry, apprehension, fear).
- Initiate at a dosage of 5 mg tid or 7.5 mg bid, with 5-mg dosage increases as needed every 2–3 days. The approved maximum dosage is 60 mg/day.
- Not widely accepted by patients previously treated with BDZs and has generally lost favor as an anxiolytic with psychiatrists. However, buspirone is finding favor as an augmenting agent when added to an SSRI for treatment-resistant depression.

■ Advantages:

- U.S. Food and Drug Administration (FDA) approved for the treatment of GAD.
- No addiction potential.
- Little to no sedation, cognitive impairment, or adverse interactions with alcohol. Occasional side effects include nausea and dizziness.
- Can be combined with BDZs.

■ Disadvantages:

- Onset is slower than with the BDZs, often requiring 7–10 days or more to become optimally effective. Regular rather than intermittent use is required.
- Patients previously treated with BDZs are less likely to be satisfied with or to respond to buspirone.
- Not effective for the treatment of panic disorder, OCD, or alcohol/BDZ withdrawal.
- Plasma levels are dramatically increased by grapefruit juice due to inactivation of cytochrome P450 (CYP) 3A metabolizing enzymes in the gastrointestinal tract.

- Contraindicated for use with monoamine oxidase inhibitors (MAOIs) secondary to the potential development of serotonin syndrome.
- Is pregnancy risk category B.

✔ SSRIs, SNRIs, and atypical antidepressants (AtypANs):

- SSRIs, venlafaxine, duloxetine, and nefazodone:
  - Effective for both psychological and somatic anxiety.
  - Because of the potential for initial worsening of anxiety symptoms, initiate treatment at a lower-than-therapeutic dose, with gradual increases as warranted.
  - Brand-name (but not generic) nefazodone is now withdrawn from the U.S. market.
  - Dosages higher than those used to treat depression may be needed.
  - One to 3 weeks may be required for optimal efficacy.

✔ Tricyclic antidepressants (TCAs):

- Clomipramine (Anafranil) is FDA approved for OCD.
- Doxepin is FDA approved for "psychoneurotic patients with depression and/or anxiety."
- Are pregnancy risk category C and D.
- Because of the potential for initial worsening of anxiety symptoms, initiate treatment at a lower-than-therapeutic dose, with gradual dosage increases as warranted.

✔ MAOIs:

- Are very effective anxiolytic agents.
- Are of significant concern for hypertensive crisis and other serious side effects, which limit their usefulness.
- Are pregnancy risk category C.

✔ Miscellaneous medications (not FDA approved) helpful alone or as adjunctive therapy in some anxiety disorders:

- Hydroxyzine pamoate:
  - Possibly effective for GAD and relatively widely used. The usual dosage range is 25–50 mg given tid–qid.
  - No potential for dependence, although possibly sedating.
  - Is pregnancy risk category C.
- Medications with GABAergic activity (e.g., topiramate, carbamazepine, lamotrigine, tiagabine, gabapentin, pregabalin).
- Beta-adrenergic antagonists (e.g., propranolol, metoprolol):
  - Propranolol (Inderal) is most helpful for reducing somatic anxiety symptoms (e.g., palpitations, tremor, sweating). The usual dosage

is 20–40 mg administered three to four times daily. Monitor pulse and blood pressure, both of which can fall. Do not use if heart rate falls below 55 bpm.

- Alpha$_2$-adrenergic agonists:
  - Clonidine (Catapres) can help reduce somatic anxiety symptoms. Usual dosage is 0.1 mg bid. A clonidine patch can also be used. Monitor pulse and blood pressure, both of which can fall.
- Alpha$_1$-adrenergic antagonists:
  - Prazosin (Minipress) can help reduce somatic anxiety symptoms. Typically dosed at 2–5 mg bid. Monitor pulse and blood pressure, both of which can fall.

➤ Psychotherapies useful for the treatment of anxiety disorders:

✔ Cognitive-behavioral therapy (CBT) is likely the most effective therapy for each of the anxiety disorders. Insight-oriented or supportive psychotherapy, interpersonal therapy, group therapy, biofeedback, yoga, meditation, and lifestyle changes (e.g., reduction of stressful environment, improved sleep hygiene, exercise) can be effective, possibly reducing or eliminating the need for medications.

➤ Medications that may worsen anxiety symptoms include bupropion, yohimbine, thyroid supplementation, and stimulants.

GENERALIZED ANXIETY DISORDER

DSM-IV-TR Diagnostic Criteria (Summary)

➤ Excessive anxiety and worry, occurring more days than not for at least 6 months, related to a number of events or activities (e.g., work, school).

➤ The person finds it difficult to control the anxiety.

➤ The anxiety and worry are associated with three or more of the following:

✔ Restlessness or feeling keyed up or on edge.

✔ Being easily fatigued.

✔ Difficulty concentrating or mind going blank.

✔ Irritability.

✔ Muscle tension.

✔ Sleep disturbance (difficulty falling or staying asleep or restless, unsatisfying sleep).

➤ The focus of the anxiety and worry is not confined to features of an Axis I disorder.

➤ The symptoms cause clinically significant distress or impairment in social, occupational, or other important areas of functioning.

➤ The symptoms are not due to a substance or a medical condition.

Clinical Issues

➤ GAD:

✔ Presents with some combination of psychological (i.e., "psychic") and/or physiological (i.e., somatic) symptoms.

■ Psychological symptoms include:

● Uncontrollable worry, apprehension, or fear, in excess of what is warranted. Worries typically relate to everyday life experiences (e.g., health, job responsibilities, finances). Worry is at least excessive and perhaps pathological in intensity and promoting functional impairment.

● Increased arousal (e.g., increased vigilance, exaggerated startle response).

■ Physiological symptoms include:

● Increased muscle tension (e.g., trembling, headaches, neck or back pain, clammy extremities).

● Increased autonomic hyperactivity (e.g., shortness of breath, sweating, palpitations, dry mouth, nausea, diarrhea, frequent urination, trouble swallowing, "lump in the throat").

● Sleep disturbance.

✔ Is a chronic disorder, with the intensity of symptoms waxing and waning over time.

✔ Is distinguished from "normal" worrying by the higher intensity of anxiety symptoms, the longer duration of the anxiety, and the resultant impairment in daily functioning.

✔ Is highly comorbid with major depressive disorder (MDD; 62%), alcohol dependence (37%), and other anxiety disorders (e.g., phobias, panic disorder). Overall, the prevalence of comorbid psychiatric disorders is impressive, ranging from 62% to 90%, depending on the study.

➤ The risk of suicide increases when severe, chronic, or ruminating anxiety accompanies MDD.

➤ Anxiety is a symptom and does not necessarily confer a diagnosis of GAD:

✔ Mild situational anxiety arising from an identifiable psychosocial stressor(s) other than a medical illness or a substance and resolving within 6 months would best be classified as an *adjustment disorder with anxiety, acute.* If symptoms last longer than 6 months after termination of the stressor(s) or if the stressor is chronic in nature, a diagnosis of *adjustment disorder with anxiety, chronic,* may be appropriate. Usually, the stressor is mild to moderate in intensity and the level of dysfunction is not severe or overly impairing.

✔ Adjustment disorder, acute stress disorder, and PTSD require an identifiable stressor. An identifiable stressor is not required for GAD but may be present.

✔ Significant anxiety resulting in impairment as a consequence of a substance of abuse or a medication is classified as a *substance-induced anxiety disorder.*

✔ Significant anxiety resulting in impairment as a consequence of a medical disorder is classified as an *anxiety disorder due to a general medical condition.*

➤ Prior to assuming a diagnosis of GAD, it is essential to *first:*

✔ Rule out medical and substance-related causes for anxiety (the possibilities are extensive).

✔ Rule out anxiety as an integral part of another psychiatric disorder (e.g., MDD, schizophrenia).

✔ Appreciate that GAD may also be comorbid with other psychiatric disorders (e.g., substance use disorders, MDD, schizophrenia).

Epidemiology

➤ Lifetime prevalence is approximately 5%. GAD is more common in females (2:1), younger individuals (average age at onset is 15–25 years), and African Americans.

Workup

➤ First assess for medical and substance-related causes of anxiety symptoms. A medical workup will typically be broad and include:

✔ Medical history, psychiatric history, and family history of medical and psychiatric disorders.

✔ Physical and neurological examination.

✔ Laboratory studies (e.g., electrolytes, complete blood count, fasting blood glucose, calcium level, hepatic function tests, renal function tests, thyroid function tests, urinalysis, drug screen).

✔ Special laboratory studies (depending on medical history and symptomatology) include:

■ Electrocardiogram (ECG) and other cardiac testing for suspected myocardial infarction or cardiac arrhythmias.

■ Chest X rays, lung perfusion scan, lung ventilation scan, or pulmonary arteriography for suspected pulmonary embolism.

- Pulmonary function tests for suspected chronic obstructive pulmonary disease.
- Electroencephalography and/or magnetic resonance imaging for abnormal neurological complaints or findings.
- Gastrointestinal studies for specific and nonspecific gastrointestinal complaints.
- Twenty-four-hour urine catecholamines and metanephrines for pheochromocytoma (tumor of the adrenal gland; low yield).
- Twenty-four-hour urine cortisol for Cushing's disease.

➤ Consider psychological testing:
 ✔ HAM-A.
 ✔ Self-rating scales:
  - Beck Anxiety Inventory.
  - State-Trait Anxiety Inventory.

Treatment

➤ BDZs:
 ✔ Are highly effective; response is almost immediate, especially when administered as an orally disintegrating dosage form (e.g., clonazepam wafer). Often preferred by patients, but can lead to the "seven D's" [p. 227]).
 ✔ Are not specifically stated as FDA approved for GAD. However, many BDZs are FDA approved for the treatment of "anxiety disorders" which most closely fit the DSM-IV-TR designation for GAD.

➤ Buspirone:
 ✔ Although FDA approved and effective, not generally preferred by patients who have previously been treated with BDZs. Is especially effective for chronic psychological anxiety.

➤ SSRIs, SNRIs, and AtypANs:
 ✔ With the exception of bupropion, these agents are highly effective and first-line choices.
 ✔ Escitalopram (Lexapro), duloxetine (Cymbalta), and venlafaxine (Effexor XR) are FDA approved.
 ✔ Bupropion can increase anxiety, especially in patients not first stabilized on an SSRI/SNRI.

➤ Alpha$_1$-adrenergic antagonists (e.g., prazocin) can be effective for somatic anxiety.

➤ Alpha$_2$-adrenergic agonists (e.g., clonidine) can be effective for somatic anxiety.

➤ Beta-adrenergic antagonists (e.g., propranolol) can be effective for somatic anxiety.

➤ GABAergic medications (e.g., divalproex, tiagabine) are gaining acceptance as effective anxiolytic agents but are not FDA approved.

➤ Hydroxyzine pamoate (Vistaril) can be effective for some patients.

➤ Psychotherapies:

 ✔ CBT can be highly effective, especially when combined with medications, and is likely considered the nonpharmacological treatment of choice.

 ✔ Individual (insight-oriented, supportive) and dynamic (analytical) therapies can be effective.

PANIC DISORDER

DSM-IV-TR Diagnostic Criteria (Summary)

➤ Recurrent unexpected panic attacks (a discrete period of intense fear or discomfort, in which four [or more] of the following symptoms developed abruptly and reached a peak within 10 minutes):

 ✔ Palpitations, pounding heart, or accelerated heart rate.

 ✔ Sweating.

 ✔ Trembling or shaking.

 ✔ Sensation of shortness of breath or smothering.

 ✔ Feeling of choking.

 ✔ Chest pain or discomfort.

 ✔ Nausea or abdominal distress.

 ✔ Dizziness, unsteadiness, light-headedness, or faintness.

 ✔ Derealization (feeling of unreality) or depersonalization (feeling of being detached from oneself).

 ✔ Fear of losing control or going crazy.

 ✔ Fear of dying.

 ✔ Paresthesias (numbness or tingling sensations).

 ✔ Chills or hot flushes.

➤ At least one of the attacks has been followed by 1 month (or more) of one (or more) of the following:

 ✔ Persistent concern about having additional attacks.

✔ Worry about the implications of the attack or its consequences.

✔ A significant change in behavior related to the attacks.

➤ Panic attacks are not due to a substance, a medical condition, or another psychiatric disorder.

➤ Panic attacks are not better accounted for by another psychiatric disorder (e.g., social phobia, OCD, PTSD).

Clinical Issues

Panic attacks:

➤ Involve the sudden onset of a constellation of physical and/or emotional symptoms, including:

✔ Autonomic hyperarousal:

■ Cardiac (e.g., palpitations, chest pain, chills/hot flushes, accelerated heart rate, sweating).

■ Neurological (e.g., dizziness, paresthesias, fainting spells, trembling, shaking).

■ Respiratory (e.g., choking sensations, feelings of smothering, shortness of breath).

■ Gastrointestinal (e.g., nausea, abdominal distress).

✔ Psychological disorganization:

■ Derealization (feeling of unreality) or depersonalization (feeling of being detached from oneself).

■ Fear of losing control, going crazy, or dying.

➤ Are a symptom and do not necessarily confer a diagnosis of panic disorder. A large number of medical disorders, psychiatric disorders, substance use disorders, and medications can induce panic attacks.

Panic disorder:

➤ Typically involves panic attacks recurring several times a week. Panic attacks typically last 5–30 minutes, peak in intensity in about 10 minutes, but on occasion can last hours.

➤ Is a chronic illness with a waxing and waning course and with varying and changing levels of symptoms.

➤ Is associated with considerable dysfunction.

➤ Is frequently "associated" with mitral valve prolapse (midsystolic click heard on auscultation; echocardiogram is diagnostic). The significance of this finding is unclear and recent studies have questioned this association. However, individuals with mitral valve prolapse typically have increased autonomic and emotional lability, just as those with panic disorder.

➤ May or may not be associated with agoraphobia (fear of being in places or situations where escape might be difficult or embarrassing, typically leading to avoidance of that place or situation):

   ✔ Recurrent panic attacks can lead to anticipatory anxiety (intense fear or dread of having another panic attack), followed by avoidance behavior and, subsequently, by agoraphobia. Common agoraphobic situations or places include crossing a bridge, traveling in vehicles, and leaving the home (i.e., fear of open spaces). Agoraphobic fears may lessen in the presence of a trusted individual.

   ✔ Panic disorder can also develop without agoraphobia and is defined in DSM-IV-TR as "panic disorder without agoraphobia." The presence or absence of agoraphobia is the only distinguishing criterion between these two disorders. Panic disorder with agoraphobia is more disabling than panic disorder without agoraphobia.

   ✔ Agoraphobia can occur without panic disorder and is described in DSM-IV-TR as "agoraphobia without history of panic disorder." Anxiety may also develop, but not to the extent of a full-blown panic attack.

Epidemiology

➤ Lifetime prevalence is between 1.5% and 3.5%, and it is more prevalent in women than men by a factor of 2:1.

➤ Onset is usually between ages 17 and 35 years. Onset after age 40 suggests an underlying medical or substance-related cause or another psychiatric diagnosis.

➤ Response to treatment is widely variable, from little to no improvement to long periods or remission.

➤ Panic disorder is highly comorbid with MDD (~60%), specific and social phobia, substance use disorders (35%), and personality disorders. Prognosis is poorer when panic disorder is comorbid with another major psychiatric disorder.

➤ Panic disorder is a risk factor for suicide. The risk of suicide further increases when panic disorder is comorbid with MDD or alcohol abuse/dependence.

➤ The consequences of panic disorder and panic attacks are far-reaching due to frequent emergency department visits, recurrent hospitalizations for physical and emotional problems, impaired marital and social functioning, a high incidence of unemployment, and a high reliance on social resources (e.g., Social Security disability, food stamps). Eighty percent of patients with panic disorder are first seen by a primary care or emergency department physician. Cardiologists are frequently consulted. Panic disorder is frequently underdiagnosed, undertreated, or remains untreated.

Etiological Formulations

➤ Dysregulation of 5-HT, NE, CRF, glutamate, and GABA has been implicated. Medications effective for panic disorder reduce excitability of the amygdala, brain-stem nuclei, and hypothalamus.

➤ A strong genetic component is evident, especially when first-degree relatives present with an anxiety or panic disorder.

➤ Anxiety is a learned response (cognitive model). CBT, therefore, can be especially effective.

➤ Anxiety represents an unsuccessful attempt to reduce anxiety-inducing stimuli (psychodynamic model). Analytical therapy can be effective.

Treatment

General considerations:

➤ Recommended somatic treatments for panic disorder include four classes of medications (i.e., SSRIs, high-potency BDZs, TCAs, MAOIs), each of which has demonstrated effectiveness, especially when combined with panic-focused CBT.

➤ Medications can reduce the frequency and intensity of panic attacks but may not, without CBT, ameliorate anticipatory anxiety or agoraphobia. Therefore, a combination of panic-focused CBT and antipanic medications is recognized as the most effective treatment.

➤ Somatic treatments may take up to 10–12 weeks to become optimally effective.

➤ Hyperventilation can induce a panic attack secondary to a decrease in blood carbon dioxide (CO_2). Treatment is to breathe deeply into a paper bag, thereby increasing $P\text{CO}_2$.

➤ Buspirone, beta-blockers (e.g., propranolol), and bupropion (Wellbutrin) are not effective treatments for panic disorder.

➤ Medications are often continued for at least 1 year, and possibly indefinitely. There is no clear consensus on this issue.

Medications:

SSRIs, SNRIs, and AtypANs:

➤ Fluoxetine (Prozac), paroxetine/paroxetine CR (Paxil), sertraline (Zoloft), and venlafaxine (Effexor XR) are FDA approved. Higher doses than those used to treat depression are often required. An expected initial worsening of anxiety symptoms at the initiation of therapy may necessitate starting the medication at a lower dose, with dosage increases as warranted.

➤ Zoloft is FDA approved to treat depression, social anxiety disorder, PTSD, panic disorder, OCD, and premenstrual dysphoric disorder (PMDD) in adults over age 18 years. It is also approved for OCD in children and adolescents ages 6–17 years.

High-potency BDZs (the most common and perhaps effective treatment):

➤ Alprazolam and clonazepam are FDA approved for the treatment of panic disorder. Lorazepam can also be as effective.

➤ The benefit of almost immediate symptom relief is unique to the BDZs. When used on a continuous basis, BDZs can eventually block the development and/or diminish the intensity of a panic attack.

➤ Orally disintegrating clonazepam (Klonopin Wafer) or alprazolam (Niravam) can speed response. A long-acting oral formulation of alprazolam (Xanax XR) is also available.

➤ The potential for abuse and for side effects should always be considered prior to initiating treatment with a BDZ.

➤ Combining a BDZ and an SSRI can be especially effective.

TCAs:

➤ Imipramine (Tofranil) and clomipramine (Anafranil) are especially effective for the treatment of panic disorder (but are not FDA approved for this indication), with clomipramine likely being more effective than imipramine. However, TCA side effects, drug interactions, and potential lethality when combined with alcohol may limit their usefulness.

➤ Initiate at a dosage of about 25–50 mg/day because of an expected initial worsening of anxiety at the start of treatment, and gradually increase the dosage as needed and as tolerated. Dosages equal to or greater than those needed for the treatment of depression may be required.

MAOIs (especially phenelzine [Nardil]):

➤ MAOIs are likely the most effective agents for the treatment of panic disorder, but adverse side effects and potentially serious drug and food interactions limit their usefulness. They are not FDA approved for the treatment of panic disorder.

Antiseizure medications:

➤ Gabapentin (Neurontin) and valproex (Depakote) can be useful but are not FDA approved for the treatment of panic disorder.

Panic-focused CBT and exposure therapy:

➤ Panic-focused CBT and exposure therapy are effective treatments (alone or in combination with antipanic medications) for panic disorder. Individuals with panic disorder tend to focus on bodily sensations that signal the onset of the next panic attack. "Panic control treatment," typically requiring approximately 12 sessions, involves cognitive restructuring, breathing techniques, and bodily sensation awareness.

Algorithm for the treatment of panic disorder (to include panic-focused CBT and/or exposure therapy):

➤ Prior to diagnosing panic disorder, assess for other causes of anxiety/panic attacks (e.g., anxiety disorder due to a general medical condition, substance-induced anxiety disorder, panic attacks secondary to a psychiatric disorder other than panic disorder). Provide treatment for the underlying problem, if present.

➤ Start with an FDA-approved SSRI, venlafaxine, or an FDA-approved BDZ:

  ✔ SSRIs and venlafaxine:

  ■ Start at somewhat lower than therapeutic dose because of an expected temporary increase in anxiety. Consider supplementing with a BDZ or hydroxyzine pamoate (Vistaril) for a short time if necessary.

  ■ Gradually optimize the dosage to perhaps somewhat higher than required for the treatment of MDD (somewhat controversial).

  ■ If there is:

   ● Only a partial response to optimization of the SSRI or venlafaxine, consider combination or augmentation strategies (e.g., an SSRI + a TCA, an SSRI + a BDZ).

   ● No response to optimization of the SSRI, consider switching between agents, to a high-potency BDZ, or to a TCA with a strong serotonergic component (e.g., clomipramine, amitriptyline, imipramine).

  ✔ BDZs:

  ■ Alprazolam or clonazepam are very effective medications. Since medications for panic disorder are often given on a long-term basis, many psychiatrists avoid this option because of the potential for developing dependence. However, for a rapid and effective response to panic symptoms, BDZs clearly provide superior results, not withstanding their potential side-effect profile and potential for abuse.

➤ If there is still a lack of an adequate response from optimization, combining, or augmenting strategies, consider a trial of phenelzine (after the appropriate waiting period). Gradually optimize the dosage to 60–90 mg/day. Selegiline transdermal (EmSam), the newest MAOI formulation, is not approved for the treatment of panic disorder.

➤ If there still is a lack of an adequate response, consider a trial of gabapentin or divalproex (neither are FDA approved).

SPECIFIC PHOBIA

DSM-IV-TR Diagnostic Criteria (Summary)

➤ Marked and persistent fear that is excessive and unreasonable, cued by the presence or anticipation of a specific object or situation.

➤ Exposure to the phobic stimulus almost invariably produces an immediate anxiety response, which may take the form of a situationally bound or a situationally predisposed panic attack.

➤ The person recognizes the fear is excessive or unreasonable.

➤ The phobic situation(s) is avoided or is endured with intense anxiety or distress.

➤ The avoided behavior significantly interferes with the person's normal routine or social or occupational functioning, or there is marked distress about having the phobia.

Clinical Issues

➤ Individuals with specific phobia:
  - ✔ Have an intense and persistent fear of a specific object or situation, which may be expressed as anxiety, fear of being harmed, fear of losing control, dizziness, or fainting spells.
  - ✔ Clearly recognize the specific object or situation as anxiogenic.

➤ Typical phobic objects or situations include animals (e.g., dogs, snakes, bugs), feeling closed in (claustrophobia), witnessing blood, heights (acrophobia), flying, driving on bridges, driving through tunnels, and being in or near a storm.

➤ Phobias are linked to the amygdala (involved with fear, alertness, and aggression).

➤ Formerly called simple phobia.

Epidemiology

➤ Lifetime prevalence is ~11%.

Treatment Considerations

➤ BDZs (not FDA approved) and CBT can be effective treatments, especially when combined. CBT should also include exposure therapy (i.e., gradual desensitization through increased exposure to the stimulus).

➤ Propranolol can reduce somatic anxiety symptoms.

➤ Behavioral therapy involves three components:

✔ *Exposure*—the patient undergoes exposure to the phobic stimuli either gradually or totally (i.e., "flooding").

✔ *Systematic desensitization*—the patient is taught relaxation techniques to be applied while mentally visualizing the phobic agent.

✔ *Participant modeling*—the treating therapist personally demonstrates that the object or situation is not dangerous; following this, the patient gradually faces the object or situation.

SOCIAL ANXIETY DISORDER (SOCIAL PHOBIA)

DSM-IV-TR Diagnostic Criteria (Summary)

➤ A marked and persistent fear of one or more social or performance situations in which the person is exposed to unfamiliar people or to possible scrutiny by others. The individual fears he or she will act in a way (or show anxiety symptoms) that will be humiliating or embarrassing.

➤ Exposure to the feared situation almost invariably provokes anxiety, which may take the form of a situationally bound or situationally predisposed panic attack.

➤ The person recognizes that the fear is excessive or unreasonable.

➤ The feared social or performance situations are avoided or endured with intense anxiety or distress.

➤ The avoided behavior significantly interferes with the person's normal routine or social or occupational functioning, or there is marked distress about having the phobia.

➤ The avoided behavior is not due to the direct physiological effects of a substance or a general medical disorder.

Clinical Issues

➤ A useful corollary for social anxiety disorder (SAD) is "a stare is a threat."

➤ DSM-IV-TR describes SAD as "avoidance limited to social situations for fear of embarrassment."

➤ Symptoms (ego dystonic) include significant uncontrollable anxiety which may develop into a panic attack.

➤ Individuals with social phobia typically:

✔ Avoid social interactions because of an intense fear of being observed, scrutinized, embarrassed, or humiliated.

✔ Tend to be hypersensitive to criticism, have low self-esteem, have poor social skills, and prefer not to make eye contact.

✔ Are markedly impaired in terms of social functioning. By definition, the impairment reaches a significant level of dysfunction (e.g., unable to attend work or school, isolation, few or no friends), or there is marked distress about having the phobia.

➤ SAD:

✔ Typically first manifests between ages 11–15, with a lifetime prevalence of ~7%.

✔ Is more prevalent in females.

✔ Is often not recognized; only 3% of patients receive treatment.

✔ Is a chronic disorder that waxes and wanes in intensity (as occurs with most anxiety disorders). Complete remission is unusual.

✔ Can be *generalized* (if the fears include most social situations) or *specific* (if the fear is limited to a single type of social situation). The generalized form is more likely to be refractory to treatment and to have a genetic basis.

➤ Typical phobias include the fear of speaking or performing in public (public-speaking phobia); the fear of shopping or eating in public; the fear of being criticized for poor school or work performance; the fear of social interaction or dating; and the fear of being observed using a public restroom ("bashful bladder"; paruresis).

➤ Despite a high lifetime prevalence, social phobia is largely unrecognized, undertreated, or remains untreated. Yet with a combination of psychotherapy and judicious use of medications, symptom improvement can be dramatic.

➤ The diagnostic criteria for social phobia and avoidant personality disorder are very similar, making it difficult to distinguish between the two. Some authorities feel the two disorders are intertwined or may be one and the same. However, the recommended treatments for the two disorders differ (i.e., psychotherapy is the treatment of choice for avoidant personality disorder).

Treatment Considerations

➤ Medications (especially when combined with CBT or cognitive-behavioral group therapy [CBGT]) can be very effective treatments:

✔ Fluvoxamine CR (Luvox CR), paroxetine, sertraline, and venlafaxine are FDA approved.

✔ MAOIs (particularly phenelzine) may provide the most effective treatment, but these agents are not FDA approved and have potentially dangerous drug and food interactions.

✔ BDZs can be helpful on an immediate-need basis but have multiple side effects, including the potential for drowsiness.

✔ Buspirone and gabapentin may be somewhat effective based on small clinical trials but are not FDA approved.

✔ Propranolol 20–40 mg taken 30 minutes before a performance or test can effectively improve "performance (test) anxiety" (e.g., for the oral board examination), but is not FDA approved.

➤ Response is best when medications are combined with CBT/CBGT.

OBSESSIVE-COMPULSIVE DISORDER

DSM-IV-TR Diagnostic Criteria (Summary)

➤ Presence of either obsessions or compulsions:

✔ Obsessions:

■ Repetitive, intrusive, persistent thoughts, ideas, impulses, or images that are recognized as excessive or senseless but cannot easily be resisted, dismissed, or ignored.

■ The symptoms cause marked anxiety or distress.

■ The thoughts, impulses, or images are not simply excessive worries about real-life problems.

■ The person attempts to ignore or suppress such thoughts, impulses, or images, or to neutralize them with some other thought or action.

■ The person recognizes that the obsessional thoughts, impulses, or images are a product of his or her own mind (i.e., not thought insertion).

✔ Compulsions:

■ Repetitive behaviors or mental acts that the person feels driven to perform in response to an obsession or according to rules that must be applied rigidly.

■ The behaviors or mental acts are aimed at preventing or reducing distress or preventing some dreaded event or situation.

■ These behaviors or mental acts either are not connected in a realistic way with what they are designed to neutralize or prevent or are clearly excessive.

➤ At some point during the illness, the person recognizes that the obsessions or compulsions are excessive or unreasonable.

➤ The obsessions or compulsions cause marked distress, are time-consuming (take more than 1 hour per day), or significantly interfere with the individual's normal routine, occupational or academic functioning, or usual social activities or relationships.

➤ The context of the obsessions or compulsions is not related to other Axis I disorders with inherent obsessions or compulsions (e.g., anorexia nervosa), and the obsessions or compulsions are not caused by the direct physiological effects of a substance or a general medical condition.

Clinical Issues

➤ The diagnosis of OCD requires *either* obsessions or compulsions.

✔ Both obsessions and compulsions are present in approximately 80% of patients. Compulsive behaviors most often follow obsessive thinking.

✔ Compulsions without obsessions are unusual but do occur.

➤ Obsessions:

✔ Are intrusive distressing thoughts or concerns that the person cannot ignore.

✔ Are often related to fears of self-contamination, doubt or uncertainty about whether an important action has been performed, or the need for organization:

■ Fear of contamination (e.g., fear that touching a doorknob or light switch might lead to an illness).

■ Fear of mistakenly harming others (e.g., hitting a bump in the road while driving generates a fear that the person has run over a pedestrian).

■ Doubt (e.g., the person fears he or she has not turned off the stove or locked the front door).

■ Fear of punishment for thinking "evil thoughts" (e.g., obscenities, sexual thoughts).

■ Need for order, exactness, or symmetry.

➤ Compulsions:

✔ Typically serve to temporarily neutralize (i.e., relieve) the anxiety created by the obsessions.

✔ Can include mental rather than physical acts (e.g., mental ordering).

✔ Commonly include:

■ Constant need for hand washing.

■ Repeated counting or mental checking.

■ Refusal to touch an object (e.g., doorknobs or light switches, shaking hands), or, alternatively, the compulsion to touch a doorknob or light switch a set number of times.

➤ The obsessions and/or compulsions are ego dystonic yet take an inordinate amount of time and energy and cause significant dysfunction or distress.

➤ Multiple and shifting patterns of obsessions and compulsions are common (e.g., the need to chant a set of words while touching a doorknob, switching from the fear of shaking hands to the fear of touching the stove).

➤ The most common obsessions (from high to low): contamination, symmetry, somatic or sexual concerns; the most common compulsion is hand washing.

➤ Primary care physicians (and many psychiatrists) rarely screen for OCD, resulting in low recognition. OCD is often a hidden disorder, in that individuals may be embarrassed to reveal symptoms for fear they may be thought of as being odd or crazy. Patients are most often seen by primary care physicians for either "anxiety" or "depression." The disorder may go undetected and untreated for years or a lifetime.

➤ Comorbidity with other psychiatric disorders is high, compounding the difficulty in establishing the diagnosis.

➤ Symptoms often are chronic, with a waxing and waning pattern (as is true with most anxiety disorders).

➤ Common features of obsessions and compulsions are:

✔ Intrusive nature of the symptoms.

✔ Ego-dystonic (i.e., unpleasant) nature of the symptoms.

✔ Recognition by the person that the obsessions and compulsions are absurd or irrational yet are difficult or impossible to resist.

➤ Psychotic symptoms are uncommon. If psychotic symptoms are present, consider a comorbid psychotic disorder or an alternative diagnosis.

➤ *Obsessive-compulsive spectrum disorders* constitute a broad category of disorders involving obsessions and/or compulsions. Included in this category are body dysmorphic disorder, some impulse-control disorders (e.g., pathological gambling, compulsive shopping, kleptomania, sexual compulsions, trichotillomania [hair pulling], bowel and urinary obsessions, compulsive skin picking, nail biting), some neurological disorders (e.g., Sydenham's chorea, Parkinson's disease, epilepsy, autism), depersonalization, eating disorders, Tourette's disorder, and hypochondriasis.

➤ OCD should be distinguished from obsessive-compulsive personality disorder (OCPD), which involves neither obsessions nor compulsions (Table 3–4).

■ **Table 3–4   Comparison of obsessive-compulsive disorder (OCD) with obsessive-compulsive personality disorder (OCPD)**

Characteristic	OCD	OCPD
Axis	I	II
Chronicity of the illness	Chronic	Chronic
Intensity of the illness	Waxes and wanes (as with other anxiety disorders)	Relatively constant (i.e., pervasive)
Obsessions	Yes	No (or not prominent)
Compulsions	Yes	No
Anxiety	Yes (severe)	No (or not prominent)
Characterization of impairments	Ego-dystonic	Ego-syntonic
Primary treatment	SSRIs combined with CBT	Psychotherapy

Note.   CBT = cognitive-behavioral therapy; SSRI = selective serotonin reuptake inhibitor.

Epidemiology

➤ Lifetime prevalence of OCD is ~2.5%, with a slightly greater incidence in females. Males have an earlier age at onset (ages 13–15 years) than do females (ages 20–24 years).

➤ As a group, the obsessive-compulsive spectrum disorders affect up to 10% of the population.

➤ OCD typically starts in adolescence or early adulthood (50% develop the disorder before age 15 years), often beginning with a stressful event (e.g., a driver of a car hits a bump in the road, and from that time onward feels compelled to return to any site at which the car hits a bump to be sure that he or she has not unknowingly run over someone).

Prognosis

➤ Prognosis is improved with:
  ✔ Obsessions without accompanying compulsions.
  ✔ Presence of a precipitating event (i.e., an abrupt onset).
  ✔ Episodic rather than chronic symptoms.
  ✔ Overall good social/occupational adjustment.
➤ Prognosis is poorer with:
  ✔ Yielding to rather than resisting the compulsion.
  ✔ Childhood onset.
  ✔ Bizarre obsessions and/or compulsions.
  ✔ Need for hospitalization because of severe symptoms.

Comorbidity

➤ Comorbid psychiatric disorders are found in more than 50% of individuals with OCD (e.g., psychotic, mood, personality, eating, substance use, Tourette's disorder, tics, as well as other anxiety disorders). MDD is possibly as high as 30%, although the prevalence of depressive symptoms can be as high as 80%.

Differential Diagnosis (Partial Listing)

➤ MDD with or without psychotic features (often mistaken for MDD).

➤ Psychotic disorders (schizophrenia, delusional disorder).

➤ Obsessive-compulsive personality disorder (rigidness, ordering).

➤ Anxiety disorders (e.g., GAD, panic disorder, PTSD).

➤ Substance use disorders.

➤ Obsessive-compulsive spectrum disorders (e.g., eating disorders, hypochondriasis, body dysmorphic disorder, depersonalization disorder, impulse control disorder).

Etiological Formulations (Noninclusive Listing)

➤ Neurotransmitter dysregulation:

  ✔ Serotonergic dysregulation is recognized as the primary causative factor. Agents that specifically increase 5-HT (e.g., SSRIs, clomipramine) effectively reduce OCD symptoms. Noradrenergic dysregulation is not felt to be causative, in that noradrenergic agonists are ineffectual in the treatment of OCD.

➤ Dopamine dysregulation and dysregulation of glutamate and GABA transmission have an impact on the development and progression of OCD.

➤ Genetic formulation:

  ✔ A genetic contribution is recognized. Approximately 35% of relatives of individuals with OCD also have the disorder.

➤ Brain changes:

  ✔ OCD involves dysfunction in a neuronal loop running from the orbital frontal cortex to the cingulate gyrus and back to the frontal cortex. Interrupting this circuit (cingulotomy) can ameliorate symptoms.

  ✔ Basal ganglia dysfunction has been suggested as an etiology of OCD. OCD and Sydenham's chorea are often comorbid.

Workup

➤ Screening questions suggestive of OCD:

  ✔ Do you have to wash your hands over and over?

  ✔ Do you have to check things repeatedly?

✔ Do you have thoughts that come into your mind that you cannot stop thinking about and that cause you distress?

✔ Do you need to complete actions over and over until they are just right or in a certain way before you can move on to the next one?

➤ The Yale-Brown Obsessive Compulsive Scale (Y-BOCS) is a 10-item severity rating scale, with scores ranging from 0 (no symptoms) to 40 (severe symptoms).

Treatment

General considerations:

➤ A combination of a potent serotonergic agent and CBT is considered the most effective treatment. The behavioral component consists of exposure and response (ritual) prevention. Exposure is more helpful for reducing obsessions, whereas response prevention is more helpful in reducing compulsive behaviors. Potent 5-HT reuptake inhibitors (SSRIs; clomipramine) are considered first-line medications for the treatment of OCD. SSRIs are preferred over clomipramine solely because of their lower propensity to cause side effects.

➤ Treatment should be individualized. Some individuals have persistent, incapacitating symptoms, whereas others have mild, non-incapacitating symptoms that typically recur under stress. Self-help methods can be beneficial for milder OCD. OCD self-help books include *Getting Control: Overcoming Your Obsessions and Compulsions,* by Lee Baer (New York, Plume, 2000), and *The OCD Workbook: Your Guide to Breaking Free From Obsessive-Compulsive Disorder,* by Bruce Hyman and Cherry Pedrick (Oakland, CA, New Harbinger Publications, 1999).

➤ Eight to 12 weeks or longer may be required for an optimal response to medications and higher dosages than used for depression or GAD are usually required. Targeted daily doses are as follows: paroxetine 40 mg, fluoxetine 40–60 mg, fluvoxamine 150–300 mg, fluvoxamine CR 100–200 mg, sertraline 100–200 mg, and clomipramine 150–250 mg.

➤ With adequate treatment, the average reduction in obsessions and compulsions is about 50%, with only 5%–10% of individuals eventually becoming symptom free. This establishes OCD as a chronic, often lifelong disorder with periods of exacerbations and partial remissions and, at best, only partially responsive to treatment modalities.

➤ Medications should be continued for a minimum of 1 year, and possibly indefinitely (controversial). Relapse is common if medications are discontinued. Maintenance doses are individually determined based on symptoms.

➤ Psychoanalysis, cognitive therapy, buspirone (as a monotherapy), noradrenergic antidepressants (e.g., desipramine), and BDZs (as a monotherapy) are not considered effective treatments. However, they can be useful as adjunctive treatments.

➤ OCD is a resilient illness with only marginally effective treatments. After the first-line treatments of SSRIs and clomipramine, additional options are limited.

Somatic therapies:

SSRIs:

➤ Fluoxetine, paroxetine, sertraline, fluvoxamine, and fluvoxamine CR are FDA approved for the treatment of OCD and are considered first-line treatments. Responsiveness generally increases with increasing dose. Lower initial doses may be needed because of a transient increase in anxiety symptoms. Citalopram, mirtazapine, venlafaxine, and duloxetine can also be effective, but are not FDA approved.

Clomipramine (Anafranil):

➤ General considerations:

✔ A tertiary-amine TCA and a potent 5-HT reuptake inhibitor FDA approved for the treatment of OCD. Clomipramine is significantly more effective than other TCAs and equal to or more efficacious than MAOIs or SSRIs.

MAOIs:

➤ Very effective, but an adverse side-effect profile and dangerous drug/food interactions limit their usefulness. They are not FDA approved for this indication.

Frequently cited augmentation strategies:

➤ Include adding the following medications to SSRIs:

✔ First- and second-generation antipsychotic medications (e.g., haloperidol, risperidone, olanzapine).

✔ Clonazepam if significant anxiety accompanies OCD.

Electroconvulsive therapy:

➤ Typically used when treatment with medications, CBT, and a combination of medications + CBT have failed.

➤ Deep brain stimulation and vagus nerve stimulation are showing promise as less invasive treatments.

Psychosurgery:

➤ Includes anterior cingulotomy (the most commonly performed surgery), tractotomy, anterior capsulotomy, and limbic leukotomy.

➤ Is an appropriate treatment for severely incapacitating (intractable) OCD in patients who remain unresponsive after trials of all available treatments.

➤ Provides significant symptom relief in 30%–67% of patients. However, options for those not responding to psychosurgery are less clear.

Nonsomatic therapies:

Cognitive-behavioral therapy (considered a first-line treatment):

➤ A very effective treatment for OCD, alone or combination with medications. The basic tenet is exposure-response prevention. As a behavioral treatment, an individual is exposed to a specific stimulus that causes distress and then works to resist engaging in compulsive rituals to reduce the anxiety.

Treatment algorithm (to include CBT):

➤ Initiate treatment with one of the four FDA-approved SSRIs, and potentially titrate to the higher approved dosage ranges ("start low, go slow").

➤ Consider augmentation with a first- or second-generation antipsychotic agent (best studied) or clonazepam.

➤ If there is no response to the SSRI, switch to another FDA-approved SSRI. There is documentation that switching SSRIs can be effective.

➤ If there is still an inadequate response to the SSRIs or augmentation of the SSRI (up to 40% of patients), switch to clomipramine or cautiously combine clomipramine with the SSRI (both significantly increase 5-HT; watch for serotonin syndrome).

➤ If there still is an inadequate response, discontinue clomipramine or the clomipramine/SSRI combination and start an MAOI (especially phenelzine), after the appropriate waiting period.

➤ If there still is an inadequate response, discontinue the MAOI and consider:

✔ Electroconvulsive therapy (variable effectiveness), especially helpful if depression is present.

✔ Novel approaches (e.g., intravenous clomipramine, antiandrogens, opioids, repetitive transcranial magnetic stimulation, vagus nerve stimulation).

➤ If there still is no response, consider psychosurgery if all of the following criteria are met:

✔ There is absolute clarification that the diagnosis is OCD.

✔ There is no response to all five medications FDA approved for OCD (with augmentation) administered at therapeutic doses for a sufficient period of time, coupled with CBT.

✔ Other causes of treatment resistance have been assessed and corrected (e.g., active substance abuse, poor compliance with medications, failure to follow prescribed behavior modifications).

✔ Symptoms are severe, intractable, incapacitating, and/or accompanied by sincere suicidal ideations or behaviors.

✔ The patient is aware of the benefits and risks and is amenable to surgery.

POSTTRAUMATIC STRESS DISORDER

DSM-IV-TR Diagnostic Criteria (Summary)

➤ The person has been exposed to a traumatic event in which both of the following are present:

✔ The person experienced, witnessed, or was confronted by an event or events that involved actual or threatened death or serious injury, or a threat to the physical integrity of self or others. Examples include personally experiencing the consequences of military combat, assault/rape, domestic violence, an automobile accident, childhood physical or sexual abuse, sudden catastrophic medical illness, or involvement with a natural disaster. However, witnessing a traumatic event or being told about a traumatic event experienced by a significant other, rather than personally experiencing the traumatic event, qualifies by DSM-IV-TR standards.

✔ The person's response involved intense fear, helplessness, or horror.

➤ The traumatic event is persistently reexperienced in one (or more) of the following ways:

✔ Recurrent and intrusive distressing recollections of the event, including images, thoughts, or perceptions.

✔ Recurring distressing dreams of the event.

✔ Acting or feeling as if the traumatic event were recurring (including a sense of reliving the experience, illusions, hallucinations, and dissociative flashback episodes, including those that occur on awakening or when intoxicated).

✔ Intense psychological distress at exposure to internal or external cues that symbolize or resemble an aspect of the traumatic event.

✔ Physiological reactivity on exposure to internal and external cues that symbolize or resemble an aspect of the traumatic event.

➤ Persistent avoidance of stimuli associated with the trauma, and numbing of general responsiveness (not present before the trauma), as indicated by three (or more) of the following:

✔ Efforts to avoid thoughts, feelings, or conversations associated with the trauma.

✔ Efforts to avoid activities, places, or people that arouse recollections of the trauma.

✔ Inability to recall important aspects of the trauma.

✔ Markedly diminished interest or participation in significant activities.

✔ Feeling of detachment or estrangement from others.

✔ Restricted range of affect (e.g., unable to have loving feelings).

✔ Sense of a foreshortened future (e.g., does not expect to have a career, marriage, children, or a normal life span).

➤ Persistent symptoms of increased arousal (not present before the trauma), as indicated by two (or more) of the following:

✔ Difficulty falling or staying asleep.

✔ Irritability or outbursts of anger.

✔ Difficulty concentrating.

✔ Hypervigilance.

✔ Exaggerated startle response.

➤ Symptoms must last longer than 1 month and cause clinically significant distress or impairment in social, occupational, or other important areas of functioning.

Clinical Issues

➤ PTSD:

✔ Is diagnosed only when all of the following five criteria are met:

■ The person is exposed to, witnesses, or is told of a traumatic event that is serious in nature (e.g., combat, sexual or physical assault or abuse, being held hostage, torture, accidents, receiving a diagnosis of a life-threatening illness), with a response of fear, helplessness, or horror.

■ The person reexperiences the traumatic event in some manner (e.g., intrusive recollections, flashbacks (while awake), nightmares (while asleep), efforts to avoid thoughts or activities associated with the trauma).

■ The person experiences increased arousal (e.g., anger outbursts, hypervigilance, difficulty sleeping, difficulty concentrating, exaggerated startle response).

■ The symptoms last longer than 1 month (to distinguish PTSD from acute stress disorder).

■ The symptoms cause clinically significant distress or functional impairment.

✔ Can be further characterized by the time of symptom onset (specifiers for PTSD):

■ Acute—duration of symptoms is less than 3 months.

■ Chronic—duration of symptoms is 3 months or more.

■ Delayed onset—onset of symptoms is at least 6 months after the stressor.

✔ Prevalence is ~8%.

✔ Is more prevalent with higher levels of trauma (e.g., war veterans: ~30%; victims of violent assault: ~20%; victims of sexual assault: ~50%; victims of traffic accident: ~10%–30%).

✔ Does not develop in everyone who experiences a traumatic event, and some individuals develop symptoms consistent with PTSD after experiencing subthreshold traumas.

✔ Increases the risk of developing another psychiatric disorder (e.g., MDD, another anxiety disorder, substance use disorder).

✔ Required differing levels of "trauma," depending on the version of DSM. DSM-III (American Psychiatric Association 1980) required the trauma to be equivalent to a life-threatening event. DSM-IV-TR (American Psychiatric Association 2000) allows less-severe traumas to qualify for a diagnosis of PTSD.

✔ Presents with characteristic findings, including:

- Psychogenic (dissociative) amnesia (inability to recall aspects of the trauma).

- Alexithymia (inability to identify or verbalize feelings).

- "Psychic numbing" (diminished responsiveness to the external world).

- Depersonalization (feeling cut off from oneself or the environment) and derealization (one and the world are not real).

- Depressive symptoms or depressive disorders.

- Impulsive, self-harming ideations/behaviors or aggressive behavior, particularly under stress or when the individual's space is invaded.

- Isolation and social withdrawal (e.g., living alone or away from others).

- "Survivor guilt" (i.e., a close friend or relative present at the time of the trauma is injured or killed).

- Significant marital (e.g., failed marriages), social (e.g., few friends), and occupational (e.g., unable to keep jobs) impairments.

✔ Has been variously described as soldier's heart (U.S. Civil War), shell shock (World War I), battle fatigue, combat neurosis, post-Vietnam syndrome, post-rape syndrome, rape-trauma syndrome, delayed stress response, abused-child syndrome, battered-wife syndrome, and accident syndrome.

✔ Experienced in Vietnam veterans is often associated with high rates of infectious illnesses (e.g., hepatitis, tuberculosis), musculoskeletal disorders (e.g., fibromyalgia, arthritis), circulatory disorders (e.g., strokes, aneurysms, hypertension, myocardial infarction), and suicides. Now recognized as having increased prevalence among returning veterans from Iraq/Afghanistan.

✔ Can be expanded to a broader classification. "Complex PTSD" is a syndrome that includes additional symptoms found in long-term trauma survivors (e.g., victims of childhood sexual abuse, survivors of political torture), such as affective dysregulation, poor impulse control, dissociation, somatization, self-destructive behaviors, and preoccupation with the perpetrator. The "Stockholm syndrome," in which kidnapped victims identify with and eventually support their captors, may also be characterized under this rubric.

✔ Various perspectives have been applied to the diagnosis, etiology, prognosis, and treatment of PTSD. Much about PTSD is unknown and unresolved. The etiology, preferred methods of treatment, length of treatment, prognosis, and whether or not this disorder belongs in the anxiety disorders group remain unsettled. In addition, there is controversy regarding how serious a traumatic event must be to satisfy criteria for PTSD. These considerations reflect the complex nature of PTSD, in that there are more unknowns than knowns about this disorder.

✔ Psychosocial treatments can be very effective and may be as helpful as medications.

Epidemiology

➤ The lifetime risk of exposure to a trauma is approximately 39%. However, the lifetime risk of developing PTSD is ~8%. There is a higher prevalence in women (up to 14%), high-risk groups (e.g., war veterans, rape victims, individuals living in countries where war and terrorism prevail), and populations with greater availability of television coverage vividly describing traumatic events.

Etiological Formulations (Poorly Understood)

Neurobiological model:

➤ A number of stress-responsive neurotransmitters (e.g., 5-HT, epinephrine, NE, cortisol, vasopressin, oxytocin, endogenous opiates) are thought to be involved in the pathogenesis of PTSD:

✔ BDZ receptor activity, thyroid functioning, and involvement of the HPA axis have been implicated.

✔ The locus coeruleus (releases NE; increases awareness and vigilance; modulates the action of the autonomic nervous system) and amygdala (processes emotions and fears) likely play a significant role in the development of PTSD.

✔ Extensive comorbidity with mood and anxiety disorders strongly implicates 5-HT and NE dysregulation.

➤ Hippocampal volume is decreased in some individuals with PTSD, suggesting brain anatomic changes as causation or consequence of PTSD.

Genetic model:

➤ A genetic predisposition increases the likelihood of developing PTSD, such that lesser traumatic events can cause PTSD in susceptible individuals.

Neurochemical associations:

➤ Stress causes release of corticotropin-releasing factor (CRF) from the hypothalamus. CRF then stimulates the pituitary to release adrenocorticotropic hormone (ACTH), which stimulates the adrenal gland to increase production of cortisol. In PTSD, CRF is increased, cortisol is decreased, and NE and epinephrine are increased. These changes result in poor adaptation to stress (low cortisol) and an exaggerated startle response (high NE and epinephrine).

Behavioral model (two-factor theory):

➤ Fear after a trauma is reinforced by subsequent avoidance of the person or the place where the trauma first occurred (classical conditioning).

Stress–diathesis model:

➤ Stress is necessary for the development of PTSD, but PTSD will occur only if additional risk factors (i.e., vulnerability) are present, such as a genetic predisposition.

Kindling model:

➤ PTSD symptoms become increasingly problematic with time (i.e., kindling effect). Antiepileptic medications (e.g., divalproex, carbamazepine, lamotrigine, phenytoin) can be beneficial treatments.

Psychodynamic factors:

➤ The trauma reactivated previous conflicts or traumas.

Threshold model:

➤ Any person will develop a stress reaction if the trauma is sufficiently intense.

Cognitive model:

➤ The patient is unable to process or rationalize the trauma that caused the event.

Comorbidity

Common comorbid disorders:

➤ Mood disorders (e.g., MDD, dysthymic disorder, bipolar disorder).
➤ Other anxiety disorders (e.g., GAD, panic disorder, OCD).
➤ Dissociative states (more common in victims of childhood abuse).
➤ Somatization disorders (extremely high comorbidity).
➤ Personality disorders (especially borderline personality disorder).
➤ Social phobia.
➤ Substance use disorders.
➤ Medical illnesses (e.g., abnormal cardiovascular function, endocrine dysregulation, altered immunosuppression).

Clinical issues related to comorbidity:

➤ Comorbidity with other psychiatric disorders is extremely high (83% of individuals with PTSD also have another psychiatric disorder). For this reason, it may be difficult to establish a diagnosis of PTSD unless the patient is asked directly about a history of traumatic events. Because of this extensive overlap with other psychiatric disorders, the etiology, treatment, and prognosis have not been as well defined as they have for other "purer" psychiatric disorders (e.g., panic disorder and OCD, which are felt to be manifestations of 5-HT dysregulation).

➤ Comorbidity with somatization disorder (i.e., physical symptoms without diagnosable physical causes) is striking. As a result, individuals with PTSD have high rates of usage of medical services and are most often seen by primary care physicians rather than by psychiatrists. This leads to a significant increase in medical costs, often without adequate treatment for the PTSD itself.

Differential Diagnosis

➤ Disorders similar to PTSD but of lesser intensity or duration:

✔ Adjustment disorder with anxiety (stressor usually not extreme; resolution usually within 6 months).

✔ Acute stress disorder (stressor required, symptoms last 1 month or less).

✔ Bereavement.

➤ Mood disorders.

➤ Phobias (avoidance behaviors).

➤ Anxiety disorders (e.g., GAD, panic disorder, OCD).

➤ Substance use disorders (especially when accompanied by hallucinations and impulsive behavior).

➤ Schizophrenia and other psychotic disorders (with hallucinations resembling flashbacks).

➤ Borderline personality disorder (especially with impulsive behavior and psychotic regressions).

➤ Neurological disorders (e.g., head injury, brain tumor, seizure disorder).

Course and Prognosis

➤ Symptom onset can be immediate or delayed:

✔ The majority of individuals exposed to a trauma do not develop PTSD, and of those who develop PTSD, a significant number recover without treatment. The onset of symptoms can be delayed for years after experiencing the traumatic event.

✔ For individuals experiencing a significant trauma, rapid intervention can potentially reduce the development of PTSD and/or facilitate recovery. However, "debriefing"(i.e., a few short therapy sessions immediately after exposure to the trauma) does not effectively protect from the development of PTSD.

➤ Once PTSD is established, the course of the disorder may become chronic, debilitating, and unrelenting.

➤ Treatment is often prompted by complaints of disturbing flashbacks, nightmares, depression, substance abuse, or work/marital problems.

➤ Symptom intensity typically waxes and wanes (as in other anxiety disorders). Symptoms may recur with exposure to situations or stimuli resembling the original trauma or on anniversaries of the trauma.

➤ Risk factors for developing PTSD include:

✔ Increasing severity of, proximity to, and duration of the traumatic event.

✔ Female gender, African American or Hispanic race/ethnicity.

✔ History of prior trauma, especially in childhood (e.g., sexual or physical abuse).

✔ History of other psychiatric disorders, especially MDD, personality disorders (especially borderline and dependent), and substance use disorders.

✔ Poor social supports (e.g., single, widowed, divorced, lower socioeconomic status).

➤ Better prognosis is indicated by:

✔ Rapid onset of symptoms, lower intensity of symptoms, and rapid intervention after the trauma. If spontaneous recovery from PTSD does not occur within the first 3 months after the trauma, a more chronic and disabling course may ensue. (Rapid intervention was provided for Gulf War veterans but not for Vietnam veterans.)

✔ Good premorbid functioning and good social supports.

✔ Absence of a psychiatric and substance abuse history.

✔ High motivation for treatment, regular attendance of therapy sessions, and absence of ongoing stressors.

Treatment

General considerations:

➤ Because of the complex nature of PTSD, treatment is usually empirical and often based on ameliorating target symptoms. As a result, there are no uniform treatment approaches.

➤ Medications and/or psychotherapy can be helpful.

Medications:

➤ Antidepressants can be useful for treating depression, anxiety, intrusive symptoms, and avoidant symptoms:

✔ SSRIs are the first-line medications for the treatment of PTSD. They reduce PTSD symptoms, treat many comorbid psychiatric disorders (e.g., MDD, panic disorder, social phobia, OCD), enhance global functioning, and reduce aggression, impulsivity, and suicidal ideations associated with PTSD. Sertraline and paroxetine are FDA approved, but other SSRIs have been shown to be effective as well (e.g., fluoxetine, fluvoxamine, citalopram).

✔ SNRIs and AtypANs (mirtazapine, nefazodone, and trazodone) can be very effective, with an early benefit of improved sleep. Trazodone is best reserved as an augmenting agent added to an SSRI. Venlafaxine and bupropion (Wellbutrin) have not been extensively studied for the treatment of PTSD.

✔ TCAs (especially amitriptyline and imipramine, but not desipramine) are effective as monotherapies (but are not FDA approved) but can be dangerous if combined with alcohol or overdosed.

✔ The MAOI phenelzine (not FDA approved) has demonstrated a robust response, with a reduction of intrusive and avoidant symptoms and an enhanced response to psychotherapy. Because of side effects, its use is generally reserved for treatment-resistant PTSD.

➤ BDZs are generally not recommended. They are not effective for many of the core PTSD symptoms, have a potential for abuse, and can be difficult to discontinue in this patient group.

➤ Mood stabilizers (e.g., carbamazepine, divalproex, lamotrigine, topiramate, gabapentin) can be helpful to control flashbacks, nightmares, impulsive behaviors, and intrusive thoughts, but have not been widely studied. Lithium has not been extensively studied, but may be helpful as an augmenting agent to reduce anger and irritability.

➤ Antipsychotic medications can be useful on a short-term basis to treat more intense and problematic symptoms (e.g., hyperarousal, hypervigilance, dissociative symptoms, aggression, and reexperiencing traumatic events).

➤ Adrenergic-inhibiting agents (reduce sympathetic-induced hyperarousal):

✔ Propranolol, a beta-adrenergic antagonist.

✔ Prazosin (Minipress), a postsynaptic alpha$_1$-receptor antagonist.

✔ Clonidine (Catapres), a presynaptic alpha$_2$-receptor agonist.

Nonpharmacological treatments:

➤ A number of therapies are effective and can be utilized with or without medications:

✔ CBTs and variants (e.g., exposure therapy, stress inoculation training, anxiety management training, virtual reality exposure, stress inoculation training).

✔ Eye movement desensitization and reprocessing (EMDR; client focuses on traumatic event while also focusing on eye movements).

✔ Individual psychotherapy, hypnosis, and psychodynamic therapy.

✔ Group therapy (especially effective for war veterans).

✔ Family/marital therapy.

➤ Debriefing (i.e., a small number of therapy sessions immediately following the trauma) is likely *not* effective for protecting against the development of PTSD, but can be effective for the treatment of acute stress disorder.

Problematic treatment issues:

➤ Achieving effective treatment can be difficult with war veterans. Missed appointments, excessive reliance on controlled substances, and poor compliance with treatment recommendations are common and can generate negative countertransference from treatment providers. Patient dropout rates and requests for help to obtain disability benefits are particularly high.

Treatment algorithm (to include CBT and/or psychotherapy):

➤ Start with paroxetine or sertraline (FDA approved).

➤ Guidelines after partial or total failure with paroxetine and sertraline are not clearly defined:

✔ For patients demonstrating partial improvement with an SSRI, augmentation with an atypical antipsychotic medication (for patients who are fearful, hypervigilant, paranoid, or psychotic), an antiadrenergic agent (for patients who are overly aroused or hyperactive or who experience dissociative episodes), or trazodone (for patients sleeping poorly) can be helpful.

✔ For patients not demonstrating improvement with SSRIs, discontinue the SSRI and consider one of the following:

■ An MAOI (particularly phenelzine).

■ A TCA (amitriptyline or imipramine, but not desipramine).

■ An antiseizure medication (e.g., carbamazepine, topiramate, lamotrigine).

■ Adrenergic-based agent (e.g., propranolol, prazosin, clonidine).

■ Inderal, if used soon after the traumatic event.

ACUTE STRESS DISORDER

➤ Acute stress disorder is defined by DSM-IV-TR as having the same qualifi-
cations as PTSD with the exception that:

   ✔ Symptom duration is 4 weeks or less.

   ✔ There is full symptom resolution.

➤ There are no FDA-approved somatic treatments available for acute stress
disorder. Treatment is targeted to symptom (e.g., insomnia, anxiety, hypervigilance, depression) relief. Psychological debriefing can be very helpful to
reduce or ameliorate symptoms and possibly to prevent the development of
PTSD.

➤ The disorder can progress to PTSD if all criteria are met.

ANXIETY DISORDER DUE TO
A GENERAL MEDICAL CONDITION

➤ The anxiety is deemed to be secondary to the consequences of a medical illness (e.g., hyperthyroidism, Cushing's syndrome).

SUBSTANCE-INDUCED
ANXIETY DISORDER

➤ The anxiety is deemed to be secondary to the effects of a substance (e.g.,
caffeine, cocaine).

ANXIETY DISORDER
NOT OTHERWISE SPECIFIED

➤ The cause of the anxiety cannot be firmly established or a sufficient number
of symptoms are not present to qualify for a known anxiety disorder.

4

SUBSTANCE-RELATED DISORDERS

Principal DSM-IV-TR Substance-Related Disorders

Substance use disorders (substance abuse and/or substance
    dependence):
    Alcohol
    Amphetamines
    Cannabis
    Cocaine
    Hallucinogens
    Inhalants
    Nicotine
    Opioids
    Phencyclidine
    Sedative, hypnotic, and anxiolytic agents
Substance-induced disorders:
    Substance intoxication:
        Alcohol
        Amphetamines
        Caffeine
        Cannabis
        Cocaine
        Hallucinogens
        Inhalants
        Opioids
        Phencyclidine
        Sedative, hypnotic, and anxiolytic agents
    Substance withdrawal:
        Alcohol
        Amphetamines
        Cocaine
        Nicotine
        Opioids
        Sedative, hypnotic, and anxiolytic agents

Substance intoxication delirium:
   Alcohol
   Amphetamines
   Cannabis
   Cocaine
   Hallucinogens
   Inhalants
   Opioids
   Phencyclidine
   Sedative, hypnotic, and anxiolytic agents
Substance withdrawal delirium:
   Alcohol
   Sedative, hypnotic, and anxiolytic agents
Substance-induced persisting dementia:
   Alcohol
   Inhalants
   Sedative, hypnotic, and anxiolytic agents
Substance-induced persisting amnestic disorder:
   Alcohol
   Sedative, hypnotic, and anxiolytic agents
Substance-induced psychotic disorder, mood disorder,
      and/or anxiety disorder:
   Alcohol
   Amphetamines
   Caffeine
   Cannabis (no mood disorder)
   Cocaine
   Hallucinogens
   Inhalants
   Opioids (no anxiety disorder)
   Phencyclidine
   Sedative, hypnotic, and anxiolytic agents
Hallucinogen persisting perception disorder (flashbacks)

Additional Substance-Related Issues

Anabolic steroids
Ephedra
Dextromethorphan
Flunitrazepam and gamma-hydroxybutyrate
Nicotine
U.S. Drug Enforcement Agency schedule classification of drugs
Street names for common drugs of abuse

SUBSTANCE USE DISORDERS

DSM-IV-TR Diagnostic Criteria for Substance Abuse (Summary)

➤ A maladaptive pattern of substance use leading to clinically significant impairment or distress, as manifested by one (or more) of the following, occurring within a 12-month period:

   ✔ Recurrent substance use resulting in a failure to fulfill major role obligations at work, school, or home (e.g., repeated absences or poor work performance related to substance use; substance-related absences, suspensions, or expulsions from school; neglect of children or household).

   ✔ Recurrent substance use in situations in which it is physically hazardous (e.g., driving an automobile or operating a machine when impaired by substance use).

   ✔ Recurrent substance-related legal problems (e.g., arrests for substance-related disorderly conduct).

   ✔ Continued substance use despite having persistent or recurrent social or interpersonal problems caused or exacerbated by the effects of the substance (e.g., arguments with spouse about consequences of intoxication, physical fights).

➤ The symptoms have never met the criteria for substance dependence for this class of substance.

DSM-IV-TR Diagnostic Criteria for Substance Dependence (Summary)

➤ A maladaptive pattern of substance use leading to clinically significant impairment or distress, as manifested by three (or more) of the following, occurring at any time in the same 12-month period:

   ✔ Tolerance, as defined by either of the following:

      ■ A need for markedly increased amounts of the substance to achieve intoxication or desired effect.

      ■ Markedly diminished response with continued use of the same amount of the substance.

   ✔ Withdrawal, as manifested by either of the following:

      ■ Characteristic withdrawal syndrome for the substance.

      ■ The same (or a closely related) substance is taken to relieve or avoid withdrawal symptoms.

   ✔ The substance is often taken in larger amounts or over a longer period than was intended.

✔ There is a persistent desire or unsuccessful efforts to cut down or control use of the substance.

✔ A great deal of time is spent in obtaining the substance (e.g., visiting multiple doctors or driving long distances), using the substance (e.g., chain-smoking), or recovering from the substance's effects.

✔ Important social, occupational, or recreational activities are given up or reduced as a result of use of the substance.

✔ The substance use is continued despite knowledge of having a persistent or recurrent physical or psychological problem that is likely to have been caused or exacerbated by the substance (e.g., current cocaine use despite recognition of cocaine-induced depression, or continued drinking despite recognition that an ulcer was made worse by alcohol consumption).

Clinical Issues Related to Substance Misuse, Substance Abuse, and Substance Dependence

Terminology:

➤ Substance misuse (not a DSM-IV-TR diagnosis) represents an overreliance on a substance for its mood-altering effects or as a means of coping with problems. However, the use does not rise to the level of abuse or dependence (i.e., a substance use disorder).

➤ DSM-IV-TR characterizes substance abuse as a pattern of *maladaptive behavior* secondary to recurrent or continued substance use. Thus, DSM-IV-TR defines substance abuse as a behavioral disorder, basing the diagnosis on the consequences rather than the amount of substance use.

➤ DSM-IV-TR characterizes substance dependence as a more problematic disorder than substance abuse in that dependence involves a greater degree of *maladaptive behavior.* Tolerance, withdrawal, and an increasing level of substance use are likely but are not required to fulfill DSM-IV-TR criteria for dependence. As with substance abuse, DSM-IV-TR defines substance dependence as a *behavioral disorder,* basing the diagnosis on the consequences rather than the amount of substance use.

➤ A useful discriminator to distinguish abuse from dependence is the concept of control:

✔ Persons who abuse but are not dependent on a substance retain control over its use, whereas persons who are dependent on a substance have lost control of their ability to stop its use.

✔ An old Japanese proverb emphasizes the issue of loss of control: "First a man takes a drink, then the drink takes a drink, then the drink takes the man."

➤ DSM-IV-TR divides substance-related disorders into substance *use* disorders (i.e., substance dependence, substance abuse) and substance-*induced* disorders (e.g., substance intoxication, substance withdrawal, substance-induced mood disorder, substance-induced psychotic disorder).

➤ By DSM-IV-TR criteria, once a person develops substance dependence, the diagnosis is retained indefinitely, even if the substance is never used again (e.g., alcohol dependence, sustained full remission).

Risk factors and prognostic issues:

➤ Substance use disorders (SUDs) are highly comorbid with virtually all categories of psychiatric disorders, especially psychotic, mood, and anxiety disorders, attention-deficit/ hyperactivity disorder, and personality disorders.

➤ Vaccines to block the reward and reinforcing effects of drugs are in development. Some promising vaccines are intended for nicotine, cocaine, methamphetamine, and phencyclidine.

➤ Stress is a strong risk factor for the initiation, continuation, and relapse of substance use disorders.

➤ Substance dependence is a relapsing illness described in treatment programs as "a disease without a cure but with effective treatments":

✔ The *total-abstinence model* states that the only acceptable goal is to completely give up the use of the substance (possibly to also include prescribed psychotropic medications [e.g., antabuse, benzodiazepines]).

✔ The *harm-reduction model* states that a reduction in substance use or transition to a safer substance rather than total abstinence represents an acceptable goal.

➤ The risk of developing a substance use disorder increases with the increasing duration and increasing amount of substance use.

➤ Prognosis for abstinence is:

✔ Poorer when:

■ The substance has been used for an extensive period of time.

■ The substance has been used at increasingly higher doses.

■ Substance use is comorbid with another psychiatric disorder.

■ There are inadequate social supports.

✔ Improved when:

■ Motivation to stop the use of the substance is high (i.e., the individual gains insight as to the magnitude and impact of his or her substance use disorder).

■ The individual is willing to engage in a 12-step program (e.g., Alcoholics Anonymous, Narcotics Anonymous).

■ Social and occupational supports are adequate and positive.

■ Stress is manageable or is maintained at a low level.

Etiological formulations for the development of a substance use disorder (more than one may be operative):

➤ Individuals who abuse substance(s) may be experiencing psychosis, anxiety, depression, or sleep problems and use substances to self-treat their symptoms.

➤ Anxiety, agitation, and depression worsen during withdrawal, thereby drawing the individual to once again utilize the substance to alleviate withdrawal symptoms.

➤ The pleasurable effects of substances are related to the release of dopamine, thereby providing reinforcement for continued abuse.

➤ The prescribed (i.e., physician-approved) use of a controlled substance may behaviorally reinforce the patient's concept of the use of a substance to satisfy emotional needs (i.e., iatrogenically induced substance use disorder).

➤ Genetics coupled with social and environmental factors have a significant impact on our likelihood to develop a substance use disorder.

Polysubstance abuse and polysubstance dependence:

➤ Always assess for the possibility of polysubstance abuse or dependence. Common examples include alcohol + nicotine, marijuana + cocaine, opioids + nicotine, and opioids + cocaine.

➤ A person stopping one substance may start another, thereby perpetuating the abuse/dependence cycle.

➤ Individuals with psychiatric disorders likely have a lower threshold for developing an SUD and should be advised of the dangers of using a mind-altering substance *in any amount.*

Dual diagnosis:

➤ Refers to comorbidity of a psychiatric disorder with a SUD. Patients with a dual diagnosis are difficult to assess accurately and difficult to treat effectively. The SUD may produce psychiatric symptoms, and the psychiatric disorder may prompt increasing substance use to "medicate" anxious, dysphoric, or psychotic symptoms. Thus, it often is difficult to establish whether the psychiatric or the substance use disorder is primary.

➤ Confers poorer treatment outcomes, higher health care utilization, and an increased risk for violence, completed suicide, child abuse/neglect, and antisocial behavior.

➤ Is difficult to treat effectively. Treatment considerations are often empirical. Despite continued substance use, patients with comorbid psychiatric disorders can likely benefit from psychotropic medications for the comorbid psychiatric disorder (very controversial). Avoid medications that can be abused (e.g., benzodiazepines).

Epidemiology and outcomes:

➤ The lifetime prevalence for developing a substance-related disorder is approximately 27% (not including nicotine-related disorders). Approximately 80% of crimes resulting in prison sentences are committed by individuals with substance-related disorders.

➤ Outcomes are inconsistent and unpredictable. Some individuals, even after years of use, are able to permanently stop their use of a substance without any formal treatment, whereas other individuals, despite repeated involvement in treatment programs, are not able to stop their substance use for any significant length of time. Substance-related disorders affect everyone who comes in contact with the user. Participation in family therapy, marital therapy, and Al-Anon–type groups are strongly encouraged.

➤ Commonly, persons with substance-related disorders are in denial about the consequences of their substance use, often underestimating the extent and impact of their substance use on their lives and the lives of people around them.

➤ Nicotine dependence (cigarette smoking) is the most prevalent substance use disorder.

➤ SUDs in the elderly (principally alcohol and benzodiazepines) are much more prevalent than is commonly appreciated by primary care providers.

SUBSTANCE-INDUCED DISORDERS

DSM-IV-TR Diagnostic Criteria for Substance Intoxication (Summary)

➤ Development of a reversible substance-specific syndrome due to recent ingestion of (or exposure to) a substance. Different substances may produce similar or identical syndromes.

➤ Clinically significant maladaptive behavioral or psychological changes that are due to the effect of the substance on the central nervous system (CNS) (e.g., belligerence, mood lability, cognitive impairment, impaired judgment, impaired social or occupational functioning) and develop during or shortly after use of the substance.

➤ The symptoms are not due to a general medical condition and are not better accounted for by another psychiatric disorder.

Clinical Issues

➤ Symptoms are reversible in that they develop as the direct consequence of using the substance and result in maladaptive behavior or consequences (e.g., substance-induced mood disorder, substance-induced anxiety disorder).

➤ In general, the larger the dose of the substance, the greater the intoxicating effects. Still-higher doses can lead to toxicity, possibly followed by death for some substances (e.g., alcohol, cocaine, heroin).

DSM-IV-TR Diagnostic Criteria for Substance Withdrawal (Summary)

➤ Development of a substance-specific syndrome due to the cessation of (or reduction in) substance use that has been heavy or prolonged.

➤ The substance-specific syndrome causes clinically significant distress or impairment in social, occupational, or other important areas of functioning.

➤ The symptoms are not due to a general medical condition and are not better accounted for by another psychiatric disorder.

Clinical Issues

➤ Withdrawal is a state of *hyperexcitability* generated by a rapid decline in the blood level of the active substance. After intoxication, abruptly stopping the substance may be followed by:

✔ No withdrawal syndrome (e.g., for alcohol, "sleeping it off").

✔ A full-blown withdrawal syndrome (e.g., for alcohol, withdrawal seizures, delirium tremens).

✔ Reversal of a developing withdrawal syndrome through reuse of the substance or through use of a cross-tolerant drug (e.g., for alcohol withdrawal, administering alcohol or chlordiazepoxide [Librium]).

➤ In general, the potential to develop a withdrawal syndrome increases the more rapidly the blood level of the substance falls after slowing or stopping its use. Thus, short-half-life agents without active metabolites (e.g., alprazolam [Xanax]) are more prone to withdrawal symptoms than longer-half-life agents with active metabolites (e.g., chlordiazepoxide). A reduction in use of a substance can be sufficient to precipitate a withdrawal syndrome if the blood level of the drug falls rapidly. Therefore, the term *abstinence syndrome* is not an accurate equivalence to withdrawal syndrome.

ALCOHOL-RELATED DISORDERS

Clinical Issues

➤ Alcohol-related neuropsychiatric disorders (Table 4–1) can produce virtually any psychiatric symptom or combination of symptoms. It is prudent to assess for alcohol-related disorders in all persons presenting with psychiatric symptoms.

▆ Table 4–1 Alcohol-related neuropsychiatric disorders

Disorder	Usual time frame for symptoms to develop	Possible signs and symptoms	Treatment
Alcohol intoxication	Immediately after use, as alcohol blood level rises	Acute intoxicating effects of alcohol (e.g., slurring of speech, incoordination, nystagmus, stupor). Impaired cognitive functioning and blackouts (memory lapses while intoxicated). Falls, hematomas, broken bones. At higher doses, respiratory depression, coma, and death. Hypothermia in cold weather death.	"Sleeping it off" (unless a withdrawal syndrome develops).
Alcohol withdrawal syndrome			
Uncomplicated withdrawal	6–18 hours after stopping drinking	Tremulousness ("shakes"), particularly of the hands, tongue, and eyelids, is the classic sign of withdrawal. Additional symptoms include nausea/vomiting, anxiety, facial flushing, elevated blood pressure, and tachycardia. Alcohol craving.	Benzodiazepines, typically oral chlordiazepoxide or diazepam. For elderly patients, lorazepam or oxazepam (no active metabolites). Thiamine 100 mg/day. Folic acid 1 mg/day. Antipsychotics can be added adjunctively if symptoms are severe or worsen.
Withdrawal seizures	6–36 hours after stopping drinking	Grand mal seizures, possibly with status epilepticus. Occur in 5%–10% of individuals experiencing alcohol withdrawal. Risk increases with previous episodes of withdrawal seizures (i.e., kindling).	Long-acting benzodiazepines are preferred. Other medications can be tried (e.g., mood stabilizers, clonidine, phenobarbital), but none are better than benzodiazepines. Thiamine 100 mg/day. Folic acid 1 mg/day. Antipsychotics can be added adjunctively if symptoms are severe or worsen.

■ Table 4–1 Alcohol-related neuropsychiatric disorders *(continued)*

Disorder	Usual time frame for symptoms to develop	Possible signs and symptoms	Treatment
Alcohol withdrawal syndrome *(continued)*			
Withdrawal delirium (delirium tremens [DTs])	1–4 days after stopping drinking	A true medical emergency. Most severe form of withdrawal. Develops in less than 5% of persons who experience alcohol withdrawal. Classic symptoms include confusion, cognitive impairment, and hallucinations. Delirium, extreme autonomic nervous system hyperactivity (tachycardia, hypertension, flushing, diaphoresis, anxiety, insomnia), hallucinations (visual, auditory, tactile [formication]), hyperactivity, agitation, poor sleep with frightening dreams, assaultive potential, suicide. Risk increases with poor physical health, prior history of DTs, and history of alcohol withdrawal seizures. Lasts approximately 15 days. Untreated, mortality can be as high as 35%.	Prevention (by using benzodiazepines early in the treatment of withdrawal). If DTs develop, increase the benzodiazepine dose and consider an antipsychotic for psychotic symptoms. Hydrate and stabilize vital signs. Improve nutritional status. Thiamine 100 mg/day. Folic acid 1 mg/day. Antipsychotics can be added adjunctively if symptoms are severe or worsen.

Table 4–1   Alcohol-related neuropsychiatric disorders (continued)

Disorder	Usual time frame for symptoms to develop	Possible signs and symptoms	Treatment
Alcohol-induced syndromes			
Alcohol-induced psychotic disorder, with hallucinations	12–48 hours after stopping drinking	Auditory hallucinations in a clear sensorium after abrupt cessation of heavy drinking. Lasts about 1 week, clears spontaneously in several months. Usually develops in patients with long-term alcohol abuse or dependence.	Benzodiazepines, improved nutritional status, and fluids. If symptoms are severe, add high-potency antipsychotics.
Alcohol-induced persisting dementia	After long-term use	Dementia (may be hard to distinguish from dementia due to other disorders and conditions [e.g., nutritional deficits, head injuries]). Global cognitive deficits. Poor nutrition and multiple medical problems are common. Brain atrophy may be evident on magnetic resonance imaging. Not universally accepted as a valid disorder secondary to likely complicating factors (e.g., poor nutrition, history of head injuries, physical illnesses) that can also produce dementia.	Rule out treatable causes of dementia. Improve physical health, nutritional status. Safety, caretaking considerations. Acetylcholine esterase inhibitors can be tried.

■ Table 4–1   Alcohol-related neuropsychiatric disorders *(continued)*

Disorder	Usual time frame for symptoms to develop	Possible signs and symptoms	Treatment
Alcohol-induced syndromes *(continued)*			
Wernicke's encephalopathy	After long-term use	Secondary to thiamine deficiency. Often precipitated by administering glucose to a malnourished alcohol-dependent individual without pretreatment with thiamine. Bilateral lesions or hemorrhages in mammillary bodies, thalamus, and hypothalamus due to thiamine deficiency. Confusion, ataxia, nystagmus, and ophthalmoplegia are classic signs. Acute disorder, reversible. Can progress to Korsakoff's syndrome.	Thiamine 100 mg/day for 25 days. Folic acid, multivitamins, improve nutritional status.
Alcohol-induced persisting amnestic disorder (Korsakoff's syndrome)	After long-term use	Secondary to thiamine deficiency. Possible consequence of Wernicke's encephalopathy, but can also occur in the absence of Wernicke's encephalopathy. Bilateral lesions or hemorrhages in mammillary bodies, diencephalon, and hippocampus. Significant anterograde amnesia in a clear sensorium. Confabulation (a hallmark finding of the disorder) is used to fill in memory gaps. Oriented to person but often not to current circumstance. Poor prognosis for recovery from amnesia (i.e., permanent damage).	Thiamine (100 mg bid–tid for 3–12 months). Folic acid, multivitamins, improve nutritional status.

Table 4–1 Alcohol-related neuropsychiatric disorders *(continued)*			
Disorder	**Usual time frame for symptoms to develop**	**Possible signs and symptoms**	**Treatment**
Alcohol-induced syndromes *(continued)*			
Alcohol idiosyncratic intoxication (not a DSM-IV-TR diagnosis; controversial diagnosis)	Onset with drinking small amounts of alcohol	Sudden onset of marked and often impulsive, dangerous, or aggressive behavior. Confusion, visual hallucinations, delusions, illusions. Followed by a prolonged sleep, with amnesia for the event. May be invoked as a legal defense.	Antipsychotic medication. Possible restraints.
Other alcohol-induced disorders		Alcohol-induced mood disorder, alcohol-induced anxiety disorder, alcohol-induced sexual dysfunction, alcohol-induced sleep disorder.	Individualized treatment dependent on the disorder.

➤ Twelve ounces of beer or wine cooler = 5 ounces of wine = 1.5 ounces of 80-proof distilled spirits = 12 grams of pure alcohol = "a drink." Proof designation equates to two times the alcohol percentage (e.g., a 160-proof beverage contains 80% alcohol).

➤ The National Institute on Alcohol Abuse and Alcoholism defines *moderate drinking* according to age and gender:

   ✔ Men younger than 65 years—no more than two drinks per day.

   ✔ Women younger than 65 years of age—no more than one drink per day.

   ✔ Individuals older than 65 years—no more than one drink per day.

➤ Individuals who are pregnant, use machinery, have liver disease, are recovering alcoholics, or who take medications that interact with alcohol should not use alcohol.

➤ Reasons individuals may give for drinking excessively:

   ✔ Pleasure from the intoxicating effects.

   ✔ Boredom and loneliness ("alcohol is my best friend").

   ✔ To treat depression (despite alcohol being a depressant).

   ✔ To treat anxiety (despite increased anxiety during the withdrawal phase).

   ✔ To treat insomnia (despite impairment of deep-sleep patterns).

   ✔ To cope with guilt and remorse (often over excessive drinking, creating a vicious cycle).

   ✔ To reduce physical pain.

   ✔ To regain a feeling of normality ("I was born a pint low").

   ✔ To come down from the effects of stimulants (e.g., cocaine, methylphenidate).

   ✔ To augment the intoxicating effects of other drugs (i.e., barbiturates, heroin, benzodiazepines).

➤ Classically, tremulousness signals the onset of an alcohol withdrawal syndrome (a hyperexcitability state). Should the process continue unabated, more severe symptoms (e.g., aggressiveness, hallucinations, delusions, grand mal seizures, delirium tremens, respiratory depression) can develop. Death can follow if symptoms are severe and/or if the person is medically compromised.

➤ Withdrawal symptoms can be reduced or eliminated by administering alcohol or cross-tolerant agents (e.g., benzodiazepines, barbiturates) or the antiseizure medications valproate or carbamazepine.

➤ Alcohol abuse and dependence may be genetically unrelated disorders, in that continued abuse may not necessarily lead to dependence.

➤ Terminology not associated with DSM-IV-TR:

   ✔ *Dry drunk syndrome* refers to a condition in which an individual's thinking and actions reflect the consequences of active drinking despite the fact that the individual is maintaining sobriety. Symptoms include grandiose behavior, impatience, compulsiveness, clouded thinking, irresponsible actions, and overreaction.

✔ *Falling off the wagon* refers to an individual's resuming drinking after a period of abstinence.

✔ *Holiday heart syndrome* refers to episodes of abnormal heart rhythm associated with alcohol withdrawal, possibly leading to sudden death.

✔ *Protracted withdrawal syndrome* refers to the persistence—potentially for a year or more after drinking has been discontinued—of autonomic hyperactivity, coupled with anxiety, depression, and sleep disturbances. The risk of relapse during this period is particularly high.

➤ Twelve-step programs (e.g., Alcoholics Anonymous) are considered an integral (if not an essential) part of the successful treatment of alcohol dependence.

➤ Distilled spirits allow for a greater intake of alcohol due to the higher concentration of alcohol. The daily consumption of a fifth of spirits (i.e., $\frac{1}{5}$ gallon; 750 mL), ¾–1 gallon of wine, or 6–24 beers is highly consistent with alcohol dependence. When alcohol is unavailable, an alcohol-dependent individual may substitute a toxic substance (e.g., methyl alcohol, isopropyl alcohol, antifreeze, Sterno), resulting in severe medical consequences and a much firmer establishment of a diagnosis of alcohol dependence.

➤ Malnutrition is a common consequence of alcohol dependence. As much as one-half of the individual's daily calories may come from alcohol, which has no true nutritional value. Excessive drinking can result in deficiencies in vitamins B (e.g., thiamine, niacin, riboflavin, pyridoxine), A, D, C, and E. Hypomagnesemia, hypoalbuminemia, and macrocytic anemia are often evident in malnourished, vitamin-deficient alcohol-dependent individuals. In an emergency setting, thiamine should be administered before or with glucose to protect against induction of Wernicke's encephalopathy.

Neurobiological Considerations

➤ The nucleus accumbens (reward center) and the neurotransmitters dopamine, gamma-aminobutyric acid (GABA), glutamate, and endogenous opiates have been implicated in alcohol abuse, dependence, intoxication, and withdrawal.

➤ Alcohol increases the activity of the inhibitory neurotransmitter GABA and decreases the activity of the excitatory neurotransmitter glutamate. When alcohol use suddenly stops after intoxication, the effects of alcohol on these two neurotransmitters are suddenly lost (GABA activity decreases and glutamate activity increases). This produces a hyperexcitable state characteristic of an alcohol withdrawal syndrome.

➤ Currently, GABAergic agents (i.e., benzodiazepines) are the primary medications used in the United States to treat alcohol withdrawal symptoms. The GABAergic agents valproate and carbamazepine are commonly used in Europe for alcohol withdrawal. However, glutamate inhibitors hold great promise as medications to reverse alcohol withdrawal states.

Health Consequences of Alcohol Use

➤ Positive effects of moderate alcohol use include:
- ✔ Reduced risk of a myocardial infarction and cerebrovascular accident, possibly due to reduced platelet stickiness. Red wine seems to have the greatest impact on these positive benefits (controversial).
- ✔ Increased levels of high-density lipoprotein (HDL) cholesterol.
- ✔ Increased bone density in women (possibly due to increased estrogen).

➤ Negative effects of moderate to severe alcohol use include:
- ✔ Alcohol intoxication:
  - ■ Clinical symptoms of alcohol intoxication develop with increasing blood levels. When the blood alcohol level rises to 0.3%–0.5% (legal driving limit is 0.08%–0.10%), respiratory depression, coma, and death can follow.
- ✔ Life-threatening hypothermia can occur when an individual is intoxicated and exposed to very cold weather because of the body's inability to constrict peripheral blood vessels and conserve body heat (e.g., a common finding in the "skid-row bum").
- ✔ Potentially severe withdrawal syndromes, especially if the individual is medically compromised, malnourished, and/or B vitamin deficient (e.g., seizures, delirium tremens).
- ✔ Medical sequelae from excessive long-term drinking (e.g., cardiovascular disease, hepatic disease, cancers, gastrointestinal bleeds, amnestic syndromes, dementia).

Epidemiology

➤ Alcohol-related disorders:
- ✔ Occur in 3%–20% of patients seen by primary care physicians but are much less often diagnosed.
- ✔ Are highly prevalent in persons involved in automobile accidents and fatalities, suicides, homicides, assaults, rapes, drownings, and child abuse.
- ✔ Result in about a 10-year reduction in life expectancy (for long-term excessive use).

✔ Are especially prevalent in:

  ■ Native Americans and Alaska Natives (as compared with Chinese Americans, Japanese Americans, and Eastern European descendants of Orthodox Jews).

  ■ Construction and food service workers.

  ■ Adolescents, young adults, and the elderly.

➤ Age factors:

  ✔ The average age at onset of abuse is 17 years and of dependence is 22 years. The lower the age when drinking begins, the greater potential for dependence to develop.

  ✔ In comparison with men, women begin drinking later in life, are more likely to hide their drinking, and are likely to develop more serious medical problems within a shorter period of time.

➤ Lifetime prevalence:

  ✔ 10% of women and 20% of men will develop alcohol abuse.

  ✔ 3%–5% of women and 13% of men will develop alcohol dependence.

  ✔ In all, the lifetime prevalence of developing an alcohol use disorder in the United States is 13.6%.

➤ Heavy use:

  ✔ Hispanics > whites > African Americans.

➤ Comorbidity:

  ✔ Alcohol use disorders are highly comorbid with other psychiatric disorders (bipolar I disorder = 46%, bipolar II disorder = 39%, schizophrenia = 34%, personality disorders = 29%, major depressive disorder = 17%, general population = 14%).

➤ Medical consequences of heavy use:

  ✔ African Americans > whites.

Adverse Systemic Effects of Acute and Chronic Alcohol Use

Neurological:

➤ Cerebellar degeneration, producing ataxia and a wide-stanced gait.

➤ Peripheral neuropathy with symptoms of paresthesias (tingling, burning) and/or pain in feet and legs ("stocking-glove" distribution).

➤ Impaired temperature regulation with increased cutaneous blood flow and decreased core body temperature (possibly leading to fatal hypothermia with exposure to cold temperatures).

➤ Dulling of taste and smell.

➤ Reduction in pain sensation that increases with increasing dose (i.e., alcohol is an anesthetic at higher doses). Sores developing from lack of sensation can become infected and progress systemically.

➤ Impairment of permanent acquisition of new information while intoxicated (anterograde amnesia), with less effect on retrieval of previously stored material (retrograde amnesia). Classically described as a blackout, information can only be recalled for a very short time, and long-term memory tracks are never laid down.

➤ Induction of sleep, but with alterations in rapid eye movement (REM) sleep patterns and a reduction in deep levels of sleeping.

➤ Dementia can develop from multiple causes, including:

  ✔ Direct toxic effects of alcohol on the brain (e.g., alcohol-induced persisting dementia).

  ✔ Hepatocerebral degeneration. Hepatic damage can lead to ammonia buildup when the liver cannot convert ammonia to urea. Ammonia is toxic to the brain, especially the basal ganglia, leading to tremors, twitching, and involuntary movements.

  ✔ Marchiafava-Bignami disease ("Italian wine-drinker's disease"). Progressive degeneration of the corpus callosum results in neurological deficits (e.g., mutism, impaired comprehension of spoken language).

  ✔ Pellagra encephalopathy (due to a dietary deficiency of niacin). Findings include the classic presentation of pellagra (the "3 D's": dementia, diarrhea, and dermatitis).

Gastrointestinal:

➤ Esophagitis.

➤ Esophageal varices (veins close to the surface of the esophagus that become dilated as a consequence of chronic drinking), which are especially vulnerable to rupturing during vomiting or retching. The resultant bleeding can be life-threatening.

➤ Throat and esophageal cancer (especially when alcohol use is combined with cigarette smoking and poor mouth hygiene).

➤ Increased stomach acid production, leading to gastritis, esophageal reflux, peptic ulcers (with production of bright-red blood from the rectum and a positive fecal blood test), and duodenal ulcers (with production of charcoal- or black-colored stools and a positive fecal blood test).

➤ Decreased absorption of nutrients (e.g., folate, vitamin B_{12}, thiamine, niacin, calcium, magnesium) due to increased intestinal motility (possibly with diarrhea) and decreased absorption from the small intestine.

➤ Hepatic injury (from direct toxic effects of alcohol and/or from chronically poor nutritional status:

  ✔ Elevated liver enzymes (aspartate transaminase [AST], alanine transaminase [ALT], gamma-glutamyltransferase [GGT]).

  ✔ Dysregulation of lipid metabolism, with elevations in triglyceride and HDL levels.

  ✔ Hypoglycemia, possibly leading to coma.

  ✔ Fatty liver (observed on physical examination as a palpable liver).

  ✔ Alcoholic hepatitis.

  ✔ Possible concurrent hepatitis C, with its negative impact on liver function.

  ✔ Cirrhosis (develops in 10%–20% of alcohol-dependent individuals), with possible consequences of jaundice, ascites, hepatic encephalopathy with some combination of asterixis (flapping tremor), portal hypertension, impaired cognition, coma, and death.

  ✔ Hepatocellular carcinoma.

  ✔ Impaired metabolism, possibly leading to production of ammonia and other toxins that can cause brain damage.

➤ Gout (due to impairment of purine metabolism, producing elevated serum uric acid)—often a clue to excessive drinking.

Hematological:

➤ Decreased serum albumin (from poor nutrition).

➤ Iron-deficiency anemia (from bone marrow suppression, gastrointestinal bleeding, poor nutrition, coagulation defects, liver disease, or portal hypertension).

➤ Morphological changes in red blood cells (e.g., elevated mean corpuscular volume [MCV]).

➤ Leukopenia (due to bone marrow suppression).

➤ Thrombocytopenia (secondary to splenic enlargement with sequestering of platelets and secondary to bone marrow suppression).

➤ Blood-sludging, secondary to blood cells clumping and blocking small blood vessels, resulting in cell death.

Muscular:

➤ Muscle weakness and muscle deterioration.

➤ Cardiomyopathy (due to direct effects of alcohol on the heart muscle and secondary to thiamine deficiency ["beriberi heart disease"]).

Renal:

➤ Reduced excretion of uric acid, possibly resulting in gout (especially in males).

➤ Renal failure as a consequence of hypertension from long-term drinking or from the direct toxic effects of alcohol on the kidney.

Pancreatic:

➤ Recurrent pancreatitis (leads to significant increases in serum amylase).

➤ Pancreatic pseudocyst.

➤ Pancreatic cancer.

Splenic:

➤ Enlarged spleen (secondary to sequestering blood cells).

Cardiovascular:

➤ Elevated blood pressure, possibly developing into sustained hypertension with subsequent cardiovascular disease.

➤ Increased pulse, possibly developing into sustained sinus tachycardia.

➤ Cardiac conduction changes or atrial fibrillation after heavy episodes of drinking ("holiday heart syndrome").

➤ Increased risk of myocardial infarction and cerebrovascular accident.

➤ Alcoholic cardiomyopathy and congestive heart failure (typically found after about 10 years of heavy alcohol use), due in part to the direct toxic effects of alcohol on the heart muscle.

Pulmonary:

➤ Increased susceptibility to tuberculosis and gram-negative infections.

➤ Chronic obstructive lung disease, reversible airway disease, and recurrent bronchitis (due to heavy rates of smoking in alcohol-dependent persons).

➤ Aspiration pneumonia during acute intoxication.

➤ Depression of pulmonary functioning during acute intoxication (additive to other pulmonary depressants [e.g., benzodiazepines, opioids]).

Infections:

➤ Decreased immunity, resulting in increased susceptibility to infections (e.g., meningitis, gram-negative pulmonary infections, tuberculosis).

Endocrinological:

➤ Hypoglycemia (after acute intoxication) and diabetes mellitus (with long-term use).

➤ In men:

  ✔ Testicular atrophy with decreased testosterone production and increased estrogen, leading to the development of female sexual characteristics (e.g., gynecomastia), loss of male secondary sexual characteristics, decreased libido, erectile dysfunction, orgasmic impairment, and decreased ability to inseminate a fertile egg.

➤ In women:

   ✔ Increased estrogen production, leading to menstrual irregularities, decreased libido, orgasmic impairment, and decreased fertility.

Oncological:

➤ Increased incidence of cancers (e.g., mouth, tongue, larynx, esophagus, stomach, liver, pancreas).

Dermatological:

➤ Facial telangiectasias, palmar erythema, rosacea, spider angiomas, white nails, plethoric facies, bruises, seborrheic dermatitis, visible abdominal wall veins, and cigarette-stained fingers or cigarette burns.

Oral:

➤ Smell of alcohol (typically associated with a blood alcohol level of greater than 0.08%).

➤ Periodontal disease.

➤ Throat cancers (the risk increases with a combination of alcohol, cigarette smoking, and poor mouth hygiene).

➤ Parotid gland enlargement ("alcoholic parotid sialadenosis").

Nutritional status:

➤ Impaired absorption of important micronutrients (e.g., vitamins, minerals).

➤ Emaciation with bloated abdomen (ascites fluid buildup) in advanced stages of dependence.

Other Adverse Effects of Acute and Chronic Alcohol Use

➤ Increased incidence of trauma (e.g., due to falls, accidents, or fights while intoxicated), possibly leading to posttraumatic stress disorder:

   ✔ Head injuries (e.g., concussions, cerebrovascular accidents, seizure disorder).

   ✔ Fractures (often evidenced on X rays as "old fractures").

   ✔ Avascular necrosis of the femoral head (more common in young adults).

➤ Increased mortality:

   ✔ The mortality rate secondary to alcohol-related disorders is three times greater than in the general population, from a wide variety of causes (e.g., accidents, cirrhosis of the liver, suicide, malnutrition, hypothermia, head injury, myocardial infarction).

➤ Fetal alcohol syndrome (alcohol-induced birth defects resulting from fetal exposure to alcohol):

   ✔ Findings include:

- Intrauterine growth retardation, smaller birth weight, and subsequent growth retardation.
- Characteristic facial anomalies, including narrow eye span, low-set ears, and microcephaly.
- Cardiac and skeletal malformations.
- Developmental delays, ADHD, learning disabilities, behavioral problems, and mental retardation.

✔ A "safe" amount of drinking during pregnancy has not been established. The incidence of fetal alcohol syndrome is 10%–15% for mothers who drink "excessively" during pregnancy. The effects on the fetus appear to increase with increasing alcohol use, especially during the first trimester. It is therefore prudent to recommend absolute avoidance of alcohol during pregnancy.

Clinical Assessment and Testing

➤ The CAGE Questionnaire is a widely used instrument for identifying problems with alcohol (2 out of 4 questions answered positively is 70%–80% indicative of alcohol dependence; 4 out of 4 questions answered positively is nearly 100% indicative of alcohol dependence):

✔ C   Cut down on drinking (unsuccessful attempts).

✔ A   Annoyed by criticism of drinking (by friends, family).

✔ G   Guilt feelings for drinking.

✔ E   Eye-opener (need to drink in the morning to reverse withdrawal symptoms).

➤ The Revised Michigan Alcoholism Screening Test is a 24-question test about drinking patterns, with a 90% sensitivity for detecting an alcohol-related problem.

➤ The Alcohol Use Disorders Identification Test is a 10-question test related to drinking patterns that reliably assesses for an alcohol-related problem in the general population (especially in women).

Psychiatric Disorders Often Comorbid With Alcohol-Related Disorders

➤ Mood disorders:

✔ Approximately 35% of individuals with alcohol-related disorders present with depressive symptoms consistent with a diagnosis of a mood disorder:

- It is important to determine if the depression is secondary to alcohol use (i.e., alcohol-induced mood disorder), a medical disorder (i.e., mood disorder due to a general medical condition), or a primary disorder (e.g., unipolar depression, bipolar depression) unrelated to alcohol use. Suicide rates are higher when mood and alcohol-related disorders are comorbid.

- ■ Depressive symptoms induced by alcohol typically clear within 2 days to 4 weeks after detoxification. If symptoms persist or if the depression predates the alcohol abuse, antidepressants (e.g., SSRIs; avoid TCAs) can be started.
- ✔ Alcohol-related disorders are frequently comorbid with bipolar disorder.
- ✔ When alcohol dependence is comorbid with a mood disorder, prognosis is poorer and suicide rates are higher than when either disorder is present alone.
- ➤ Anxiety disorders:
  - ✔ Approximately 25%–50% of persons with alcohol-related disorders also meet the criteria for an anxiety disorder (most often panic disorder and social phobia). Suicide rates are higher when alcohol dependence and an anxiety disorder are comorbid.
- ➤ Other substance-related disorders (e.g., nicotine, marijuana, cocaine, heroin).
- ➤ Personality disorders (particularly borderline and antisocial personality disorders).
- ➤ ADHD or conduct disorder.
- ➤ Schizophrenia.

Etiological Formulations of Alcohol-Related Disorders

Genetic/familial formulations:

- ➤ Alcohol-related disorders are more prominent in individuals with a family history of alcohol-related disorders.
- ➤ Men and women differ in their ability to detoxify alcohol, possibly due to differences in lean body mass, liver size, or the activity of enzymes that metabolize alcohol in the liver.
- ➤ Genetic polymorphism (variability) in rates of metabolism and the magnitude of dopamine release from the ventral tegmental area can lead to widely variable effects in different races.

Behavioral and learning formulations:

- ➤ Alcohol-related disorders develop because the individual learns by observing, during the developmental years, family members who drink.

Social and cultural formulations:

- ➤ Certain social settings predispose to excessive drinking (e.g., college campuses, military bases).
- ➤ Certain cultural groups predispose to excessive drinking (e.g., adolescents, Hispanics, Native Americans).

Psychological formulations:

➤ Alcohol is used to self-medicate (e.g., psychosis, anxiety, depression, insomnia).

Developmental formulations:

➤ Individuals with alcohol-related disorders have a greater likelihood of having a personality disorder, ADHD, or conduct disorder.

Psychoanalytic formulations:

➤ Alcohol reduces stress caused by an overpunitive superego (e.g., to reduce self-imposed guilt over heavy drinking).

➤ Alcohol reduces inhibition (i.e., the superego "dissolves" in alcohol), and as a consequence, drinking continues.

Physiological Consequences of Drinking Alcohol

Alcohol blood levels and absorption:

➤ One drink raises the blood alcohol concentration (BAC) an average of 0.015%–0.02%. Alcohol enters the body water, such that the higher the body fat–to–lean muscle ratio, the higher the BAC per drink.

➤ Absorption is rapid (more so for women), with 20% absorbed from the stomach and 80% absorbed from the small intestine.

➤ Carbonation increases and food decreases the rate of alcohol absorption.

Metabolism of alcohol:

➤ Ninety percent of ethyl alcohol is metabolized by oxidation in the liver, and 10% is excreted unchanged in urine, sweat, and expired air (thereby providing the basis for the Breathalyzer Test).

➤ Alcohol dehydrogenase (at least nine forms are recognized) is responsible for the breakdown of alcohol to acetaldehyde. Acetaldehyde (a toxic substance) is then metabolized by aldehyde dehydrogenase to acetic acid. Disulfiram (Antabuse) blocks this latter conversion, with the resultant buildup of toxic acetaldehyde. Also, acetaldehyde is felt to be partially responsible for the hangover.

➤ Women may have lower levels of aldehyde dehydrogenase in gastric stomach lining than men, resulting in a greater potential for intoxication when using equal amounts of alcohol as men.

➤ The rate of metabolism is relatively constant, at approximately 1 drink/hour (~0.15% BAC/hour). However, at higher blood alcohol levels, the rate of metabolism is significantly slowed, resulting in a much longer period of intoxication and possibly alcohol toxicity.

➤ When methyl alcohol (commonly used to denature ethanol, rendering it undrinkable) is substituted for ethyl alcohol, it is converted to formaldehyde by alcohol dehydrogenase. Formaldehyde is extremely toxic and, along with methyl alcohol, can result in permanent blindness.

BAC and resultant physiological effects in alcohol-naive persons:

➤ 0.01%–0.03%—generally not intoxicated (feeling of well-being, tranquility; skin flushed; decreased inhibitions).

➤ 0.03%–0.08%—mild to moderate intoxication (e.g., mild to moderate cognitive impairment, poor coordination), alcohol smell on breath (~0.08%).

➤ 0.08%–0.2%—obvious intoxication, increasing cognitive deficits, ataxia, and slurred speech.

➤ 0.2%–0.4%—variable effects (e.g., sleep, unconsciousness, inability to constrict arterial blood vessels in the cold, incontinence, lowered body temperature, poor respiratory effort, fall in blood pressure, anesthesia, coma, death).

➤ 0.4%–0.5%—death in about 50% of users (median lethal dose [LD_{50}]), often from respiratory failure and/or asphyxiation from aspirated regurgitated gastric contents. This LD_{50} may be operative for alcohol-dependent persons as well.

➤ The absence of observable intoxicating effects at blood alcohol levels above 0.1% is suggestive of alcohol dependence, whereas intoxicating effects in non–alcohol-dependent individuals can occur at blood levels significantly below the legal driving limit (typically defined as 0.08–0.10%).

General Patterns of Alcohol Dependence

➤ Heavy drinking can be defined as having more than two drinks a day for men and more than one drink a day for women.

➤ Binge drinking is drinking sufficiently to bring the BAC to 0.08% within a short period of time (~2 hours).

➤ Male pattern:
  ✔ Alcohol use develops insidiously, often starts in the mid- to late teens, is not recognized as a problem until age 30 or later, and has an association with antisocial behavior. Men are more likely than women to binge-drink and become heavy drinkers.

➤ Female pattern:
  ✔ Alcohol use generally starts later in life, spontaneous remissions are less likely, and there is a greater potential for significant medical sequelae in a shorter period of time.

Treatment of Alcohol Withdrawal Syndrome (Detoxification)

➤ Administer an oral long-acting benzodiazepine (e.g., chlordiazepoxide, diazepam) or oral short-acting benzodiazepine (e.g., lorazepam, oxazepam), with the dosage and frequency of administration based on a monitoring scale such as the Clinical Institute Withdrawal Assessment for Alcohol—Revised (CIWA-Ar), a 10-item scale for assessing the intensity of withdrawal symptoms and treatment response:

✔ Treatment is safer on an inpatient unit than as an outpatient and typically lasts 2–6 days.

✔ Longer-acting benzodiazepines provide greater protection from breakthrough symptoms during withdrawal, reduce the potential for developing withdrawal seizures and delirium tremens, and provide a smoother withdrawal, but pose a greater risk of sedation (especially in patients who are elderly or have liver disease) than do the shorter-acting benzodiazepines. Diazepam has the added benefit of being available in intravenous dosage (IV) form (intramuscular [IM] administration can produce erratic results).

✔ A typical starting daily dose of chlordiazepoxide ranges from 25 mg tid to 100 mg qid (or more), with a gradual daily downward titration. A rigid schedule (i.e., no dosing adjustments), a flexible dosing schedule (i.e., prn use), and front-loading (high initial dosing until calming is evident) are common treatment protocols.

➤ Barbiturates (particularly phenobarbital), clonidine, beta-blockers, phenothiazines, and antiepileptic medications (e.g., phenytoin, carbamazepine, divalproex, gabapentin) are not widely advocated as primary agents for alcohol withdrawal, although some are used extensively outside the United States for this purpose.

➤ Administer adjunctive medications during detoxification to treat specific symptoms:

✔ Antipsychotic medications can help reduce psychotic symptoms (e.g., hallucinations) or persistent or escalating anxiety or agitation.

✔ Alpha$_2$-adrenergic agonists (e.g., clonidine) can help reduce excessive autonomic hyperactivity (e.g., elevated blood pressure, elevated pulse).

✔ Beta-blockers (e.g., propranolol) can help reduce excessive autonomic hyperactivity and somatic anxiety.

➤ For persons experiencing withdrawal seizures, an antiepileptic drug (e.g., phenytoin [Dilantin]) is often used and then continued for maintenance.

Treatment After Detoxification

General considerations:

➤ Patients come to treatment as a result of outside pressure (e.g., spouse, parent, employer, the legal system) or of their own accord. Success for recovery is significantly reduced if the patient does not truly want to stop drinking.

➤ Complete abstinence is the ultimate goal of treatment. However, some patients:

   ✔ Experience multiple failures at sustaining abstinence before reaching this goal.

   ✔ Never experience an extensive period of abstinence.

   ✔ Benefit from a harm-reduction model, where the goal is decreased consumption rather than absolute abstinence (controversial).

Treatment options:

Somatic treatments:

➤ Disulfiram (Antabuse):

   ✔ Constitutes aversion therapy (i.e., does not reduce craving for alcohol).

   ✔ Is suitable for patients who:

     ■ Are in good physical health.

     ■ Have normal, near-normal, or normalizing liver enzymes.

     ■ Are highly motivated to stop drinking.

     ■ Are able to fully cooperate with the treatment protocol.

     ■ Have adequate control over the potential for impulsive drinking and function in a near-normal fashion with good work and social supports.

   ✔ Dosage is 250–500 mg in the morning, thereby eliminating for that day the consideration of drinking alcohol. Wait at least 24–48 hours after the last drink before starting disulfiram.

   ✔ Effectiveness reportedly lasts 10–14 days after disulfiram is stopped, although some individuals can drink alcohol sooner or can drink alcohol without an adverse reaction while taking disulfiram:

     ■ If the patient on disulfiram drinks, buildup of acetaldehyde can produce facial flushing, diaphoresis, nausea, vomiting, confusion, and *hypo*tension. Alcohol's interaction with disulfiram can be lethal in severe cases, and some patients can be adversely affected by alcohol vapors from sources such as cologne or aftershave lotions containing alcohol. Nonalcoholic substitutes are available for most products intended for external or internal use.

   ✔ Side effects (while not drinking) include confusion and psychotic symptoms (more likely at higher dosages).

✔ Is a partial dopamine agonist (inhibits the breakdown of dopamine to norepinephrine). The confusion and psychosis occasionally developing secondary to antabuse may be due to this effect.

✔ Can be combined with naltrexone.

➤ Naltrexone (oral: ReVia; IM: Vivitrol):

✔ Is a mu opioid antagonist FDA approved for the treatment of alcohol dependence. The IM form removes the variability associated with poor compliance. Be certain that the patient is not using narcotics when initiating naltrexone. Dosing is 50–100 mg/day (oral) or 380 mg/month (IM; gluteal muscle).

✔ Is effective in reducing alcohol cravings in about 50% of patients and is effective in reducing the intensity of the intoxicating effects of alcohol if patients continue to drink.

✔ The Combining Medications and Behavioral Interventions (COMBINE) study (2006) demonstrated that naltrexone was effective as a stand-alone medication for the treatment of alcohol dependence without adjuunctive psychotherapy.

✔ Side effects are typically minimal (e.g., nausea, anxiety).

➤ Acamprosate calcium (Campral):

✔ FDA-approved for the maintenance of abstinence from alcohol in persons with alcohol dependence who are abstinent at the initiation of acamprosate therapy.

✔ Reduces the frequency of drinking, especially when used in conjunction with psychosocial and behavioral therapies. Effects seem to be specific for alcohol. However, the COMBINE study did not find acamprosate better than placebo (unlike results from European studies).

✔ No additional danger if patients drink alcohol while using acamprosate.

✔ Tablets are enteric coated to provide for absorption from the small intestine rather than from the stomach to reduce gastrointestinal side effects.

✔ Side effects include gastrointestinal disturbance (e.g., nausea, vomiting), appetite increase with subsequent weight gain, sedation, and decreased libido.

✔ Dosage is 666 mg tid.

➤ Non-FDA-approved agents showing promise to reduce alcohol craving include:

✔ Dopamine antagonists (clozapine, olanzapine).

✔ SSRIs (fluoxetine, sertraline).

✔ Antiseizure medications inhibiting glutamate (topiramate, gabapentin).

✔ Corticotropin-releasing factor anatagonists (in development; may also play a role as future antidepressants).

✔ Cannabinoid receptor antagonists (rimonabant [Complia]).

✔ Lithium.

✔ Kudzu root.

Psychosocial treatments:

➤ Psychotherapy (cognitive-behavioral therapy [CBT], individual, marital, and group) can be very helpful. The COMBINE study established that combining somatic and psychosocial interventions is advantageous.

➤ Support meetings:

✔ Alcoholics Anonymous and Alateen are 12-step programs focusing on total abstinence, reduction of stress, and a "one day at a time" philosophy. Frequent meetings (e.g., "30 meetings in 30 days") and a sponsor who has been alcohol-free for at least 1 year are recommended. The first step is to acknowledge lack of power over drinking.

✔ Al-Anon provides support for spouses and family members of individuals with drinking problems.

✔ Adult Children of Alcoholics (ACOA), pioneered by Dr. Janet Woititz, provides support for adult children of a parent or parents who are alcohol dependent.

➤ After detoxification, recommendations include one of the following:

✔ Continued treatment on an outpatient basis.

✔ Continued treatment in a 21- to 28-day inpatient treatment program (helpful for patients who fail to stop drinking after repeated attempts at detoxification), possibly followed by a 6- to 24-month program in a long-term treatment facility.

COCAINE-INDUCED DISORDERS

DSM-IV-TR Diagnostic Criteria for Cocaine Intoxication (Summary)

➤ Recent use of cocaine.

➤ Clinically significant maladaptive behavioral or psychological changes (e.g., euphoria or affective blunting; changes in sociability; hypervigilance; interpersonal sensitivity; anxiety, tension, or anger; stereotyped behaviors; impaired judgment; impaired social or occupational functioning) that developed during or shortly after use of cocaine.

➤ Two (or more) of the following, developing during or shortly after cocaine use:

✔ Tachycardia or bradycardia.

✔ Pupillary dilation.

✔ Elevated or lowered blood pressure.

✔ Perspiration or chills.

✔ Nausea or vomiting.

✔ Evidence of weight loss.

✔ Psychomotor agitation or withdrawal.

✔ Muscle weakness, respiratory depression, chest pain, or cardiac arrhythmias.

✔ Confusion, seizures, dyskinesias, dystonias, or coma.

DSM-IV-TR Diagnostic Criteria for Cocaine Withdrawal (Summary)

➤ Cessation of (or reduction in) cocaine use that has been heavy and prolonged.

➤ Dysphoric mood and two (or more) of the following physiological changes, developing within a few hours to several days after cessation or reduction in use:

✔ Fatigue.

✔ Vivid, unpleasant dreams.

✔ Insomnia or hypersomnia.

✔ Increased appetite.

✔ Psychomotor retardation or agitation.

➤ The symptoms cause clinically significant distress or impairment in social, occupational, or other important areas of functioning.

Clinical Issues Related to Cocaine Intoxication and Withdrawal

➤ Cocaine:

✔ Is a natural psychostimulant produced from the leaves of the coca plant from South America.

✔ Is used legally (as a topical anesthetic [e.g., nasal]) and illegally (as a euphoric agent).

✔ Produces its effects by blocking monoamine reuptake (serotonin, norepinephrine, and dopamine) by presynaptic neurons and possibly by promoting the release of these neurotransmitters from the presynaptic neuron.

✔ Is administered by smoking (freebasing [cocaine base] or crack cocaine), inhaling (snorting or "tooting"), injecting subcutaneously (skin-popping), or injecting intravenously (shooting up). Speedballing is the practice of injecting intravenously a combination of heroin and cocaine.

✔ Is readily available as crack cocaine, a highly addictive, potent, and cheap form of cocaine. When cocaine is mixed with bicarbonate, crack cocaine is produced. When smoked, crack cocaine produces a crackling sound as freebase cocaine is regenerated. The freebase cocaine is rapidly absorbed after smoking and produces an almost immediate euphoria lasting about 15 minutes.

✔ Elimination half-life is 30–90 minutes. Its primary metabolite, benzoylecgonine, is inactive and detectable in the urine for 2–5 days and forms the basis for urine testing.

✔ Is intensified in its effects when combined with alcohol (cocaethylene).

✔ Is a powerful reinforcer for recurrent use and is extremely addictive. Dependence can develop over a weekend of heavy use. The short duration of stimulant activity promotes an almost insatiable drive to use more cocaine to again experience euphoria. The increase in dopamine in the nucleus accumbens after release from the ventral tegmental area is thought to be responsible for its pleasurable and reinforcing effects. When the "reservoir" of neurotransmitters runs low from repeated use:

■ Depression can develop.

■ The individual may dramatically increase the dosage of cocaine to achieve the desired euphoric effect, potentially precipitating a fatal cardiac arrythmia.

✔ Is frequently abused by individuals with bipolar disorder to induce or sustain a prolonged high and by individuals with opioid dependence to reinforce or modulate the effects of the narcotic.

✔ Can induce serious consequences as the dose progressively increases. The presentation includes increased wakefulness, increased activity, decreased appetite, and rapid weight loss. At higher doses, euphoria, nasal septum defects from continued snorting, and chronic cough or bronchitis from repeated smoking can develop. At still higher doses, the person can experience frank psychosis (paranoid delusions, visual and tactile hallucinations). Psychosis significantly increases the risk of aggression or violence. Further dose increases can generate a fatal cardiac arrhythmia, a myocardial infarction, or a cerebrovascular accident.

✔ Can induce significant emotional and physical problems for infants born to mothers who used cocaine during their pregnancy ("cocaine babies"). Symptoms include low birth weight, startle reactions, agitation, frequent crying, restlessness, learning difficulties, and lower IQ.

Treatment of Cocaine Intoxication, Dependence, or Withdrawal

➤ Treatment is typically supportive—there are no FDA-approved treatments for any of the nine cocaine-related disorders described by DSM-IV-TR:

✔ Medications can ease withdrawal symptoms:

■ Benzodiazepines can be helpful to reduce anxiety and agitation and are the preferred treatment. Antipsychotic medications can be added if psychosis or excessive agitation develops.

■ Antipsychotic medications can be helpful to reduce psychotic symptoms or excessive agitation.

✔ Medications potentially effective for reducing cocaine craving (not FDA approved) include:

■ Antidepressants (desipramine, fluoxetine, bupropion).

■ Dopaminergic agonists (amantadine, selegiline, bromocriptine, disulfiram).

■ Opioid-related agents (buprenorphine).

■ Antiseizure medications (topiramate, gabapentin).

■ Baclofen.

■ Cocaine vaccine (in development).

■ Prometa (flumazenil + hydroxyzine + gabapentin)—highlighted on *60 Minutes* (CBS).

✔ CBT can help sustain abstinence.

AMPHETAMINE-INDUCED DISORDERS

DSM-IV-TR Diagnostic Criteria for Amphetamine-Induced Disorders (Summary)

➤ The DSM-IV-TR classification of and diagnostic criteria for amphetamine-induced disorders are identical to those for cocaine. Other stimulants (e.g., methylphenidate [Ritalin]) are included in this group.

Clinical Issues Related to Amphetamine Intoxication and Withdrawal

➤ Amphetamine ("speed") and methamphetamine ("ice") are psychostimulants that:

✔ Can be administered orally (swallowed, chewed), by snorting, by smoking, or by IV injection.

✔ Are cheaper than cocaine, are extremely addictive, and are much longer lasting in their effects than cocaine (15–20 minutes for cocaine vs. 2–14 hours for methamphetamine).

✔ Can be produced (as methamphetamine) in a home laboratory, utilizing anhydrous ammonia (obtained from large farms) and pseudoephedrine or ephedrine (restricted availability):

- Formulas for manufacturing methamphetamine are readily available on the Internet.
- Dangerous explosions are possible during the manufacture of methamphetamine.
- Selling the raw ingredients in large quantities sufficient to provide production of methamphetamine is illegal.

✔ Increase serotonin, norepinephrine, and dopamine in the synaptic cleft by blocking their reuptake and possibly by promoting their release into the synaptic cleft.

✔ Can induce serious consequences as the dose progressively increases. The presentation includes increased wakefulness, increased activity, decreased appetite, and rapid weight loss, progressing to euphoria and "tweaking," and then to frank psychosis (paranoid delusions, visual and tactile hallucinations). Psychosis significantly increases the risk of violence. Further dose increases can generate a cardiac arrhythmia, a myocardial infarction, or a cerebrovascular accident.

✔ Are considered at least as powerful as cocaine because:

- Users will go days without sleeping or eating.
- Psychosis can develop quickly, with prominent paranoid delusions and visual/tactile hallucinations. Users may develop excoriations from scratching at nonexistent bugs (i.e., formication).

➤ Methamphetamine produces a much longer "high" than cocaine because of slower metabolism and because of its metabolism to active amphetamine. Alkalinization of the urine can further increase the duration of action.

➤ Tweaking occurs when the user has gone for days without sleep, is irritable, is highly paranoid, and is prone to obsessive and erratic behavior (e.g., takes electronic items apart with no knowledge of how to put them back together).

➤ Abuse of methylphenidate is problematic, with significant dangers from intoxication (e.g., alterations in vital signs, arrhythmias, myocardial infarction, cerebrovascular accidents, psychosis, violence). Methylphenidate tablets are typically crushed, followed by snorting or IV use to produce a rapid and intense high. The longer-acting sustained-release preparations taken orally at the prescribed dosage do not produce the intense high.

Treatment of Amphetamine Intoxication, Dependence, or Withdrawal

➤ Treatment considerations for amphetamines are basically the same as for cocaine. Please refer to previous section on cocaine for treatment considerations.

CANNABIS-INDUCED DISORDERS

DSM-IV-TR Diagnostic Criteria for Cannabis Intoxication (Summary)

➤ Recent use of cannabis.

➤ Clinically significant maladaptive behavioral or psychological changes (e.g., impaired motor coordination, euphoria, anxiety, sensation of slowed time, impaired judgment, social withdrawal) that developed during or shortly after cannabis use.

➤ Two (or more) of the following signs, developing within 2 hours of cannabis use:

  ✔ Conjunctival injection.

  ✔ Increased appetite.

  ✔ Dry mouth.

  ✔ Tachycardia.

Clinical Issues Related to Cannabis Intoxication

➤ Intoxication is rapid, beginning with euphoria (a high), often accompanied or followed by:

  ✔ Uncontrollable laughter.

  ✔ Impairment in short-term memory, attention span, insight, and judgment.

  ✔ Distorted sensory perceptions, impaired motor performance, and the sensation that time is passing slowly.

  ✔ Conjunctival injection (bloodshot eyes, scleral injection, "red eyes") due to dilation of blood vessels in the eye.

  ✔ Poor physical coordination.

  ✔ Depression.

  ✔ Increased blood pressure and pulse.

  ✔ Mild sedation.

  ✔ Increased appetite and/or thirst (i.e., "the munchies"), with dry mouth.

  ✔ Hypothermia.

  ✔ "Bad trips," with anxiety, delusions, and hallucinations (at high doses).

Clinical Issues Related to Cannabis Abuse and Dependence

➤ The psychoactive ingredient of the Indian hemp plant is delta-9-tetrahydrocannabinol (THC), although other cannabinoids likely also have THC-like activity.

➤ THC is usually administered by smoking but can also be administered orally (e.g., made into a tea, prescribed [Schedule III] as dronabinol [Marinol]). Dronabinol is administered to reduce nausea in cancer patients receiving chemotherapy and to improve appetite in patients with AIDS.

➤ "Medical marijuana" (i.e., physician-authorized prescriptions for marijuana cigarettes) is promoted for relieving nausea associated with cancer, reducing intraocular pressure in persons with glaucoma, and stimulating appetite in patients with AIDS or cancer. At this time, its use in the United States is generally illegal (Schedule I), although some states provide regulation for its use under strict guidelines.

➤ Marijuana is commonly abused with other substances, especially cocaine, alcohol, and cigarettes. A marijuana cigarette (a joint) or cigar (a blunt) may be unknowingly "spiked" with phencyclidine or cocaine.

➤ Marijuana does not produce physical dependence, and therefore there is no physical withdrawal syndrome. However, psychological dependence can develop. Marijuana can exacerbate symptoms of schizophrenia and induce psychosis at higher doses.

➤ THC can be found in the urine for up to 10 days after a single use and up to 30 days with chronic use (an important consideration for drug testing).

➤ Individuals who abuse cocaine and heroin are more likely to have previously abused marijuana and, prior to marijuana, to have abused alcohol or developed nicotine dependence.

➤ Controversial issues regarding long-term marijuana abuse:

✔ Marijuana can induce mood disorders, can precipitate schizophrenia, can impair cognition, can produce an amotivational syndrome, and can cause throat and lung cancer (from smoking).

✔ There is a growing tendency to disregard or discount marijuana as an abusive drug, even with regard to substance abuse treatment programs.

Treatment of Cannabis Intoxication

➤ Allow the individual to sleep, with "talking down" if agitation or anxiety occurs. Medications are seldom needed except if the patient is delusional (treat acutely with a low-dose antipsychotic medication) or presents with severe anxiety (treat acutely with a benzodiazepine). Typically, the intoxicating effects last 2–3 hours and are followed by sleepiness.

➤ Medications aimed at the cannabinoid-1 receptor (CB_1) may, in the future, provide benefit for a wider range of psychiatric and physical disorders. Currently, dronabinol (Marinol) is indicated for the treatment of nausea in cancer chemotherapy patients and rimonabant (Acomplia) is indicated for the treatment of obesity.

HALLUCINOGEN-INDUCED DISORDERS

Common Hallucinogens

➤ Lysergic acid diethylamide (LSD).

➤ Mescaline (peyote cactus).

➤ Methylenedioxymethamphetamine (MDMA; "ecstasy," "love drug") and methylenedioxyamphetamine (MDA; "Eve").

➤ Psilocybin (mushrooms)—metabolized to the active hallucinogen psilocin.

➤ Dimethyltryptamine (DMT).

Clinical Issues Related to Hallucinogen-Induced Disorders

➤ Hallucinogens:
   ✔ Can produce unusual sensory perceptions (e.g., feeling of heaviness, increased auditory sensations, enhancement of colors), frank hallucinations, or synesthesias (e.g., the "hearing" of a color) in a clear sensorium.
   ✔ Are Schedule I drugs.
   ✔ Are at times combined with each other to produce "designer" effects.
   ✔ Likely produce their psychological effects by inducing the release of serotonin from the presynaptic vesicles. Also, reuptake of serotonin may be blocked. This results in overwhelming postsynaptic serotonin receptor activity for 4–8 hours. Serotonin is more associated with an "empathetic" response than a pleasurable response characteristic of dopamine release.
   ✔ Differ in the rate of onset, duration, and intensity of effects (e.g., LSD is 200 times as potent as psilocybin and 5,000 times as potent as mescaline).
   ✔ Under controlled conditions, the active ingredients may be helpful in the treatment of obsessive-compulsive disorder and body dysmorphic disorder.

➤ Lysergic acid diethylamide (LSD):
   ✔ Is one of the most potent and the most commonly abused hallucinogens. The typical street dose of LSD producing intoxicating effects ranges from 30 to 200 μg.
   ✔ Has been associated with the onset of active-phase symptoms of schizophrenia, although LSD is not necessarily causative of schizophrenia. LSD intoxication and the active phase of schizophrenia can present with nearly identical symptoms.

➤ MDMA, MDA, and DMT are "designer drugs," in that they were synthesized to produce specific stimulant, hallucinogenic, and/or euphoric effects. These drugs can cause permanent neurotoxicity (e.g., Parkinson's disease) possibly due to the direct effects of the active ingredient, to serotonin excess, or due to contaminants in the formulation. MDA and MDMA possess both stimulant and hallucinogenic properties and therefore are very desirable as substances of abuse.

➤ MDMA (prototype of this group):

✔ Is a ring-substituted amphetamine.

✔ Produces more prominent stimulation than hallucinogenic effects.

✔ Was used in trials to enhance psychotherapy in the 1980s (psychedelic psychotherapy) and in trials to treat PTSD in 2001.

✔ Regulated to U.S. Drug Enforcement Administration Schedule I in 1985.

Hallucinogen Intoxication

DSM-IV-TR diagnostic criteria for hallucinogen intoxication (summary):

➤ Recent use of a hallucinogen.

➤ Clinically significant maladaptive behavioral or physiological changes (e.g., marked anxiety or depression, ideas of reference, fear of losing one's mind, paranoid ideation, impaired judgment, impaired social or occupational functioning) that developed during or shortly after hallucinogen use.

➤ Perceptual changes occurring in a state of full wakefulness and alertness (e.g., subjective identification of perceptions, depersonalization, derealization, illusions, hallucinations, synesthesias) that developed during or shortly after hallucinogen use.

➤ Two (or more) of the following signs, developing during or shortly after hallucinogen use:

✔ Pupillary dilation.

✔ Tachycardia.

✔ Sweating.

✔ Palpitations.

✔ Blurring of vision.

✔ Tremors.

✔ Incoordination.

Clinical issues related to hallucinogen intoxication:

➤ The first 4-hour period after administration is described as a "trip." The effects can be intense and include physical, perceptual, and "psychic" changes:

✔ Physical changes include elevations in vital signs (blood pressure, pulse, body temperature), dilated pupils, restlessness, dizziness, paresthesias, tremors, weakness, blurred vision, and incoordination.

✔ Perceptual changes include alteration or intensification of any of the five senses, illusions, hallucinations, delusions, and synesthesias.

✔ "Psychic" changes include dreamlike feelings, altered sense of time, depersonalization, derealization, and changes in mood.

➤ "Bad trips" occur when the administration of a hallucinogen produces frightening hallucinations, alarming delusions, significant anxiety, panic attacks, and/or an increased potential for violence. Treatment options for a "bad trip" include:

✔ Symptom-targeted interventions, such as:

■ "Talking down" to diminish the need for medications and to reduce self-injurious or aggressive behaviors.

■ Minimizing stimulation by keeping the patient in a quiet, darkened room.

■ Benzodiazepines, particularly lorazepam (Ativan) and diazepam (Valium), to reduce anxiety, agitation, and panic attacks when talking down is not effective.

■ High-potency antipsychotic medications, to reduce severe agitation. Haloperidol (Haldol) alone or combined with lorazepam in an intramuscularly administered formulation can be very effective. Chlorpromazine (Thorazine) has been linked to deaths when used to reduce agitation associated with some of the hallucinogens.

Hallucinogen Persisting Perception Disorder (Flashbacks)

DSM-IV-TR diagnostic criteria for hallucinogen persisting perception disorder (summary):

➤ The reexperiencing, following cessation of use of a hallucinogen, of one or more of the perceptual symptoms that were experienced while intoxicated with the hallucinogen (e.g., geometric hallucinations, false perceptions of movement in the peripheral visual fields, flashes of color, intensified colors, trails of images of moving objects, positive afterimages, halos around objects, macropsia, micropsia).

➤ The symptoms cause clinically significant distress or impairment in social, occupational, or other important areas of functioning.

➤ The symptoms are not due to a general medical condition (e.g., anatomic brain lesions, infections of the brain, seizure disorder with accompanying visual hallucinations) and are not better accounted for by another psychiatric condition (e.g., delirium, dementia, schizophrenia) or hypnopompic hallucinations.

Clinical issues related to hallucinogen persisting perception disorder:

➤ Flashbacks:

  ✔ Are phenomena occurring while awake in which intoxication-type symptoms are reexperienced after (perhaps years after) the use of the hallucinogen has been discontinued.

  ✔ Have also been reported for chronic abusers of amphetamine and methamphetamine.

INHALANT-INDUCED DISORDERS

Commonly Abused Inhalants

➤ Airplane glue (e.g., toluene, ethyl acetate).

➤ Spray paint (e.g., toluene, butane, propane).

➤ Hair sprays (e.g., butane, propane).

➤ Cleaning agents (e.g., trichloroethylene).

➤ Solvents (e.g., acetone, toluene, butane, gasoline).

➤ Food products (e.g., nitrous oxide in whipped cream dispensers).

➤ Room "odorizers" (e.g., amyl nitrite, butyl nitrite).

➤ Correction fluid (e.g., petroleum naphtha).

➤ Permanent markers (xylene).

➤ Home welding kits (butane).

➤ Carburetor starting fluid (diethyl ether [ether]).

➤ Nail polish remover (acetone).

DSM-IV-TR Diagnostic Criteria for Inhalant Intoxication (Summary)

➤ Recent intentional use of or short-term, high-dose exposure to volatile inhalants (excluding anesthetic gases and short-acting vasodilators).

➤ Clinically significant maladaptive behavioral or psychological changes (e.g., belligerence, assaultiveness, apathy, impaired judgment, impaired social or occupational functioning) that developed during or shortly after use of or exposure to volatile inhalants.

➤ Two (or more) of the following signs, developing during or shortly after inhalant use or exposure:

✔ Dizziness.

✔ Nystagmus.

✔ Incoordination.

✔ Slurred speech.

✔ Unsteady gait.

✔ Lethargy.

✔ Depressed reflexes.

✔ Psychomotor retardation.

✔ Tremor.

✔ Generalized muscle weakness.

✔ Blurred vision or diplopia.

✔ Stupor or coma.

✔ Euphoria.

Clinical Issues Related to Inhalant Intoxication

➤ Inhalants can be inhaled directly (e.g., sniffing gasoline) or inhaled from an aerolized source (i.e., sprayed into a paper bag, which is then placed over the nose and mouth).

➤ Inhalants typically produce an almost immediate but short-lived euphoria (at times with giddiness) that rapidly turns to drowsiness, disinhibition, agitation, and/or light-headedness. With increasing dose, ataxia, dizziness, and disorientation may occur. With still higher doses, sleeplessness, general muscle weakness, dysarthria, nystagmus, hallucinations, and disruptive or violent behavior may ensue. Blindness, neuropathy, and "sudden sniffing death" (i.e., cardiac arrhythmias, asphyxiation) have also been reported.

➤ Chronic use can result in permanent neurological damage, including encephalopathy, cerebellar ataxia, ototoxicity, optic neuropathy, peripheral neuropathy, intellectual impairment, and permanent hepatic damage.

➤ Subtle signs of inhalant intoxication include the smell of solvents on the person's breath or on clothes and a rash around the mouth or nose ("glue sniffer's rash").

➤ The peak age of inhalant abuse is 14–15 years. The "average" inhalant abuser is male and white, Hispanic, or Native American.

➤ Activity seems to be related to a balance between NMDA antagonism and GABA agonism. For example, ether is more effective as an NMDA antagonist and ethyl alcohol is more effective as a GABA agonist.

➤ Chloroform, diethyl ether, and nitrous oxide are effective as anesthetics for medicinal purposes. Only nitrous oxide is currently used (as a dental anesthetic) and therefore is readily accessible for abuse.

OPIOID-INDUCED DISORDERS

Opioids (Narcotics)

➤ Morphine (the primary analgesic component of opium).

➤ Heroin (diacetylmorphine; synthesized from morphine).

➤ Hydromorphone (Dilaudid).

➤ Meperidine (Demerol).

➤ Methadone.

➤ Fentanyl (including the transmucosal Actiq, which is supplied as a lollipop).

➤ Propoxyphene (Darvon).

➤ Codeine (derived from opium; metabolized to morphine).

➤ Levomethadyl (LAAM)—no longer in use, in part due to QTc increases.

➤ Buprenorphine (Subutex).

Clinical Issues Related to Opioids

➤ Opium is extracted from the plant *Papaver somniferum,* yielding the natural (i.e., nonsynthetic) opioids morphine and codeine.

➤ Pain is recognized when a stimulus acts on nociceptors, travels afferent pathways to the spinal cord, and induces the release of substance P. Substance P then binds with receptors in the spinal cord to send pain impulses to the brain. Opioids (either exogenously administered or naturally produced [e.g., beta-endorphins, enkephalins, dynorphin]) inhibit the release of substance P, thereby reducing pain. However, in time, tolerance may develop, necessitating higher doses to achieve the same degree of pain relief (or euphoria).

➤ Risk factors for developing opioid dependence include chronic pain syndromes treated with opioids, family history of substance abuse, younger age, male, and access to opioids (e.g., health care professionals).

➤ Potential consequences of IV abuse of opioids include HIV infection, hepatitis, osteomyelitis, tetanus, and subacute bacterial endocarditis.

➤ Opioids:

✔ Are characterized as agonists (bind to and activate opioid receptors) or antagonists (bind to but do not activate opioid receptors). Partial agonists/antagonists (properties of both) are commonly used clinically and may reduce the potential for dependence.

✔ Are classified as naturally occurring alkaloids (e.g., codeine, morphine thebaine, oripavine), semisynthetic (e.g., oxycodone, heroin, hydromorphone, hydrocodone), or synthetic (e.g., methadone, fentanyl, meperidine, propoxyphene, buprenorphine). Additionally, naturally body-produced opioid peptides include endorphins, enkephalins, dynorphins, and endomorphins.

✔ Can be administered by injection (IV, IM, subcutaneous), by snorting, by smoking, and orally, depending on the particular opioid.

✔ Can be classified as short-acting (e.g., morphine, heroin, meperidine) or longer-acting (e.g., methadone, levomethadyl, buprenorphine).

✔ Produce many of their pharmacological effects by interacting with specific receptors (mu, kappa, sigma, epsilon, and delta):

■ Mu, kappa, and delta receptors are involved with analgesia, but mu and delta receptors also influence mood, respiration, blood pressure, endocrine, and gastrointestinal functioning. The mu receptor is the most studied and is especially crucial to the rewarding and addictive properties of opioids.

■ Sigma receptors mediate dysphoria, hallucinations, and psychosis.

■ Opioid antagonists (e.g., naloxone, naltrexone) antagonize the effects of opioids, rendering them nonfunctional and can precipitate an immediate withdrawal syndrome.

✔ Produce a wide range of pharmacological effects, including:

■ Analgesia (a desired clinical effect).

■ Suppression of the cough reflex (a desired clinical effect).

■ Feeling of well-being or euphoria (desirable for abuse). When opioids are abused, the euphoria (described as a "rush") is due (at least in part) to the release of dopamine.

■ Decreased peristalsis, with possible constipation.

■ Decreased pupil size (miosis).

■ Vasodilation of skin vessels and pruritus secondary to release of histamine.

■ Lack of pain recognition (e.g., gums, diabetic foot ulcers), leading to undesired consequences (e.g., gingivitis and poor dentition, foot ulcers in diabetic individuals).

■ Impotence.

■ CNS depression, with findings of decreased vital signs (e.g., blood pressure, pulse, respiration, core body temperature), possibly leading to death.

Opioid Intoxication

DSM-IV-TR diagnostic criteria for opioid intoxication (summary):

➤ Recent use of an opioid.

➤ Clinically significant maladaptive behavioral or psychological changes (e.g., initial euphoria followed by apathy, dysphoria, psychomotor agitation or retardation, impaired judgment, or impaired social or occupational functioning) that developed during or shortly after opioid use.

➤ Pupillary constriction (or pupillary dilation due to anoxia from severe overdose) and one (or more) of the following signs, developing during or shortly after opioid use:

✔ Drowsiness or coma.

✔ Slurred speech.

✔ Impairment in attention or memory.

Clinical issues related to opioid intoxication:

➤ Heroin:

✔ Is synthesized from morphine. Heroin (a prodrug) is metabolized by the liver to 6-monoacetylmorphine (an active opioid), which in turn is metabolized back to morphine. Morphine is then metabolized to the mostly inactive normorphine.

✔ Is relatively inexpensive. Black tar heroin is from Mexico and white heroin is from South America.

✔ Can be administered by IV injection ("mainlining"), IM or subcutaneous injection, smoking ("chasing the dragon"), snorting, sniffing liquefied heroin intranasally ("shabanging"), and orally.

✔ Is significantly more lipid soluble than morphine and therefore has greater access to the CNS. As a consequence, lower amounts produce the desired euphoria without producing significant histamine side effects (a major benefit for the opioid abuser).

✔ Is illegal to produce, possess, use, or sell in the United States (a Schedule I medication).

✔ Can be combined with cocaine ("speedballing") or snorted in an alternate manner with cocaine ("crisscrossing"). It is also commonly abused along with diazepam, alcohol, and/or cigarette smoking.

✔ Is seven times more toxic than morphine. Many deaths from heroin occur from intoxication after IV use, especially when heroin is mixed with benzodiazepines and/or alcohol or when the individual again uses heroin at a prior dosage after completing detoxification and tolerance has been reduced.

✔ When administered at lower-than-toxic doses, is followed within seconds by euphoria ("rush"), at times likened to "whole body" sexual orgasm. Additional findings include nausea with possible vomiting (indicative of "good" heroin), head falling to the chest ("nodding"), slurred speech, constricted or pinpoint pupils (a clinical sign of opioid intoxication in emergency settings), and peripheral vasodilation.

✔ When administered at toxic doses, may be followed by stupor leading to coma, significant hypotension, respiratory failure, pulmonary edema, and death.

✔ Intoxication:

■ Presents with three classic signs:

● Coma.

● Respiratory depression.

● Pinpoint pupils.

■ Can be life-threatening:

● Respiration slows, blood pressure falls, seizures can develop with resulting rhabdomyolysis, coma develops, and death can ensue due to respiratory failure or aspiration.

● Emergency treatment with naloxone (Narcan) 0.4 mg intravenously, followed by a second dose of 1–2 mg intravenously in 3–5 minutes if needed, can be lifesaving. Ventilation for respiratory failure is usually needed as well.

✔ IV administration with "dirty" needles or poor injection techniques can cause or induce the spread of a variety of serious ailments (e.g., HIV, hepatitis, bacterial endocarditis, septicemia, meningitis, osteomyelitis).

Opioid Withdrawal

DSM-IV-TR diagnostic criteria for opioid withdrawal (summary):

➤ Either of the following:

✔ Cessation of (or reduction in) opioid use that has been heavy and prolonged (several weeks or longer).

✔ Administration of an opioid antagonist after a period of opioid use.

➤ Three (or more) of the following, developing within minutes to several days after cessation of the opioid:

✔ Dysphoric mood.

✔ Nausea and vomiting.

✔ Muscle aches.

✔ Lacrimation or rhinorrhea.

✔ Pupillary dilation, piloerection (goose bumps), or sweating.

✔ Diarrhea.

✔ Yawning.

✔ Fever.

✔ Insomnia.

Clinical issues related to opioid withdrawal:

➤ For heroin, symptoms of opioid withdrawal include intense flulike symptoms that begin within hours of the last dose of heroin. Symptoms can last about 1 week, are accompanied by opioid craving, and are unlikely to be life-threatening. Additional signs and symptoms of opioid withdrawal include:

  ✔ Increased vital signs (hypertension, tachycardia, and hyperventilation)—the opposite of opioid intoxication.

  ✔ Piloerection.

  ✔ Dilated pupils (the opposite of opioid intoxication).

  ✔ Nausea and diarrhea.

  ✔ Yawning.

  ✔ Muscle cramps/back aches.

  ✔ Anxiety and/or irritability.

➤ The time of onset of withdrawal symptoms depends on the half-life of the opioid and/or its active metabolite(s). Typical half-lives are 6–12 hours for heroin (includes the active metabolite morphine), and 24–36 hours for methadone.

➤ The intensity of withdrawal can be assessed with the 11-item Clinical Opiate Withdrawal Scale (CIWA). Higher numbers are indicative of more severe withdrawal.

➤ Treatment of opioid withdrawal is symptomatic. Unlike opioid intoxication, opioid withdrawal is rarely life-threatening. Benzodiazepines, muscle relaxents (e.g., cyclobenzaprine), and clonidine (oral, patch) can reduce the intensity of withdrawal symptoms.

➤ "Rapid detoxification" involves the induction of withdrawal by IV injection of naloxone after the patient is anesthetized. The treatment typically requires only 24–48 hours to complete and is expensive ($5,000–$10,000). The safety of this procedure is controversial, and craving after physical detoxification is unabated. An incremental (stepped) rapid detoxification uses smaller, subcutaneous doses of naloxone along with an oral dose of naloxone to ease withdrawal symptoms.

➤ After withdrawal is complete, naloxone can be taken orally to block euphoria if opioids are again used.

Opioid Dependence

Clinical issues related to opioid dependence:

➤ Opioid dependence likely develops from a combination of factors, including:

  ✔ Positive reinforcement due to the pleasurable response from repetitive opioid use involving the ventral tegmental area and nucleus accumbens.

✔ Reversing the very long and unpleasant withdrawal syndrome associated with reducing or stopping the opioid.

✔ The development of tolerance and an ever-growing need to increase the dose to achieve the desired euphoria.

✔ Self-treatment of anxiety, depression, or other psychiatric symptoms. However, long-term use can lead to depression.

➤ Heroin dependence is increasing in higher-educational-level groups as a result of the increased purity (allowing a high from snorting rather than injecting), abundant availability, and decreased cost.

➤ Psychiatric comorbidities are high:

✔ Comorbid drug dependencies—20% to 25%. Comorbid nicotine dependence is as high as 90%.

✔ Comorbid depression—35% to 50% (lifetime prevalence).

✔ Comorbid antisocial personality disorder—25%.

Treatment of opioid dependence other than acute withdrawal:

➤ Opioid-dependent individuals can possibly benefit from long-acting opioids if they have repeatedly failed to "stay clean" after detoxification. However, patients who use dirty needles, are promiscuous, or are pregnant are prime candidates for treatment with long-acting opioids. Methadone is preferred over street heroin during pregnancy.

➤ Methadone (full agonist), buprenorphine (partial agonist), and buprenorphine/naloxone are prescribed to replace street opioids but are not intended for pain management when prescribed under the auspices of an opioid addiction treatment program.

➤ The end point of treatment is the ultimate withdrawal of the replacement opioid (e.g., methadone, buprenorphine). The decision of when (or whether) to withdraw the replacement opioid can be difficult to assess and/or accomplish.

Methadone:

➤ Methadone (a full opioid agonist that binds to the mu receptor) maintenance is an accepted (albeit controversial) treatment for opioid dependence that purposely perpetuates the addiction, utilizing a longer-acting opioid (half-life can be as long as 190 hours) in a strictly supervised setting of a methadone maintenance clinic. Methadone is very inexpensive and is typically dispensd as a liquid formulation to protect against cheeking the drug and then selling it on the street.

➤ Methadone (Schedule II) is started at 10–30 mg/day (based on an approximate equivalence of 8–10 mg of methadone per bag of heroin injected). The dosage may be gradually increased and typically ranges between 30 and 200+ mg/day in most clinics. Methadone is usually administered once daily but may be given in divided daily doses for "fast" metabolizers.

➤ Side effects include the entire plethora of opioid side effects and increased QTc interval with potential for *torsades de pointes*.

➤ Urine is routinely monitored for illicit drug use (i.e., "dirty urine"). Continual dirty urines may necessitate discontinuation from the methadone treatment program, whereas clean urines are rewarded with "take home" doses (reduces contact with the clinic).

➤ For individuals who repeatedly fail at staying clean from illicit opioids while taking methadone, treatment in a long-term treatment center may be needed.

➤ Additional supportive measures are often beneficial and at times mandated, including attending individual and group psychotherapy sessions, participation in Narcotics Anonymous, and seeking and maintaining employment where possible. A critical aspect of the physician's assessment is to determine whether the methadone is truly being used by the patient for treatment or is being used as a means of propagating the abuse because of the euphoria it can continue to promote.

Buprenorphine (Subutex) and buprenorphine/naloxone combination (Suboxone):

➤ Buprenorphine is a partial opioid agonist that binds to the mu receptor and can serve as a sublingually administered substitute for other opioids. Buprenorphine was a Schedule V medication but is now Schedule III. The prescribing program is unique, in that with special approval from the U.S. Drug Enforcement Agency, individual practitioners (after a special training course) can prescribe buprenorphine and buprenorphine/naloxone combination from their offices rather than from a methadone maintenance treatment center:

✔ Physician requirements include a physician certification through an 8-hour training course, routine urine checks, and substance abuse counseling.

✔ The half-life of buprenorphine is rather long (~37 hours), and the usual detection methods for morphine and opiates will not detect buprenorphine.

✔ Initially, 30 patients may be treated by one physician at one time. After 1 year, up to 100 patients can be treated.

✔ When given to patients actively taking opioids, buprenorphine can induce an opioid withdrawal syndrome.

✔ Buprenorphine blocks the mu receptor sufficiently to protect against withdrawal and reduce craving but does not generally produce euphoria.

✔ IM/IV (Buprenex) buprenorphine is not FDA approved for the treatment of opioid dependence but is approved for pain management.

✔ Combining buprenorphine with benzodiazepines (especially when one or both are administered intravenously) can be life threatening because of possible respiratory depression.

➤ Initiate dosing with sublingual buprenorphine/naloxone (Suboxone) or sublingual buprenorphine (Subutex). Naloxone guards against euphoria from attempts at IV abuse and will precipitate immediate withdrawal if the patient is currently using opioids. Patients must be in a moderate phase of self-imposed detoxification before starting buprenorphine.

➤ Urine testing is necessary to assure compliance with a "drug free" environment.

➤ Prescriptions can be filled at a community pharmacy. Ensure that the pharmacy will maintain an adequate supply of the medication, to protect against unintended withdrawal if the patient is in need of a refill.

➤ Ideally, detoxification from buprenorphine should be undertaken (desirable time frame for buprenorphine use is at least 1 year), thereby "ending" the dependence on opioids.

Naltrexone:

➤ Although naltrexone is not FDA approved for the treatment of opioid dependence, some patients can be adequately treated with naloxone (oral, IM; FDA approved for alcohol dependence).

➤ For highly motivated patients, knowing that the use of an opioid while taking naltrexone will precipitate an immediate withdrawal syndrome is sufficient in itself to protect from future opioid use.

PHENCYCLIDINE-INDUCED DISORDERS

DSM-IV-TR Diagnostic Criteria for Phencyclidine Intoxication (Summary)

➤ Recent use of phencyclidine (or a related substance).

➤ Clinically significant maladaptive behavioral changes (e.g., belligerence, assaultiveness, impulsiveness, unpredictability, psychomotor agitation, impaired judgment, impaired social or occupational functioning) that developed during or shortly after phencyclidine use.

➤ Within an hour (less when smoked, "snorted," or used intravenously), two (or more) of the following signs:

✔ Vertical or horizontal nystagmus.

✔ Hypertension or tachycardia.

✔ Numbness or diminished response to pain.

✔ Ataxia.

✔ Dysarthria.

✔ Muscle rigidity.

✔ Seizures or coma.

✔ Hyperacusis.

Clinical Issues Related to Phencyclidine Intoxication

➤ Phencyclidine ("angel dust"; PCP):

✔ Was marketed as an anesthetic but is no longer used for this purpose.

✔ Is considered a dissociative anesthetic (i.e., gives a feeling of being disconnected from one's body and environment and/or produces a dreamlike state) secondary to N-methyl-D-aspartate (NMDA) receptor antagonism. Dextromethorphan, an over-the-counter antitussive, also acts as a dissociative hallucinogen when abused at high doses.

✔ Ketamine, a derivative of phencyclidine, is used as a veterinary anesthetic. When abused, ketamine produces effects similar to those of phencyclidine.

➤ PCP and ketamine act by antagonizing the NMDA receptor.

➤ Typical use involves smoking cigarettes or marijuana to which phencyclidine has been added ("laced") or adding the phencyclidine to a sugar cube, a gelatin cube, or blotter paper.

➤ Increasing levels of intoxication can produce life-threatening physiological toxicity secondary to cardiovascular, neurological, respiratory, or muscular (e.g., rhabdomyolysis) effects. Hypertension, agitation, and muscle spasms are common physical findings; frank psychotic symptoms are common mental health findings.

➤ Considerations for treatment of a "bad trip":

✔ The intensity of neurological and physical symptoms increases with increasing dose. Rhabdomyolysis can result in permanent renal failure and is a bad prognostic sign.

✔ Death can occur from hyperthermia and/or autonomic instability.

✔ "Talking down" may exacerbate symptoms, and a quiet room with little sensory stimulation is recommended. The use of physical restraints should be avoided if possible, to minimize the development of rhabdomyolysis.

✔ Muscle spasms and anxiety can be treated with benzodiazepines.

✔ Hypertension can be treated with phentolamine (Vasomax).

✔ Persistent psychotic symptoms can be treated with high-potency antipsychotic medications.

✔ Acidification of urine (e.g., ammonium chloride, vitamin C, cranberry juice) can promote the urinary excretion of phencyclidine.

SEDATIVE-, HYPNOTIC-, OR ANXIOLYTIC-RELATED DISORDERS

Classification

➤ High therapeutic-to-toxic ratio agents:

✔ Benzodiazepines.

➤ Low therapeutic-to-toxic ratio agents:

✔ Barbiturates (e.g., phenobarbital, pentobarbital, butabarbital)—Schedule II and III.

✔ Ethchlorvynol (Placidyl)—Schedule IV.

✔ Methaqualone (Quaalude)—Schedule I.

✔ Meprobamate (Miltown, Equanil)—Schedule IV.

✔ Glutethimide (Doriden)—Schedule II.

✔ Chloral hydrate (a "Mickey" when combined with alcohol)—Schedule IV.

✔ Gamma-hydroxybutyrate (GHB)—Schedule I.

Sedative, Hypnotic, or Anxiolytic Abuse and Dependence

➤ Abuse potential of these agents is relatively high (less so for phenobarbital). Tolerance and dependence can develop rapidly. The risk of dependence increases with higher doses and longer periods of use and is greater in individuals with a history of substance abuse (especially alcohol or narcotics). At times, physicians may iatrogenically induce benzodiazepine dependence through too-casual prescribing habits.

➤ Benzodiazepines may be abused in combination with other substances ("polyaddiction"). They are frequently abused to reduce unpleasant withdrawal symptoms of other drugs (e.g., heroin, alcohol), to reduce side effects of drug intoxication (e.g., cocaine, amphetamine), to experience a relaxing or numbing effect, to induce sleep, or to enhance the effects of other drugs (e.g., heroin, marijuana, alcohol).

➤ Zolpidem (Ambien) and zaleplon (Sonata) are hypnotics with very short half-lives. These agents are structurally unrelated to benzodiazepines, although their pharmacology and binding to GABA receptors are relatively similar to those of the benzodiazepines. Tolerance does not seem to develop as quickly as with the benzodiazepines, perhaps because the very short half-life promotes total elimination of the drug from the body prior to the next dose, thereby reducing the potential for dependence. Additional studies are needed to assess abuse and dependence issues with these agents.

Sedative, Hypnotic, or Anxiolytic Intoxication

DSM-IV-TR diagnostic criteria for sedative, hypnotic, or anxiolytic intoxication (summary):

➤ Recent use of a sedative, hypnotic, or anxiolytic agent.

➤ Maladaptive behavioral or psychological changes (e.g., inappropriate sexual or aggressive behavior, mood lability, impaired judgment, impaired social or occupational functioning) that developed during or shortly after sedative, hypnotic, or anxiolytic use.

➤ One (or more) of the following, developing during or shortly after sedative, hypnotic, or anxiolytic use:

✔ Slurred speech.

✔ Incoordination.

✔ Unsteady gait.

✔ Nystagmus.

✔ Impairment in attention or memory.

✔ Stupor or coma.

Clinical issues related to sedative, hypnotic, or anxiolytic intoxication:

➤ Most agents in this group are cross-tolerant with one another and with alcohol.

➤ In terms of morbidity and mortality, intoxication is somewhat safer with benzodiazepines than with the other agents listed. All of these agents are especially dangerous when combined with other cross-tolerant agents or with alcohol. Death can result from respiratory failure, CNS depression, and/or cardiovascular collapse.

Sedative, Hypnotic, or Anxiolytic Withdrawal

DSM-IV-TR diagnostic criteria for sedative, hypnotic, or anxiolytic withdrawal (summary):

➤ Cessation of or reduction in use of a sedative, hypnotic, or anxiolytic agent.

➤ Two (or more) of the following, developing within several hours to a few days after cessation of or reduction in use:

✔ Autonomic hyperactivity (e.g., sweating or pulse rate greater than 100 beats per minute).

✔ Increased hand tremor.

✔ Insomnia.

✔ Nausea and vomiting.

✔ Transient visual, tactile, or auditory hallucinations or illusions.

✔ Psychomotor agitation.

✔ Anxiety.

✔ Grand mal seizures.

Clinical issues related to sedative, hypnotic, or anxiolytic withdrawal:

➤ Withdrawal is a state of *hyperexcitability* producing some combination of anxiety, restlessness, agitation (at times with aggression or violence), insomnia, delirium, psychosis (delusions, hallucinations), grand mal seizures, respiratory depression, and/or hypertension. Death can follow. Withdrawal symptoms are more likely when the substance is used at a high dose, is used for a long period of time, has no active metabolites, and has a short half-life. Anxiety is the most prominent symptom of a mild withdrawal syndrome.

➤ Withdrawal from benzodiazepines can be dangerous, though it is somewhat safer than from barbiturates. Flumazenil (Romazicon), 0.2 mg administered intravenously, is indicated for the management of benzodiazepine withdrawal or overdose. Generally, a slow taper on an outpatient basis can be effective if the patient is cooperative and is not medically compromised.

➤ Withdrawal from barbiturates can be dangerous, and overdoses can be lethal. Some authorities recommend that barbiturate detoxification be undertaken only on an inpatient basis at a much slower rate than with benzodiazepines. To detoxify from barbiturates, utilize a "pentobarbital challenge" to determine the extent of barbiturate intoxication and then slowly detoxify with phenobarbital.

ANABOLIC STEROIDS

➤ Anabolic steroids (testosterone derivatives, "roids") are abused by men and women athletes to increase muscle mass, body weight, and endurance. They are classified as Schedule III drugs. Anabolic steroids are masculinizing. They increase muscle mass, muscular strength, and endurance. They are banned by all professional sports.

➤ Characteristic effects/side effects include increased sex drive, acne, elevated liver enzymes, male pattern baldness, hirsutism and deepening of the voice (in females), and testicular atrophy (in males). More serious adverse side effects include hepatic damage possibly leading to hepatocellular cancer, increases in low density lipoprotein (LDL), decreases in high density lipoprotein (HDL), cardiovascular damage, myocardial infarction, and sudden cardiac-related death.

➤ Irritability, anger, and violence ("roid rage") have been attributed to anabolic steroid abuse (controversial) and may continue for months after stopping the drug. Lithium and antidepressants (SSRIs) can be helpful to reduce symptoms (anecdotal reports).

➤ When used illicitly, administration is most commonly by the IM route.

EPHEDRA

➤ Ephedra (contains ephedrine and pseudoephedrine; also known as ma huang) is contained in a variety of products intended for a variety of uses (e.g., weight loss, to improve energy, to improve athletic performance). Ephedra is both a stimulant and a thermogenic ("fat burning") agent.

➤ Ephedrine and pseudoephedrine stimulate the release of norepinephrine and stimulate alpha- and beta-adrenergic receptors. This nonspecific stimulation of adrenergic receptors induces bronchodilatation (desired) but also adversely increases heart rate and blood pressure while decreasing circulation to the renal system and other parts of the body.

➤ Adverse events reported with ephedra products include insomnia, irritability, and agitation. At higher doses, myocardial infarction, cerebrovascular accidents, and psychosis have been reported.

➤ The FDA has now banned the sale of ephedra as a supplement, although the active ingredients are still available by prescription, as over-the-counter medications containing synthesized ephedrine, and as Chinese herbal remedies or herbal teas.

DEXTROMETHORPHAN

➤ Dextromethorphan is:

✔ The dextro isomer of levomethorphan, a semisynthetic morphine derivative.

✔ An NMDA receptor antagonist like that of PCP and ketamine via its primary metabolite dexorphan.

✔ An antitussive without analgesic properties found in many over-the-counter cough suppressants (formulations with names including "DM" or "Tuss").

✔ Widely used as a cough suppressant (e.g., Alka-Seltzer Plus, Children's Vicks NyQuil Cold/Cough Relief, Coricidin HBP Cough & Cold Tablets, Robitussin DM, Vicks Formula 44, Sudafed Cough Syrup).

✔ Abused to induce a high, but can also produce manic-like symptoms, euphoria, psychosis (e.g., paranoid delusions, florid visual hallucinations), dissociation, and confusion.

✔ Is considered to be a "cheap high," and its potential for abuse is often not recognized. Dextromethorphan can be combined with inhalants (e.g., aerosol paint) to produce an LSD-like effect ("Robo Fire").

✔ At higher doses or in the presence of 2D6 inhibitors, produces hallucinogenic effects much like that of ketamine and PCP via antagonism at the NMDA receptor. Dextromethorphan is metabolized by cytochrome P450 (CYP450) 2D6. 2D6 inhibitors (e.g., paroxetine, fluoxetine) can raise blood levels substantially. Additionally, 10%–15% of Caucasians are slow metabolizers, further increasing the risk. Deaths have been reported.

✔ Can produce serotonin syndrome when combined with other serotonergic medications.

FLUNITRAZEPAM AND GAMMA-HYDROXYBUTYRATE

➤ General considerations:

✔ Flunitrazepam (Rohypnol) and gamma-hydroxybutyrate (GHB) are abused:

■ For their intoxicating or bodybuilding effects.

■ To take sexual advantage of another person without his or her consent (i.e., "date rape" drugs):

● Congress passed the Drug-Induced Rape Prevention and Punishment Act of 1996, increasing the federal penalties for the use of any controlled substance to aid in sexual assault. It is also a federal crime to give someone a controlled substance without the person's knowledge.

● An increasing number of individuals are receiving long prison sentences for the unlawful use of these agents as date-rape drugs.

➤ Flunitrazepam (Rohypnol):

✔ Is a very potent benzodiazepine (10 times as potent as diazepam) that can produce intoxication, deep sedation, respiratory distress, and blackouts.

✔ Can rapidly produce tolerance, dependence, and life-threatening withdrawal symptoms.

✔ Intoxication can result in death, especially when mixed with cross-tolerant agents, including alcohol.

✔ Is not a scheduled drug; is not legal for possession, sale, or use in the United States but is readily available over the Internet from other countries.

➤ Gamma-hydroxybutyrate (GHB):

✔ Is a CNS depressant abused for its euphoric, sedative, and anabolic (i.e., body building) effects.

✔ Is a Schedule I drug; is not legal for possession, sale, or use in the United States but is readily available over the Internet from other countries.

✔ Can produce anterograde amnesia, analgesia, hallucinations, and possibly loss of consciousness at doses of 10–20 mg. Unpleasant side effects include nausea, vomiting, and vertigo. Higher doses can produce anesthesia, seizures, respiratory depression, coma, and death. The effects are increased when GHB is combined with alcohol.

✔ Acute withdrawal can be severe and life-threatening (as with benzodiazepines).

NICOTINE

➤ Is absorbed from the lungs, mucus membranes of the mouth or nose, and skin. When inhaled, nicotine reaches the brain in 8–11 seconds.

➤ Induces release of dopamine (much like cocaine), rapidly produces dependence, and has perhaps the most difficult and problematic withdrawal syndrome.

➤ Genetic influences appear to be operable with regard to the initiation, propagation, and the development of nicotine dependence.

➤ Induces release of epinephrine (elevates blood pressure, respiration, and heart rate; increases alertness), reduces the release of insulin (leading to mild hyperglycemia), dulls the sense of smell and taste, causes arterial vasoconstriction (leading to wrinkling of the skin), and leads to long-term medical sequelae (e.g., myocardial infarction; cerebrovascular accident; emphysema; cancer of the mouth, throat, and lungs).

➤ Reduces anxiety, has antidepressant effects, improves cognition in Alzheimer's disease and mild cognitive impairment, and may help ameliorate some of the symptoms of schizophrenia. It is very likely that some individuals smoke to relieve various psychological symptoms.

➤ Withdrawal generates irritability, anxiety, depressive symptoms, headache, fatigue, weight gain, and intense craving for nicotine.

➤ Treatment of dependence is most effective when somatic and psychosocial modalities are combined.

　✔ FDA-approved medications:

　　■ Bupropion (reduces the craving for smoking). Side effects (see Table 2–3).

　　■ Varenicline (Chantix), an alpha-4 beta-2 nicotine acetylcholine receptor partial agonist, reduces the craving for smoking. Recent anecdotal reports of depression/suicidal behavior as well as other adverse effects not fully delineated.

　　■ Nicotine replacement (patch, lozenge, gum, transdermal patch, inhaler, nasal spray).

　✔ Non-FDA-approved medications:

　　■ Clonidine (reduces somatic side effects of withdrawal).

　　■ Gradually reduce the nicotine content of cigarettes for gradual detoxification.

　✔ Psychosocial treatments include Nicotine Anonymous (12-step program), short-term (7-day) residential treatment, and CBT.

U.S. DRUG ENFORCEMENT AGENCY SCHEDULE CLASSIFICATION OF DRUGS

Schedule I—high abuse potential, no current "approved" medical use

➤ Examples are heroin, MDMA, GHB, LSD, and marijuana:

　✔ Some states provide for the legal prescribing of marijuana ("medical marijuana") and place it in a category not recognized by the U.S. Drug Enforcement Agency (e.g., Schedule VI).

Schedule II—high potential for severe psychological or physiological dependence

➤ Examples are most narcotics, most barbiturates, cocaine/amphetamine/methamphetamine, and phencyclidine.

Schedule III—lower abuse potential than Schedule I or II drugs

➤ Examples are aspirin or acetaminophen with codeine, paregoric, anabolic steroids, buprenorphine, and the oral formulation of THC (Marinol).

Schedule IV—lower abuse potential than Schedule III drugs

➤ Examples are benzodiazepines, zaleplon, zolpidem, and meprobamate.

Schedule V—lower abuse potential than Schedule IV drugs

➤ Examples are antitussives with codeine.

STREET NAMES FOR COMMON DRUGS OF ABUSE

➤ Cocaine—coke, blow, crack, powder, sugar, nose candy, rock, base.

➤ Heroin—horse, lady, smack, white girl, black tar, brown sugar, goods, H, junk.

➤ Fentanyl transmucosal—percopop.

➤ LSD (lysergic acid diethylamide)—acid, beast, blue cheer, blue heaven, dot, Lucy in the sky with diamonds.

➤ Marijuana—pot, weed, reefer, herb, green, Mary Jane, MJ, joints, bong, toke.

➤ Methamphetamine—meth, crank, speed, crystal, go-fast, go, zip, chris, cristy, ice.

➤ MDMA (methylenedioxymethamphetamine)—ecstasy, X, XTC, Adam, wonder drug, euphoria, E. Commonly used at large parties, described as "raves."

➤ MDA (methylenedioxyamphetamine)—Eve.

➤ Dextromethorphan—robo, skittles, Vitamin D, dex, tussin.

➤ GHB (gamma-hydroxybutyrate)—liquid ecstasy, liquid X, Georgia home boy, goop, gamma-OH, grievous bodily harm.

➤ Rohypnol (flunitrazepam)—rophies, roofies, roach, rope, rape, date rape drug, Mexican Valium.

➤ PCP (phencyclidine)—angel dust, ozone, wack, rocket fuel. When combined with marijuana—killer joints, crystal supergrass.

➤ Ketamine—special K, vitamin K, purple, super C.

➤ Inhalants—sniffing, glue sniffing, huffing.

5

PERSONALITY DISORDERS

DSM-IV-TR Personality Disorders

Cluster A personality disorders:
  Paranoid personality disorder
  Schizoid personality disorder
  Schizotypal personality disorder
Cluster B personality disorders:
  Antisocial personality disorder
  Borderline personality disorder
  Histrionic personality disorder
  Narcissistic personality disorder
Cluster C personality disorders:
  Avoidant personality disorder
  Dependent personality disorder
  Obsessive-compulsive personality disorder
Personality disorder not otherwise specified
Personality change due to a general medical condition

GENERAL CONCEPTS

DSM-IV-TR Diagnostic Criteria (Summary)

➤ An enduring pattern of inner experience and behavior that deviates mark-edly from the expectations of the individual's culture. This pattern is mani-fested in two (or more) of the following areas:

✔ Cognition (i.e., ways of perceiving and interpreting self, other people, and events).

✔ Affectivity (i.e., the range, intensity, lability, and appropriateness of emo-tional response).

315

✔ Interpersonal functioning.

✔ Impulse control.

➤ The enduring pattern is inflexible and pervasive across a broad range of personal and social situations.

➤ The enduring pattern leads to clinically significant distress or impairment in social, occupational, or other important areas of functioning.

➤ The pattern is stable and of long duration, and its onset can be traced back at least to adolescence or early adulthood.

➤ The enduring pattern is not better accounted for as a manifestation or consequence of another psychiatric disorder.

➤ The enduring pattern is not due to the direct physiological effects of a substance (e.g., a drug of abuse, a medication) or a general medical condition (e.g., head trauma).

Clinical Issues

➤ Personality disorders (PDs):

✔ Encompass impairments in personality (i.e., character) that are maladaptive, pervasive, deeply ingrained, inflexible, and enduring. These impairments start in early childhood or adolescence and are not caused by another psychiatric disorder, a substance (i.e., drug of abuse, medication), or a medical illness.

✔ Can be grouped by the similarity (clusters) of symptoms:

■ Cluster A—paranoid, schizoid, and schizotypal PDs are characterized as the "odd or eccentric" group.

■ Cluster B—histrionic, narcissistic, antisocial, and borderline PDs are characterized as the "dramatic, emotional, or erratic" group.

■ Cluster C—obsessive-compulsive, dependent, and avoidant PDs are characterized as the "anxious or fearful" group.

✔ Can be assessed by administering psychological tests:

■ Objective testing (restricted response format [e.g., "yes" or "no" responses], standardized scoring, large database for scoring):

• Minnesota Multiphasic Personality Inventory–II (MMPI-II): 567 true-false questions—see Chapter 1 ("Schizophrenia and Other Psychotic Disorders").

• Millon Clinical Multiaxial Inventory—III (MCMI-III): 157 true-false questions; testing specifically directed toward elucidating personality traits or PDs as well as other clinical scales (e.g., anxiety, posttraumatic stress disorder [PTSD], substance abuse).

• The Narcissistic Personality Inventory is used to identify narcissistic traits.

- The Borderline Personality Organization Scale can elucidate traits of borderline personality disorder.
- The Structured Clinical Interview (SCID-II) is based on DSM-IV-TR criteria for elucidating personality traits.
- The Multidimensional Anger Inventory helps identify angry attitudes.
- Projective testing—uses unstructured or ambiguous material; response is dynamic (e.g., stories, meanings):
  - Rorschach ("inkblot") test.
  - Thematic Apperception Test (stories developed after viewing black-and-white pictures).

✔ Differ from personality traits (i.e., features of a personality that do not reach the threshold for a PD). A diagnosis of a PD is warranted only when personality traits:

- Are inflexible, maladaptive, and enduring.
- Start in early childhood or adolescence.
- Cause significant functional impairment or subjective distress.

✔ Are highly prevalent (15% of the adult population have at least one PD).

✔ Are ego-syntonic, in that the person is not overly bothered by the behavior and blames others for his or her conflicts (i.e., alloplastic defenses). However, others must endure the consequences of interacting with the person on the person's terms. The individual typically has poor insight as to how and why the behavior is maladaptive. As a result, the maladaptive behaviors are repeated, leading to recurrent and at times continual problems. Dysfunctional relationships are a consistent finding.

✔ Encompass ten individual PDs and the catch-all *personality disorder not otherwise specified* (PDNOS). It is fairly easy to meet criteria for more than one PD, and it is possible that two individuals meeting a given PD diagnosis may not share any common criteria (e.g., obsessive-compulsive personality disorder requires four out of eight symptoms to make the diagnosis).

✔ Are poorly understood in terms of etiology. Most likely, some combination of developmental, environmental, and genetic influences play a role.

✔ Typically present with poor emotional maturity, with peak emotional development achieved in adolescence. Early traumatic experiences are common findings.

✔ Historically are treated with long-term insight-oriented or psychodynamic therapy with a goal of changing fundamental personality traits. However, a number of clinical trials and anecdotal reports suggest that medications (e.g., selective serotonin reuptake inhibitors [SSRIs], monoamine oxidase inhibitors [MAOIs], typical [i.e., first-generation antipsychotic medications (FGAs)] and atypical [i.e., second-generation antipsychotic medications (SGAs)] antipsychotic agents, mood stabilizers) can be quite efficacious for treating some of the core features of PDs, especially for persons with borderline, schizotypal, and obsessive-compulsive PDs.

✔ Typically present with difficult-to-treat patients. Persons with PDs tend to be alloplastic in their thinking, believing that society (but not them) should change to make things better. Their difficulty with maintaining relationships is mirrored in their therapy.

✔ Are relatively poorly studied in comparison to Axis I diagnoses. Borderline PD is the most studied.

✔ May demonstrate anatomical changes. Antisocial PD can present with decreased prefrontal gray matter and borderline PD can present with changes in the amygdala.

✔ Are viewed pejoratively by health insurance companies as being non-fixable and ever lasting, with a reluctance for approval for long-term treatment.

➤ Cautions:

✔ "Personality-disordered behavior" is not synonymous with having a PD. For example, a person presenting with repeated acts of self-harming behavior should not, without satisfying the other diagnostic criteria, be labeled as having borderline PD.

✔ DSM-IV-TR does not allow for a classification of substance-induced PD.

✔ If you suspect a PD, include the diagnosis in your differential but indicate that a longer period of assessment (e.g., two to five therapy sessions), possibly to include psychological testing and collateral information sources, would be needed to make a definitive diagnosis. This allows the examiners to appreciate that you suspect a PD but recognize that a short interview typically does not provide sufficient time to firmly establish the diagnosis.

✔ Although you may be reasonably certain that a patient has a PD, it is often difficult to determine with certainty which PD is present. The diagnostic criteria of the PDs often overlap. For example, distinguishing among borderline, histrionic, narcissistic, and antisocial PDs can be difficult (if not impossible after a short interview). Compounding this difficulty is the trend toward the more frequent diagnosis of borderline or histrionic PD in women and of antisocial or narcissistic PD in men when clinical presentations are nearly identical.

✔ Current studies are demonstrating significant value of cognitive-behavioral therapy (CBT) for the treatment of PDs. The focus is on the core beliefs that are the foundation of the maladaptive behavior.

Risk Factors (Not Consistent From Study to Study)

➤ Young adult.

➤ African American or Native American.

➤ Low socioeconomic status.

➤ Widowed, divorced, separated, or never married.

Etiological Considerations

Genetic formulations:

➤ A genetic predisposition has been implicated. Some PDs are more prevalent in monozygotic twins than in dizygotic twins.

➤ The Cluster A grouping of PDs (paranoid, schizoid, schizotypal) may:

✔ Have a genetic link to schizophrenia.

✔ Present as the prodromal phase for schizophrenia.

➤ Family members of schizophrenic patients are more likely to present with paranoid and schizoid PDs.

Childhood factors:

➤ An increased prevalence of childhood central nervous system dysfunction (e.g., head injury) is found in persons with antisocial and borderline PDs.

➤ Children with attention-deficit/hyperactivity disorder are at greater risk of developing antisocial PD.

➤ Females with a history of sexual abuse are at greater risk of developing borderline PD.

Endocrinological formulations:

➤ Impulsive traits in persons with antisocial PD may be linked to higher levels of testosterone.

➤ Thyroid dysfunction is more common in individuals with borderline PD.

Neurological formulations:

✔ Smooth-pursuit eye movements may be abnormal in schizotypal PD (as well as in schizophrenia).

✔ Increased slow-wave activation may be found on the electroencephalograms (EEGs) of persons with antisocial and borderline PDs.

Neurotransmitter formulation:

➤ Changing levels of serotonin may influence personality traits, depression, impulsivity, and aggression.

➤ Low levels of serotonin may predispose to borderline PD.

Psychodynamic and psychological formulations:

➤ The patient is fixated (i.e., stops further maturation) at one of the psychosocial stages of development:

✔ Fixation at the oral stage results in an individual with passive and dependent traits.

✔ Fixation at the anal stage results in an individual who is stubborn, rigid, and compulsive.

✔ Failure to separate and individuate from parents leads to the development of borderline PD.

Defense mechanisms:

➤ Defense mechanisms are unconscious processes utilized to reduce anxiety associated with unmet instinctive desires or needs.

➤ Common defense mechanisms (usually unhealthy) include:

✔ Fantasy—imaginary lives are created (schizoid PD). The person is fixated (i.e., stops further maturation) at one of the psychosocial stages of development.

✔ Dissociation—unpleasant affects are replaced with pleasant ones (histrionic PD).

✔ Isolation—characteristic of an orderly, controlled person who shows little affect (obsessive-compulsive PD).

✔ Projection—unacknowledged feelings are attributed to others (borderline PD, paranoid PD, and schizoid PD).

✔ Projective identification—aspects of self are projected onto someone else. The projector tries to coerce the other person to identify with what has been projected. As a result, the recipient of the projection and the projector feel a sense of oneness (borderline PD).

✔ Passive aggression—anger toward others is acted out passively.

✔ Acting out—the display of previously inhibited emotions (often in actions rather than words).

✔ Regression—fleeing adult issues by assuming a younger or infantile state.

✔ Reaction formation—unconscious development of attitudes and behavior that are the opposite of unacceptable repressed desires and impulses (e.g., advocating strict morality is a reaction formation used by an individual to hide his or her own desire to act on a strong sexual drive).

✔ Denial—denial of the existence of painful thoughts.

✔ Conversion—repression of emotional conflicts by converting them into physical symptoms that have no organic basis.

✔ Splitting—an object (e.g., person) is viewed as either all good or all bad, sometimes alternating between the two (borderline PD).

✔ Undoing—a symbolic means of negating or making amends for unacceptable thoughts or feelings (e.g., repetitively washing hands as an unconscious gesture of "washing away" the guilt for something the person has done).

➤ Common defense mechanisms (usually healthy):

✔ Anticipation—thinking ahead to events that might occur in the future and considering realistic responses or solutions.

✔ Affiliation—seeking out others for emotional support or physical help.

✔ Altruism—doing good and kind things for others, rather than worrying about one's own immediate satisfaction or fears.

✔ Humor—noticing the amusing or ironic aspects of something rather than the unpleasant aspects.

PARANOID PERSONALITY DISORDER

Essential Characteristics

➤ Extreme suspiciousness. There is an unwarranted tendency to interpret the actions or motives of others as threatening (malevolent). However, the suspiciousness does not rise to the level of a paranoid delusion.

DSM-IV-TR Diagnostic Criteria (Summary)

➤ A pervasive distrust and suspiciousness of others such that their motives are interpreted as malevolent, beginning by early adulthood and present in a variety of contexts, as indicated by four (or more) of the following:

✔ Suspects, without sufficient basis, that others are exploiting, harming, or deceiving him or her.

✔ Is preoccupied with unjustified doubts about the loyalty or trustworthiness of friends or associates.

✔ Is reluctant to confide in others because of unwarranted fear that the information will be used maliciously against him or her.

✔ Reads hidden demeaning or threatening meanings into benign remarks or events.

✔ Persistently bears grudges (i.e., is unforgiving of insults, injuries, or slights).

✔ Perceives attacks on his or her character or reputation that are not apparent to others and is quick to react angrily or to counterattack.

✔ Has recurrent suspicions, without justification, regarding fidelity of spouse or sexual partner.

Clinical Issues

➤ Characteristically, persons with paranoid PD:

✔ Expect exploitation or harm by others, interpret benign statements or acts as threatening, hold grudges, and are unforgiving. As a result, persons with paranoid PD live in a malevolently hostile world of their own making.

✔ Tend to isolate themselves as a means of protection from the hostile world.

✔ Question the loyalty and trust of friends, co-workers, and family. They may not confide in others, fearing that the information will be used against them.

✔ Often rely on the legal system to correct the injustice or associate with groups who share a similar ideology (e.g., antigovernment groups desiring to overthrow the country).

✔ May experience transient psychotic symptoms under stress, but not to the extent of qualifying for a diagnosis of delusional disorder, persecutory type. However, this differentiation can be very difficult to make, especially after a short interview.

✔ Utilize projection as the primary defense mechanism.

➤ Paranoid PD may represent a prodromal phase for the eventual development of schizophrenia.

Epidemiology

➤ Prevalence is ~4% of the general population; more common in males.

Etiology

➤ Not fully established, but an association with schizophrenia spectrum disorders has been proposed.

➤ A genetic influence is supported by a greater prevalence of paranoid PD in relatives of individuals with paranoid PD.

Common Comorbidities

➤ Substance use disorders.

➤ Major depressive disorder.

➤ Panic disorder.

➤ Obsessive-compulsive PD.

Prognosis

➤ Generally poor. Paranoid thinking (at either the nonpsychotic level or the psychotic level) is perhaps the most difficult psychiatric symptom to effectively ameliorate.

Differential Diagnosis

➤ Delusional disorders—delusions are not typically present in paranoid PDs (except transiently under stress). But, deciding if falsehood is an ideation or delusion can be difficult.

➤ Schizophrenia, paranoid type—psychotic features (e.g., hallucinations, delusions, disorganization) are not typical features of PDs.

➤ Mood disorder (major depressive disorder, bipolar disorder).

➤ PDs (particularly Cluster A):

  ✔ Borderline PD—tumultuous relationships are more likely in borderline PD.

  ✔ Antisocial PD—repeated antisocial behaviors are not prevalent in paranoid PD.

  ✔ Narcissistic PD—greater level of entitlements in narcissistic PD.

  ✔ Schizoid, schizotypal, and avoidant PDs can appear to have paranoid traits.

Treatment

➤ Individuals are not eager for treatment, in that they believe their paranoid thinking is justified. The therapist can quickly become included in the patient's inherent belief of a malevolent world.

➤ Support and crisis stabilization are the primary treatment goals. Rarely is there a full remission.

➤ Supportive psychotherapy (individual, cognitive therapy) is the principal treatment, with honesty and absolute reliability of the therapist. An overly friendly and warm approach is not appropriate. Because trust is a fundamental problem, individual rather than group therapy is more likely to be accepted by the patient.

➤ Medications can be used to target comorbid symptoms or disorders (e.g., antipsychotic medication for psychotic episodes, antidepressants for depression, anxiolytic medications for anxiety). However, because patients do not believe they are ill, compliance with medications is often problematic.

SCHIZOID PERSONALITY DISORDER

Essential Characteristics

➤ Withdrawn and aloof behaviors. Individuals prefer aloneness over companionship.

DSM-IV-TR Diagnostic Criteria (Summary)

➤ A pervasive pattern of detachment from social relationships and a restricted range of expression of emotions in interpersonal settings, beginning by early adulthood and present in a variety of contexts, as indicated by four (or more) of the following:

✔ Neither desires nor enjoys close relationships, including being part of a family.

✔ Almost always chooses solitary activities.

✔ Has little, if any, interest in having sexual experiences with another person.

✔ Takes pleasure in few, if any, activities.

✔ Lacks close friends or confidants other than first-degree relatives.

✔ Appears indifferent to the praise or criticism of others.

✔ Shows emotional coldness, detachment, or flattened affectivity.

Clinical Issues

➤ Characteristically, persons with schizoid PD:

✔ Are socially withdrawn, aloof, affectively restricted, emotionally cold, and introverted. They prefer solitary activities, rarely marry, feel discomfort with human interactions, and show little or no desire for intimacy.

✔ May be described by others as "robotic."

✔ Lack normal social skills and have difficulty expressing feelings.

✔ Highly value nonhuman interests (e.g., mechanical or electronic devices) or show an unusual interest in animals.

✔ Typically prefer to adhere to rigid and predictable behaviors (i.e., "creatures of habit").

✔ Excessively daydream and develop an extensive fantasy life.

➤ Schizoid PD may represent a prodromal phase for the eventual development of schizophrenia.

➤ Common defenses include projection and fantasy.

Epidemiology

➤ Prevalence is ~3% of the general population (poorly documented); no difference in frequency between the sexes.

Etiology

➤ Not established, but an association with the TaqAl allele of the dopamine D_2 receptor has been identified.

➤ Familiar patterns of introversion strongly suggest a genetic basis.

Prognosis

➤ Unknown. Some patients respond quite well to psychotherapy and are able to develop closer personal relationships. Others can only be helped to learn to adapt to a reclusive lifestyle.

Differential Diagnosis

➤ Schizophrenia—persistent psychotic symptoms are not present in schizoid PD.

➤ Delusional disorder—psychotic symptoms are not present in schizoid PD.

➤ PDs:

✔ Cluster A:

■ Paranoid PD—not eccentric, not odd.

■ Schizotypal PD—more oddities are usually present in schizotypal PD, but the differentiation can be difficult.

✔ Cluster B:

■ Borderline PD—desire for rather than fleeing from intimacy.

■ Narcissistic PD—feelings of entitlement prevail, without excessive oddness.

✔ Cluster C:

■ Avoidant PD—want to associate but retreat due to excessive anxiety.

Treatment

➤ Psychotherapy (individual, group) is the treatment of choice, as with other PDs. Take into account the defenses of projection and fantasy.

➤ Medications can be used to target comorbid symptoms or disorders (e.g., antipsychotic medication for psychotic episodes, antidepressants for depression, anxiolytic medications for anxiety).

SCHIZOTYPAL PERSONALITY DISORDER

Essential Characteristics

➤ Odd, strange, and eccentric behaviors coupled with magical thinking, peculiar ideation, ideas of reference, illusions, and derealization.

DSM-IV-TR Diagnostic Criteria (Summary)

➤ A pervasive pattern of social and interpersonal deficits marked by acute discomfort with, and reduced capacity for, close relationships as well as by cognitive or perceptual distortions and eccentricities of behavior, beginning by early adulthood and present in a variety of contexts, as indicated by five (or more) of the following:

✔ Ideas of reference (excluding delusions of reference).

✔ Odd beliefs or magical thinking that influences behavior and is inconsistent with subcultural norms (e.g., superstitions, belief in clairvoyance, telepathy, or "sixth sense").

✔ Unusual perceptual experiences, including bodily illusions.

✔ Odd thinking and speech (e.g., vague, circumstantial, metaphorical, overelaborate, stereotyped).

✔ Suspiciousness or paranoid ideation.

✔ Inappropriate or constricted affect.

✔ Behavior or appearance that is odd, eccentric, or peculiar.

✔ Lack of close friends or confidants other than first-degree relatives.

✔ Excessive social anxiety that does not diminish with familiarity and tends to be associated with paranoid fears rather than negative judgments about self.

Clinical Issues

➤ Characteristically, persons with schizotypal PD:

✔ Have odd beliefs, magical thinking, unusual perceptual experiences, and illusions, as if they had a "sixth sense."

✔ May report supernatural experiences (e.g., clairvoyance, telepathy, out-of-body voyages).

✔ Use unusual wording or odd phrasing, at times consistent with a private language.

✔ Show eccentric behavior and/or odd dress (e.g., may dress as a gypsy).

✔ Have no or few close friends and may show excessive social anxiety. When around others, they may show inappropriate or constricted affect.

✔ Can have paranoid ideation and ideas of reference. Typically, patients are convinced that they are continually being criticized, gossiped about, or mocked by others. Paranoid delusions can develop in extreme cases.

✔ May be involved with cults, the occult, and other strange religious practices.

➤ Schizotypal PD:

✔ May represent a prodromal phase for the eventual development of schizophrenia.

✔ Is very culture bound in its diagnosis. Many of the behaviors cited are normal in certain cultures and subcultures, at times making the diagnosis difficult to establish.

Epidemiology

➤ Prevalence is 2%–5% of the general population (poorly documented); more common in males.

Etiology

➤ Possibly related to schizophrenia.

➤ Familiar patterns of "introversion" strongly suggest a genetic basis.

Prognosis

➤ Unknown. Some patients can respond quite well to psychotherapy.

Differential Diagnosis

➤ Schizoid PD—excessive overt oddities are not typically seen in schizoid PD, although isolation is common in both disorders. Can be difficult to differentiate from schizotypal PD.

➤ Avoidant PD—overt oddities are not seen in avoidant PD.

➤ Paranoid PD—suspiciousness may be present in both disorders, but overt oddities are not present in paranoid PD.

➤ Borderline PD—may at times meet the criteria for schizotypal PD.

➤ Schizophrenia—persistent psychotic symptoms are not present in schizotypal PD.

➤ Delusional disorder—psychotic symptoms are not present in schizotypal PD.

Treatment

➤ Psychotherapy (individual, group) is the treatment of choice, as with all PDs.

➤ Medications can be used to target comorbid symptoms or disorders (e.g., antipsychotic medication for psychotic episodes, antidepressants for depression, anxiolytic medications for anxiety).

➤ Approximately 10% of persons with schizotypal PD eventually commit suicide.

ANTISOCIAL PERSONALITY DISORDER

Essential Characteristic

➤ An inability to conform to social norms, with repeated exploitations and criminal acts for material gain.

DSM-IV-TR Diagnostic Criteria (Summary)

➤ A pervasive pattern of disregard for and violation of the rights of others occurring since age 15 years, as indicated by three (or more) of the following:

✔ Failure to conform to social norms with respect to lawful behaviors, as indicated by repeatedly performing acts that are grounds for arrest.

✔ Deceitfulness, as indicated by repeated lying, use of aliases, or conning others for personal profit or pleasure.

✔ Impulsivity or failure to plan ahead.

✔ Irritability and aggressiveness, as indicated by repeated physical fights or assaults.

✔ Reckless disregard for safety of self or others.

✔ Consistent irresponsibility, as indicated by repeated failure to sustain consistent work behavior or honor financial obligations.

✔ Lack of remorse, as indicated by being indifferent to or rationalizing having hurt, mistreated, or stolen from another.

➤ The individual is at least 18 years of age.

➤ There is evidence of conduct disorder with onset before age 15 years.

Clinical Issues

➤ Characteristically, individuals with antisocial PD:

✔ Develop symptoms in childhood or adolescence, first as oppositional defiant disorder, progressing to conduct disorder, and then progressing to antisocial PD (the usual progression). By definition, symptoms of conduct disorder must begin by at least age 15 years.

✔ Have an inflexible doctrine that the rules of society do not apply to them. They are unable to see how their behavior affects victims and often lack remorse or concern for others who have been injured or have sustained losses by their behaviors.

✔ May be highly manipulative and fit the designation of a "con man" (i.e., one who promotes unethical, quick, and easy schemes for the victim to make a lot of money at someone else's expense). Lying, stealing, and harming others for personal gain are characteristic findings.

✔ View others as objects to be manipulated to gain control of their money or other possessions.

✔ Often act impulsively without thinking of long-term consequences. Legal issues are common.

✔ Present with a high potential for a wide range of inappropriate behaviors (e.g., promiscuity, spousal and child abuse).

✔ May present with "soft" neurological deficits or other psychiatric difficulties (e.g., abnormal EEG, attention-deficit/hyperactivity disorder, learning disabilities).

➤ Individuals with antisocial PD were previously labeled (somewhat pejoratively) as psychopaths or sociopaths. Some authorities do not feel that antisocial PD is a true psychiatric disorder.

➤ Individuals with antisocial PD can be difficult to treat effectively. They show little regard for the rights of others. Missing appointments, outright lying, not paying for treatment, malingering to avoid legal issues or work, altering prescriptions, and having poor compliance with treatment recommendations are common behaviors.

➤ Antisocial acts, in and of themselves, do not necessarily qualify for a diagnosis of antisocial PD. *Adult antisocial behavior* (a DSM-IV-TR diagnosis) describes antisocial acts (e.g., criminal activity undertaken for gain) that are not accompanied by the personality features of antisocial PD.

➤ There is an increased risk of early death, often due to association with other individuals with antisocial PD, who also show little regard for the rights of others.

➤ Common defense mechanisms include intellectualization and projective identification at a primitive level.

Epidemiology

➤ Prevalence is 3%–4% in males and 1% in females.

➤ Prevalence ranges from 40% to 75% in prison populations.

➤ Males tend to show symptoms earlier than do females.

Comorbidity

➤ Substance abuse disorders (extremely high).

➤ Other Cluster B PDs.

➤ Impulse-control disorders (e.g., intermittent explosive disorder, pathological gambling).

Etiology

➤ A genetic contribution to the development of antisocial PD has been proposed (e.g., adopted children of antisocial birth parents are more likely to develop antisocial PD than are adopted children of nonaffected birth parents).

➤ Environmental factors (e.g., dysfunctional family structure, learned behavior, lack of adequate discipline as a child) likely play a role in the development of antisocial PD.

➤ Brain abnormalities secondary to injury to the prefrontal cortex and amygdala may produce impairment in ability to make appropriate moral judgments and to feel remorse for inappropriate behaviors.

Prognosis

➤ Poor up to approximately age 40 years. Individuals with antisocial PD are more likely to:

✔ Have failed marriages.

✔ Be imprisoned for illegal activities (e.g., assaults, robberies, rape, murder, "con man").

✔ Die at an earlier age (e.g., substance abuse, AIDS, violence perpetrated against them by others with antisocial PD, suicide, accidents).

➤ Guarded after age 40 years, with some natural burnout of antisocial behavior expected. By age 45 years, 80% no longer meet diagnostic criteria. This "evolution" is not appreciated by the legal system.

Differential Diagnosis

➤ Adult antisocial behavior and antisocial behavior secondary to substance abuse, neurological or medical causes, or mental retardation.

➤ Other PDs, particularly those in Cluster B.

➤ Manic or hypomanic episodes of bipolar disorder.

➤ Medical disorders (e.g., frontal lobe head injury, brain tumor).

Treatment

➤ Psychotherapy is the treatment of choice, as with all PDs. Limit setting is a must.

➤ Medications can be used to target comorbid symptoms or disorders (e.g., antipsychotic medication for psychotic episodes, antidepressants for depression, anxiolytic medications for anxiety). Especially avoid prescribing controlled substances (high likelihood of being abused or sold).

BORDERLINE PERSONALITY DISORDER

Essential Characteristic

➤ Instability ("stably unstable") with regard to impulsivity, anger, affect, identity, and interpersonal relationships.

DSM-IV-TR Diagnostic Criteria (Summary)

➤ A pervasive pattern of instability of interpersonal relationships, self-image, and affects, and marked impulsivity beginning by early adulthood and present in a variety of contexts, as indicated by five (or more) of the following:

✔ Frantic efforts to avoid real or imagined abandonment, not including suicidal or self-mutilating behavior.

✔ A pattern of unstable and intense interpersonal relationships characterized by alternating between extremes of idealization and devaluation.

✔ Identity disturbance: markedly and persistently unstable self-image or sense of self.

✔ Impulsivity in at least two areas that are potentially self-damaging (e.g., spending, sex, substance abuse, reckless driving, binge eating), not including suicidal or self-mutilating behavior.

✔ Recurrent suicidal behavior, gestures, or threats, or recurrent self-mutilating behavior.

✔ Affective instability due to a marked reactivity of mood (e.g., intense episodic dysphoria, irritability, or anxiety, usually lasting a few hours and only rarely more than a few days).

✔ Chronic feelings of emptiness.

✔ Inappropriate, intense anger or difficulty controlling anger (e.g., frequent displays of temper, constant anger, recurrent physical fights).

✔ Transient, stress-related paranoid ideation or severe dissociative symptoms.

Clinical Issues

➤ Characteristically, persons with borderline PD:

✔ Are repeatedly, if not chronically, in a state of crisis.

✔ Present with marked and persistent identity disturbance (identity diffusion). This includes uncertainty about life issues, self-image, sexual orientation, and long-term goals (e.g., career choices).

✔ Form intense but unstable (and thus short-lived) relationships. Relationships typically are at first highly valued (idealized). In time, with disappointments (e.g., feelings of abandonment, disagreements), the person may develop depression, anger, resentment, and hostility (devaluation). Individuals are unusually demanding with their involvement in relationships and with their therapists, feel both dependent and hostile in relationships, and typically have tumultuous interpersonal conflicts. In this regard, there is a "narcissistic" quality evident—an ever-present need to find acceptance and valuation from others when the person with borderline personality disorder has very low self-esteem and low self-worth and a belief that the person(s) they depend on will ultimately abandon them.

✔ Show affective instability with marked and rapid mood shifts (e.g., depression, irritability, hypomania, anger, rage). Often, the anger is far in excess of what is warranted (inappropriate anger).

✔ Describe extreme feelings of emptiness and boredom, with inappropriate behaviors (e.g., one-night stands, suicidal threats) to avoid abandonment (real or imagined) or to gain attention.

✔ Regress under stress with depersonalization, derealization, or brief psychotic episodes.

✔ Engage in impulsive, reckless, and self-harming behaviors (e.g., self-cutting, cigarette burning, sexual improprieties [e.g., unsafe sex, one-night stands], substance abuse, gambling, binge eating, antisocial acts) as a means of diffusing internal painful affects, to gain attention, or to control another individual. Self-mutilation or self-harming behaviors enacted as a means of diffusing anger or painful affects are termed *parasuicide.* Although often manipulative in nature, such behaviors must be taken seriously. Individuals with borderline PD may act on suicidal threats, with suicide attempts and, at times, completed suicides.

✔ Shift rapidly between depression and euphoria, anxiety and self-confidence, calmness and rage attacks, often depending on the immediacy of the circumstance with regard to acceptance or rejection.

✔ View themselves as helpless and needing to trust in another person, who, they believe, will ultimately abandon them.

Components of Borderline Personality Disorder

➤ Affective (e.g., labile affect, mood instability, irritability, depression).

➤ Impulsive (e.g., self-mutilation, suicidal behavior, substance abuse, promiscuity, assaults, antisocial acts).

➤ Ego and interpersonal (e.g., abandonment issues, intense interpersonal relationships, identity disturbance, chronic feelings of emptiness).

➤ Psychotic or near-psychotic (e.g., transient psychotic episodes, "psychotic micro-episodes," derealization, depersonalization, ideas of reference, dissociation, reality distortion, illusions, magical thinking).

➤ Cognitive (e.g., distorted views of self, the world, the future).

➤ Anxiety (e.g., the constant search for affirmation and assurance of self-worth).

Metaphor for Borderline Personality Disorder[1]

➤ "Borderline PD patients perceive themselves as balancing precariously at the peak of a mountain. They are at the mercy of the wind and rain, and at any time they can fall off the mountain and die. All of their energy goes into keeping themselves from falling off the mountain, and they grasp at whatever is readily available to them, even if what they grasp does them or others harm."

Etiological Formulations

Historical considerations:

➤ The term *borderline* reflects an early categorization of patients who were felt to be on the border between neurosis (i.e., excessive anxiety) and psychosis (possibly schizophrenia).

Biological considerations:

➤ Mood disorders may play an etiological role, as evidenced by a high comorbidity with depression, increased prevalence of major (but not bipolar) depression in relatives, electroencephalographic patterns similar to those found in depressed individuals, and similar response patterns to some (but not all) antidepressants.

Genetic, psychodynamic, and psychosocial formulations:

Trauma hypothesis:

➤ There are pathological similarities in early childhood traumas that lead to the development of borderline PD and PTSD (e.g., childhood physical and sexual abuse issues).

Meissner's perspective:

➤ Borderline PD is organized along a spectrum from psychosis to mood disorder (hysteroid dysphoria). The psychotic and affective spectrum may be genetically related.

Gunderson's perspective:

➤ Intense and unstable relationships, self-destructive behavior, hypersensitivity, impulsive behavior, and poor social adaptation are the foundations of borderline PD.

Mahler and Masters' perspective:

➤ Borderline PD is a consequence of developmental problems related to the separation–individuation stage. Here, the child does well in the symbiotic

---

[1]Yeomans, Kernberg, and Clarkson: *A Primer of Transference Focused Psychotherapy for the Borderline Patient.* Lanham, MD, Jason Aronson, 2002.

phase (second to fifth months of life), but in the separation–individuation stage (about 2 years of age), the child is unable to separate and, therefore, unable to individuate. In healthy development, the good-enough mother usually provides an adequate environment (holding environment) that fosters separation–individuation. It is this rapprochement subphase of development that is impaired in borderline PD.

Kernberg's perspective:

➤ Excessive aggression in early childhood does not allow integration of mother as both good and bad. This results in splitting (a primitive defense) as a means to decrease anxiety. Here, the person can see others only as either all good or all bad, but not with both qualities simultaneously. Also, who is good and who is bad can quickly change, often depending on whether or not the person's needs are being met. Although persons with borderline PD are not usually psychotic, there is impaired ego integration. Fundamentally, persons with borderline PD use primitive defenses (e.g., splitting, magical thinking, projective identification) to deal with anxiety. Kernberg defined *borderline personality disorganization* as reflecting an impaired sense of identity while maintaining reality-testing capacity.

Linehan's perspective:

➤ The development of borderline PD can be explained by a stress–diathesis model, in which a punishing or invalidating environment (stress) interacts with poorly modulated emotionality (diathesis). For example, a child's emotional feelings are invalidated by a sexually abusive parent who convinces the child that the sexual behavior is proper. The child does not learn to trust his or her own feelings, resulting in the instability and identity diffusion of borderline PD. Linehan theorized that persons with borderline PD are born with a poor ability to deal with and recover from stress. Linehan's model is validated by the success of dialectical behavior therapy (DBT; teaches adaptive behaviors to learn to appropriately deal with stress, resulting in a reduction of impulsive and suicidal behaviors, improved coping skills, and improved relationships).

Family hypothesis:

➤ Early parental loss or abrupt and traumatic separations from parents are often found in individuals with borderline PD (i.e., a high degree of family dysfunction). Also, there is a high incidence of parental abuse and neglect of a child who later develops borderline PD. In addition, there are findings of frequent Axis II disorders and alcohol/drug abuse among first-degree relatives. There is typically severe psychopathology in both mothers and fathers of persons with borderline PD. Mothers are typically depressed, and fathers are typically detached.

Epidemiology

➤ Borderline PD is found in approximately 2.5% of the general population, 10% of psychiatric outpatients, and 15%–25% of psychiatric inpatients. Individuals with borderline PD account for about 50% of all persons with PDs.

➤ Prevalence is three times greater in females than in males.

➤ A history of childhood physical and/or sexual abuse is frequently present in individuals with borderline PD.

Outcome

➤ Eight percent to 10% of persons with borderline PD complete suicide, often after multiple prior attempts. In general, the more closely an individual meets criteria for borderline PD (DSM-III [American Psychiatric Association 1980]), the higher the risk of suicide (e.g., 35% of persons presenting with all eight diagnostic criteria listed by DSM-III eventually commit suicide).

➤ Early in therapy, acting-out behaviors are frequent and generate a significant measure of negative countertransference (anger directed from the therapist to the patient). Patients will miss appointments, yet call after hours demanding time with the therapist. Often, they are inconsistent with compliance with treatment recommendations (e.g., to stop inappropriate sexual behaviors, to stop substance abuse).

➤ Patients may, through projective identification, cast the therapist in a particular role (e.g., parent, lover, rescuer). Because of the intensity of the therapeutic relationship, the therapist may inappropriately assume one or more of these roles, potentially violating the physician–patient relationship (e.g., sexual activity between patient and physician). However, as time progresses, if the physician–patient relationship remains appropriate, a stabilizing quality that comes with treatment, increasing age, and possibly a tendency for natural burnout of the disorder ensues. At such a time, there can be significant emotional reward for having worked with such difficult and unusually demanding patients.

➤ Prognosis is improved for patients who have:
  ✔ A high IQ and higher educational achievement.
  ✔ Never being jailed.
  ✔ No history of substance abuse.
  ✔ No history of sexual or physical abuse.

Comorbidity

➤ Substance abuse (especially alcohol).

➤ Mood disorders, such as major depression, atypical depression (hysteroid dysphoria), or bipolar II disorder.

➤ Histrionic, antisocial, or schizotypal PD (50% of patients also present with one of these disorders).

➤ Neurological disorders (e.g., seizure disorder).

➤ Anxiety disorders:

✔ PTSD (due to high rates of childhood physical and sexual abuse).

✔ Panic disorder and other anxiety disorders.

Common Defenses

➤ Splitting:

✔ People are seen as either all good or all bad, with frequent shifts between these two idealizations. There is a diminished ability to view people in shades of gray (i.e., a mixture of good and bad qualities).

➤ Projective identification:

✔ Intolerable aspects or feelings of self are projected onto others, and the other person is induced to fulfill that role. If such projection is successful, the patient and the other person "feel as one."

➤ Magical thinking:

✔ The belief that thoughts can cause events to occur.

Differential Diagnosis

Schizophrenia:

➤ Affect is blunted, flat, or inappropriate in schizophrenia, whereas in borderline PD, affect is typically intense and unstable.

➤ Schizophrenic individuals often prefer isolation from others, whereas individuals with borderline PD show compulsive and intense desire for relationships (including therapy).

➤ Schizophrenic individuals have prolonged psychotic episodes, whereas individuals with borderline PD typically have short-lived psychotic episodes.

Other PDs (borderline PD overlaps criteria of many other PDs):

➤ Histrionic PD:

✔ There may be significant overlap between histrionic PD and borderline PD. Individuals with histrionic PD typically rarely experience regression to transient psychotic states, as occurs in borderline PD. Also, persons with histrionic PD are not as destructive and do not chronically complain of loneliness and abandonment.

➤ Antisocial PD:

✔ There is a greater emphasis on exploitation for material rather than emotional gain in antisocial PD. Men are more likely to be diagnosed with antisocial PD, and women are more likely to be diagnosed with borderline PD (when both have nearly similar presentations). However, stealing, lying, and a disregard for the rights of others is also found in borderline PD.

➤ Narcissistic PD:

✔ Narcissistic PD and borderline PD may have significant symptom overlap, and it may be difficult to distinguish between them. Men are more likely to be diagnosed with narcissistic PD, and women are more likely to be diagnosed with borderline PD (when both have nearly similar presentations).

➤ Schizotypal PD:

✔ Individuals with schizotypal PD show marked peculiarities of thinking, strange ideation, and ideas of reference to a degree not typically found in individuals with borderline PD.

➤ Dependent PD:

✔ Persons with dependent PD are less intensive with relationship issues. When threatened with abandonment, persons with dependent PD are much less destructive and more willing to develop a new relationship.

➤ Paranoid PD:

✔ The extreme level of suspiciousness in individuals with paranoid PD helps distinguish this disorder from borderline PD. However, paranoid ideation, ideas of reference, and at times paranoid delusions can develop in borderline PD.

Depressive disorders (e.g., major depression, dysthymic disorder, atypical depression):

➤ Affect is stable (but depressed) in individuals with depressive disorders but labile (at times appearing manic or hypomanic) in individuals with borderline PD. It is often difficult to distinguish between borderline PD and depressive disorders. Both should be included in your differential diagnosis.

Bipolar disorder (especially bipolar II disorder and cyclothymia):

➤ Affect and impulsivity can be labile and intense in both bipolar II disorder and borderline PD. It is often difficult to distinguish between bipolar II disorder and borderline PD. Include both in your differential diagnosis.

Treatment

Psychotherapy (the cornerstone of treatment for borderline PD):

➤ Patients with borderline PD are a challenge to treat. Importantly, patients are very willing to be treated and readily attach to the therapist. Therefore, an unusually high percentage of patients with borderline PD are seen in both outpatient and inpatient psychiatric settings.

➤ Maintain honesty, reliability, and a professional demeanor and insist on limit setting. Maintain objectivity to protect against developing a personal or overly attached relationship with the patient.

➤ Individual (usually supportive), group, and, if appropriate, family therapy can be helpful:

✔ Transference-focused psychotherapy—a psychodynamic therapy designed to help patients with serious PDs.

✔ Cognitive-behavioral therapy.

✔ Dialectical behavior therapy (DBT)—a psychosocial treatment for borderline PD that is becoming an accepted (if not expected) treatment in conjunction with other types of psychotherapy. DBT involves fundamental skills training, teaches patients to improve coping skills, and helps patients learn to appropriately manage anger and to tolerate stress (i.e., DBT applies a broad array of cognitive-behavioral strategies).

➤ Cautions:

✔ Projective identification (the patient tries to coerce the therapist to act out a particular type of behavior) is often covert and can result in negative countertransference or, alternatively, compliance with the patient's wishes (e.g., to bail them out of jail, to engage in sexual relations).

✔ Frequent regressions are common in early years of treatment. Depression, "rage attacks," brief psychotic episodes, and acting out of impulses (e.g., sexual indiscretions, suicide attempts) are common.

✔ Exercise due caution "uncovering" early traumas. Childhood sexual abuse issues are common in patients with borderline PD, and uncovering memories may result in regression and acting-out behaviors. Alternatively, "false memory syndrome," in which allegations are made against the therapist for inducing in the patient false memories of sexual abuse (often with satanic overlays), is a relevant concern from a therapeutic and legal (malpractice and possibly criminal) perspective.

Medication issues:

Depression:

➤ The "quality" of depression in borderline PD is often different from that of major depression. In borderline PD, depression is often characterized by:

✔ Feelings of chronic emptiness and loneliness, periods of anger or rage, and repeated suicidal gestures and/or attempts.

✔ Excessive concern for relationship losses, separation, or abandonment.

✔ Atypical features (e.g., sensitivity rejection, increased sleep).

➤ Antidepressants are typically less effective when depression and borderline PD are comorbid.

Affective instability (i.e., lability):

➤ Antidepressants: Avoid tricyclic antidepressants secondary to the potential for overdose.

➤ Mood stabilizers (e.g., lithium, carbamazepine [Equetro], divalproex [Depakote]).

➤ Low-dose antipsychotic medications: Affective instability is an accepted indication for short-term use of an antipsychotic medication for a nonpsychotic state.

Anger, hostility, self-destructive behavior, or rage:

➤ Antidepressants:

✔ Fluoxetine (Prozac) reduces anger and hostility distinct from its antidepressant effect.

➤ Antipsychotic medications.

➤ Mood stabilizers (e.g., lithium, carbamazepine, divalproex sodium).

Psychotic or regressed state:

➤ Antipsychotic medications (on a short-term basis).

Anxiety:

➤ Buspirone (BuSpar) and cautious use (if at all) of benzodiazepines (secondary to concerns for disinhibition and the potential for abuse).

Hospitalization:

Indications:

➤ Consider short-term hospitalization for a life-threatening crisis, a transient psychotic episode, a relapse into drug abuse, persistent depressive symptoms, or a severe transference reaction during outpatient treatment.

➤ Try to avoid hospitalization when it represents a repeat of a treatment that has repeatedly failed or when the patient is malingering (e.g., to avoid legal consequences, to stop a lover from leaving). However, suicidal threats must be taken seriously.

Ward management:

➤ Maintain close communication between staff to avoid splitting (propensity of patients with borderline PD to divide staff into those who strongly defend and support the patient and those who are angered at the patient and want the patient discharged).

✔ Provide a consistent treatment plan.

✔ Set firm limits.

Provision of structure after discharge:

➤ Consider discharge to home if supports are healthy. If sexual abuse issues were elements of the home environment, alternative living arrangements should be considered.

➤ For patients with severe impairment from borderline PD with a longer-term need for a more structured treatment program, a shorter inpatient hospital stay (until dangerousness issues are resolved) can be followed by transition to residency in a "quarter-way house," where the patient can live close to the hospital and receive individual, behavior, and/or group therapy. This placement would possibly be coupled with medications for treating depression, mood lability, aggression, and/or psychotic regressions and, if appropriate, involvement in Alcoholics Anonymous/Narcotics Anonymous.

HISTRIONIC PERSONALITY DISORDER

Essential Characteristic

➤ An extreme need to receive attention, with a dramatic flair (i.e., "drama queen").

DSM-IV-TR Diagnostic Criteria (Summary)

➤ A pervasive pattern of excessive emotionality and attention seeking, beginning by early adulthood and present in a variety of contexts, as indicated by five (or more) of the following:

✔ Is uncomfortable in situations in which he or she is not the center of attention.

✔ Often interacts with others in a manner characterized by inappropriate sexually seductive or provocative behavior.

✔ Displays rapid shifting and shallow expression of emotions.

✔ Consistently uses physical appearance to draw attention to self.

✔ Has a style of speech that is excessively impressionistic and lacking in detail.

✔ Shows self-dramatization, theatricality, and exaggerated expression of emotion.

✔ Is suggestible (i.e., easily influenced by others or circumstances).

✔ Considers relationships to be more intimate than they actually are.

Clinical Issues

➤ Characteristically, persons with histrionic PD:

✔ Are colorful, dramatic, extroverted, and overly concerned with physical attractiveness. Individuals express emotion with great, and at times inappropriate, exaggeration. Often, they emphasize issues to a greater extent than is warranted by their true importance. A "theatrical" presentation, with exaggerated gestures and emotions, is common.

✔ Need to be the center of attention, requiring constant reassurance and admiration. Individuals are self-centered and show little tolerance for delayed gratification. They may seek attention, and at times sensation, through inappropriate behaviors, such as temper tantrums, substance abuse, or promiscuous behavior (although sexual dysfunction may be present).

✔ Are at increased risk of abusing alcohol and drugs.

✔ Go from relationship to relationship when they eventually deplete the "narcissistic reserve" of the other person.

✔ Often use physical appearance and attire to gain access to a new relationship, later terminate the relationship when their narcissistic needs are no longer being met.

Epidemiology

➤ Prevalence is ~2% of the general population (poorly documented), with the disorder more common in females.

Etiology

➤ Genetic influence includes an increased risk of histrionic PD in other genetically close family members.

➤ Cultural effects (i.e., learned behavior) have been proposed.

Prognosis

➤ Patients can benefit from psychotherapy. There appears to be some burnout of the disorder as the patient ages (as with borderline PD and antisocial PD).

Differential Diagnosis

Borderline personality disorder:

➤ It may be difficult to distinguish between the two disorders. Patients with borderline PD have a greater suicide potential, more identity issues, and a greater potential for brief psychotic episodes.

Antisocial personality disorder:

➤ The goal is for material rather than emotional gain in antisocial PD.

Narcissistic personality disorder:

➤ Individuals are self-centered in both disorders, but persons with narcissistic PD are more preoccupied with grandiose ideation, envy, and having their needs met. However, differentiation between narcissistic PD and histrionic PD can be especially difficult.

Somatization disorder (Briquet's syndrome):

➤ Individuals with somatization disorder complain more of physical illness than persons with histrionic PD, although both disorders can coexist.

Treatment

➤ Psychotherapy is the treatment of choice, as with all PDs:

✔ Individual psychotherapy, both long-term and for crisis stabilization.

✔ Group therapy.

✔ Marital therapy.

✔ Behavioral therapy (avoid giving into patient demands, react appropriately to suicidal gestures, and do not reinforce demands for attention [e.g., missing an appointment but calling after office hours for therapy]).

➤ Medications can be targeted to specific symptoms or comorbid disorders (e.g., antidepressant medications or mood stabilizers for mood disorders, anxiolytics for anxiety, antipsychotic medications for emergent psychotic symptoms). Avoid controlled substances, especially benzodiazepines and opioids, due to an increased likelihood to develop a dependence on prescribed medications.

NARCISSISTIC PERSONALITY DISORDER

Essential Characteristics

➤ An exaggerated sense of entitlement, a need to be admired, feelings of being special, and lack of empathy for others.

DSM-IV-TR Diagnostic Criteria (Summary)

➤ A pervasive pattern of grandiosity (in fantasy or behavior), need for admiration, and lack of empathy, beginning by early adulthood and present in a variety of contexts, as indicated by five (or more) of the following:

✔ Has a grandiose sense of self-importance (e.g., exaggerates achievements and talents, expects to be recognized as superior without commensurate achievements).

✔ Is preoccupied with fantasies of unlimited success, power, brilliance, beauty, or ideal love.

✔ Believes that he or she is special and unique and can only be understood by, or should only associate with, other special high-status people (or institutions).

✔ Requires excessive admiration.

✔ Has a sense of entitlement (i.e., unreasonable expectations of especially favorable treatment or of automatic compliance with his or her expectations).

✔ Is interpersonally exploitative (i.e., takes advantage of others to achieve his or her own ends).

✔ Lacks empathy (i.e., is unwilling to recognize or identify with the feelings and needs of others).

✔ Is often envious of others or believes that others are envious of him or her.

✔ Shows arrogant, haughty behaviors or attitudes.

Clinical Issues

➤ Characteristically, persons with narcissistic PD:

✔ Show an extreme sense of unwarranted entitlement, a grandiose sense of self-importance, and a strong tendency to exploit others to meet their needs. Because of self-idealization, persons with narcissistic PD demand to be recognized as superior and believe that they can only be understood by or associate with other unique or special persons.

✔ Exaggerate achievements and talents, with feelings that he or she is special and unique, to be admired by all.

✔ Are preoccupied (and possibly obsessed) with fantasies of unlimited success, power, brilliance, beauty, or ideal love, yet are envious of others.

✔ May feel that they have unequalled brilliance (the "cerebral narcissist"), extraordinary greatness (the superior narcissist), and/or exceptional physical beauty or sexual abilities (the "somatic narcissist").

✔ Are interpersonally exploitative, frequently lie, and use others to fulfill their needs.

✔ Lack empathy for others.

✔ Have a tendency to view others in one of two ways (which may alternate):

■ The other person is seen as satisfying the patient's needs and is coveted for that reason.

■ The other person is seen as not satisfying the patient's needs or as blocking the patient's ability to have his or her needs met. As a consequence, there is little desire to associate with that person, or, in extreme cases, there may be an actual act of pushing (possibly physically) the other person out of the way.

✔ Basically, see themselves as superior and others as inferior.

Epidemiology

➤ Prevalence is less than 1% of the general population (poorly documented), with the disorder more common in males (50%–75%).

Etiology

➤ Psychodynamic formulations posit that the individual had unmet needs in childhood and subsequently developed narcissistic thinking to regain the lost sense of importance.

➤ Cultural effects (i.e., learned behavior) have been proposed.

Prognosis

➤ Patients can benefit from psychotherapy. There appears to be some burnout of the disorder as the patient ages (as with other Cluster B PDs).

Differential Diagnosis

➤ Cluster B PDs:

   ✔ Borderline PD.

   ✔ Histrionic PD.

   ✔ Antisocial PD.

Treatment

➤ Psychotherapy is the treatment of choice, as with all PDs.

➤ Medications can be targeted to specific symptoms or comorbid disorders (e.g., antidepressant medications or mood stabilizers for mood disorders, anxiolytics for anxiety, antipsychotic medications for emergent psychotic symptoms). Avoid controlled substances, especially benzodiazepines and opioids, due to an increased likelihood for substance abuse and dependence.

AVOIDANT PERSONALITY DISORDER

Essential Characteristic

➤ Avoidance manifesting as an extreme sensitivity to rejection, often leading to a socially withdrawn life.

DSM-IV-TR Diagnostic Criteria (Summary)

➤ A pervasive pattern of social inhibition, feelings of inadequacy, and hypersensitivity to negative evaluation, beginning by early adulthood and present in a variety of contexts, as indicated by four (or more) of the following:

   ✔ Avoids occupational activities that involve significant interpersonal contact, because of fears of criticism, disapproval, or rejection.

✔ Is unwilling to get involved with people unless certain of being liked.

✔ Shows restraint within intimate relationships because of the fear of being shamed or ridiculed.

✔ Is preoccupied with being criticized or rejected in social situations.

✔ Is inhibited in new interpersonal situations because of feelings of inadequacy.

✔ Views self as socially inept, personally unappealing, or inferior to others.

✔ Is unusually reluctant to take personal risks or to engage in any new activities, because they may prove embarrassing.

Clinical Issues

➤ Characteristically, persons with avoidant PD:

✔ Want companionship but avoid relationships and activities that increase contact with others, for fear of not being accepted, being embarrassed, or being criticized.

✔ Need acceptance, are easily hurt by criticism, and are devastated by disapproval.

✔ Will only accept relationships when there is absolute assurance of acceptance without rejection.

✔ View themselves as socially inept, personally unappealing, or inferior to others (i.e., inadequate).

✔ Are anxious or fearful of developing close friendships and outwardly seem shy.

✔ Utilize avoidance as a means to cope with life.

Epidemiology

➤ Prevalence is 2%–3% of the general population (poorly documented), with the disorder more common in females.

Etiology

➤ Unknown.

Prognosis

➤ Patients can benefit from psychotherapy.

Differential Diagnosis

Schizoid personality disorder:

➤ Individuals with schizoid PD also present with extreme social isolation but have no inherent desire for social involvement.

Schizotypal personality disorder:

➤ Individuals with schizotypal PD are also reclusive with few or no friends, but additionally present with odd or unusual speech, behavior, and dress.

Phobias:

➤ Individuals with phobias typically avoid situations or objects, not relationships. However, it may be difficult to distinguish between social phobia and avoidant PD, and the two disorders may actually be intertwined.

Treatment

➤ Psychotherapy (e.g., individual, group, family, cognitive-behavioral), as with all PDs, is the treatment of choice. Individuals with avoidant PD are likely to have the best response of all the PDs to psychotherapy.

➤ Medications can be targeted to specific symptoms or comorbid disorders (e.g., antidepressant medications or mood stabilizers for mood disorders, anxiolytics for anxiety, antipsychotic medications for emergent psychotic symptoms).

➤ Avoidant PD and social phobia share similar features, and some authorities feel that they are one and the same. However, if there is a stronger consideration for social phobia, treatment options are much greater (e.g., treatment with SSRIs).

DEPENDENT PERSONALITY DISORDER

Essential Characteristic

➤ An extreme sense of neediness, with an overdependence on others to direct some or all aspects of their lives (i.e., codependency).

DSM-IV-TR Diagnostic Criteria (Summary)

➤ A pervasive and excessive need to be taken care of that leads to submissive and clinging behaviors and fears of separation, beginning by early adulthood and present in a variety of contexts, as indicated by five (or more) of the following:

✔ Has difficulty making everyday decisions without an excessive amount of advice and reassurance from others.

✔ Needs others to assume responsibility for most major areas of his or her life.

✔ Has difficulty expressing disagreement with others because of fear of loss of support or approval.

✔ Has difficulty initiating projects or doing things on his or her own (because of a lack of self-confidence in judgment or abilities rather than a lack of motivation or energy).

✔ Goes to excessive lengths to obtain nurturance and support from others, to the point of volunteering to do things that are unpleasant.

✔ Feels uncomfortable or helpless when alone, because of exaggerated fears of being unable to care for himself or herself.

✔ Urgently seeks another relationship as a source of care and support when a close relationship ends.

✔ Is unrealistically preoccupied with fears of being left to take care of himself or herself.

Clinical Issues

➤ Characteristically, persons with dependent PD:

✔ Are unable to make trivial or everyday decisions without first seeking advice or reassurance from others.

✔ Prefer to transfer the authority for decision making to others.

✔ Avoid being alone, are fearful of abandonment, and feel devastated if a close relationship ends.

✔ Are easily hurt by criticism and rejection and have low self-esteem.

✔ Are preoccupied with fears of having to take care of themselves.

✔ Go to excessive lengths to obtain nurturance, acceptance, and support from others, at times to the point of volunteering to do things that are unpleasant to them (codependency).

✔ Basically, believe they are helpless and in dire need of others to direct their lives.

➤ The diagnosis of dependent PD should be assigned only when cultural factors are not the cause of the dependency (e.g., women in cultures that do not permit women to work will naturally become dependent on their husbands for financial support).

Epidemiology

➤ Prevalence is 2%–4% of the general population (poorly documented), with the disorder more common in females.

Etiology

➤ A genetic influence has been proposed.

➤ Cultural effects (i.e., learned behavior) have been proposed, in that parents reward submissiveness but punish attempts at independence.

Prognosis

➤ Unknown. Patients can benefit from psychotherapy.

Differential Diagnosis

➤ Other disorders with a likelihood of dependency issues (e.g., major depression, schizophrenia, panic disorder with agoraphobia).

Treatment

➤ Psychotherapy is the treatment of choice, as with all PDs.

➤ Medications can be targeted to specific symptoms or comorbid disorders (e.g., antidepressant medications or mood stabilizers for mood disorders, anxiolytics for anxiety, antipsychotic medications for emergent psychotic symptoms).

OBSESSIVE-COMPULSIVE PERSONALITY DISORDER

Essential Characteristic

➤ A pattern of perfectionism and inflexibility.

DSM-IV-TR Diagnostic Criteria (Summary)

➤ A pervasive pattern of preoccupation with orderliness, perfectionism, and mental and interpersonal control, at the expense of flexibility, openness, and efficiency, beginning by early adulthood and present in a variety of contexts, as indicated by four (or more) of the following:

   ✔ Is preoccupied with details, rules, lists, order, organization, or schedules to the extent that the major point of the activity is lost.

   ✔ Shows perfectionism that interferes with task completion (e.g., is unable to complete a project because his or her own overly strict standards are not met).

   ✔ Is excessively devoted to work and productivity to the exclusion of leisure activities and friendships (not accounted for by obvious economic necessity).

   ✔ Is overconscientious, scrupulous, and inflexible about matters of morality, ethics, or values (not accounted for by cultural or religious identification).

✔ Is unable to discard worn-out or worthless objects even when they have no sentimental value.

✔ Is reluctant to delegate tasks or to work with others unless they submit to exactly his or her way of doing things.

✔ Adopts a miserly spending style toward both self and others; money is viewed as something to be hoarded for future catastrophes.

✔ Shows rigidity and stubbornness.

Clinical Issues

➤ Characteristically, persons with obsessive-compulsive PD:

✔ Show preoccupation with detail and perfectionism to a level that actually interferes with completion of the task and lack flexibility and efficiency.

✔ Have an excessive devotion to work, to the exclusion of leisure and family time ("workaholic"). There is usually a strong effort to please those in higher authority.

✔ Are insistent that others do things their way; otherwise, they are reluctant to allow others to work with them.

✔ Are extremely preoccupied with lists, rules, organization, and the need for perfection to the point of virtual paralysis.

✔ Show an excessive level of indecisiveness due to fear of making a mistake.

✔ Show a lack of generosity and are considered to be cheap. They often will not discard old or worn-out objects. The fear of change can be so intense that the person is unable to deviate from a familiar route to work, rearrange the furniture in his or her house, change jobs, move to a new home, or spontaneously embark on a new activity.

✔ Have a restricted ability to express affection, limited interpersonal skills, and a tendency to alienate others.

✔ Present with neither obsessions nor compulsions.

Epidemiology

➤ Prevalence is ~8% of the general population (poorly documented); no differences in frequency between the sexes. Obsessive-compulsive PD is the most prevalent PD.

Etiology

➤ A genetic influence has been proposed.

➤ Cultural effects (i.e., learned behavior) have been proposed.

Prognosis

➤ Unknown. Patients can benefit from psychotherapy.

Differential Diagnosis

➤ Obsessive-compulsive disorder (Axis I). For a detailed differentiation, see Table 3–4 ("Comparison of obsessive-compulsive disorder [OCD] with obsessive-compulsive personality disorder [OCPD]") in Chapter 3 ("Anxiety Disorders").

➤ Narcissistic PD:

  ✔ Persons with obsessive-compulsive PD can be so preoccupied as to appear to be narcissistic.

➤ Schizoid/avoidant PD:

  ✔ Persons with obsessive-compulsive PD tend to isolate themselves and have few friends.

Treatment

➤ Psychotherapy is the treatment of choice, as with all PDs.

➤ Medications can be targeted to specific symptoms or comorbid disorders (e.g., antidepressant medications or mood stabilizers for mood disorders, anxiolytics for anxiety, antipsychotic medications for emergent psychotic symptoms).

PERSONALITY DISORDER NOT OTHERWISE SPECIFIED

➤ Use this designation when the personality features do not meet criteria for any specific PD (i.e., "mixed personality") or fit criteria for a proposed classification (e.g., depressive PD, passive-aggressive PD).

PERSONALITY CHANGE DUE TO A GENERAL MEDICAL CONDITION

Essential Characteristics

➤ Especially suspect a medical cause for a change in personality when there is an abrupt personality or behavioral change in a person without a prior psychiatric history, particularly when coupled with emotional lability and impaired impulse control. Medical disorders associated with a change in personality include:

✔ Head trauma (probably the most common cause), cerebrovascular accident, and brain tumor.

✔ Frontal lobe syndrome ("frontal lobe personality"):

■ Classic findings include indifference, apathy, temper outbursts, and violent behavior (disinhibition) secondary to injury to the frontal/prefrontal lobes. Family members may complain that the person is "no longer like his [her] old self."

■ Additional findings include excessive talkativeness, inappropriate joking, childlike silliness (moria), sexual inappropriateness (e.g., exhibitionism), elevated mood, and antisocial behavior.

✔ Temporal lobe epilepsy:

■ Classic findings include humorlessness, hypergraphia, hyperreligiosity, aggressiveness during seizures, and altered sexuality. Psychosis of a type consistent with schizophrenia may be observed, with the exception of "preserved affective warmth."

■ Neurologically, the clinical manifestations include olfactory hallucinations, flashbacks or déjà vu, staring, and automatisms (e.g., repeated buttoning and unbuttoning of clothes, chewing movements).

✔ Infections (e.g., AIDS, neurosyphilis).

✔ Demyelinating diseases (e.g., multiple sclerosis).

✔ Cortical and subcortical dementias.

✔ Endocrine disorders.

✔ Heavy metal poisoning.

GENERAL CONSIDERATIONS REGARDING PERSONALITY DISORDERS

➤ "Personality change due to a substance" is not, unfortunately, a valid DSM designation for a personality classification. Personality changes secondary to long-term substance abuse are well recognized.

➤ Potential transitions between disorders:

✔ Oppositional defiant disorder (childhood) → conduct disorder (childhood/adolescence) → antisocial PD (adult).

✔ Avoidant disorder of childhood → avoidant PD.

✔ Identity disorder → borderline PD.

✔ Schizoid/schizotypal/paranoid PD → schizophrenia.

Common Comorbidities

➤ Substance abuse is common among individuals with Cluster B PDs.

➤ Anxiety disorders are common among individuals with dependent and avoidant PDs.

6

COGNITIVE DISORDERS

Principal DSM-IV-TR Cognitive Disorders

Delirium
Dementia
Amnestic disorders
Cognitive disorder not otherwise specified (NOS)

GENERAL CONCEPTS

➤ Cognitive impairment:
- ✔ Is a cardinal feature of delirium, dementia, amnestic disorders, and cognitive disorder not otherwise specified (NOS).
- ✔ Is defined as the significant loss of the intellectual functioning in areas of thinking, reasoning, and remembering, to the extent that the affected person has difficulty with activities of daily living (i.e., a dysfunctional course).
- ✔ Includes to varying degrees:
  - ■ Memory impairment: Defined as the inability to learn new material or the forgetting of previously learned material (delirium, dementia, amnestic disorders).
  - ■ Attention deficits: Defined as the inability to sustain concentration or focus on a task (delirium).
  - ■ Aphasia: Defined as the inability to comprehend or produce spoken or written language (delirium, dementia).
  - ■ Apraxia: Defined as the inability to execute purposeful (skilled) movements despite intact motor functioning (dementia, delirium).
  - ■ Agnosia: Defined as the inability to recognize or identify common objects (dementia, delirium).
  - ■ Executive functioning deficits: Defined as an impaired ability to think abstractly, plan, sequence, and carry out complex behaviors or tasks; also characterized as an impairment in "working memory" (dementia, delirium).

➤ Dementia, delirium, and depression (the "three D's") are the most common causes of cognitive impairment in the elderly. Table 6–1 provides a comparison of the DSM-IV-TR cognitive disorders.

■ **Table 6–1   Comparison of delirium, dementia, and amnestic disorders**

Disorder	Cognitive impairment	Disturbance of consciousness (i.e., "clouded" consciousness)
Delirium	Yes (although DSM-IV-TR allows for a perceptual disturbance in lieu of cognitive impairment)	Yes
Dementia	Yes (multiple impairments, but must also include memory loss)	No
Amnestic disorders	Yes (memory loss only)	No

➤ Cognitve impairment is NOT synonymous with memory impairment. It is possible to have good memory recall despite cognitive impairment, such as is found in the early stages of subcortical dementia.

➤ Testing for cognitive impairment:

✔ The Alzheimer's Disease Assessment Scale—Cognitive Subscale (ADAS-Cog) is a comprehensive assessment of memory, orientation, language, and functionality measured on a 70-point scale that increases in numerical value as the level of dementia worsens.

✔ The Mini-Mental State Examination (MMSE) is a rapid and convenient 11-question test to determine the degree of cognitive impairment. Higher scores (on a scale of 0–30) are indicative of better functioning. The examination includes questions for orientation, registration, attention, calculation, recall, language, and construction ability. The MMSE does not distinguish between dementia and delirium but is sensitive to the trend of cognitive functioning over time. Scores are influenced by age and educational level. Scoring:

■ 24–30 = within normal limits.

■ 18–23 = mild to moderate cognitive impairment.

■ 0–17 = severe cognitive impairment (likely unsafe for the patient to live alone).

✔ The Short Portable Mental Status Questionnaire (SPMSQ) is a 10-question examination testing orientation, current date, presidents, mother's maiden name, and subtraction of serial 3s from 20. Higher numbers are indicative of greater cognitive impairment.

DELIRIUM

DSM-IV-TR Diagnostic Criteria (Summary)

➤ Disturbance of consciousness (i.e., reduced clarity of awareness of the environment) with reduced ability to focus, sustain, or shift attention.

➤ A change in cognition or the development of a perceptual disturbance that is not better accounted for by a dementia.

➤ The disturbance develops over a short time period (usually hours to days) and tends to fluctuate during the course of the day.

➤ The disturbance is caused by the direct physiological consequences of a general medical condition, substance intoxication, substance withdrawal, use of a medication, toxin exposure, or some combination of these causes.

Clinical Issues

➤ Delirium:

- ✔ Is defined by DSM-IV-TR as a disturbance in consciousness accompanied by a change in cognition or the development of a perceptual disturbance that is not better accounted for by preexisting or evolving dementia. The disturbance develops over a short period of time and symptoms fluctuate over the course of a 24-hour day.

- ✔ Is always referenced as to causation and never only as "delirium":
  - ■ Delirium due to a medical condition.
  - ■ Substance intoxication delirium.
  - ■ Substance withdrawal delirium.
  - ■ Delirium due to multiple etiologies.
  - ■ Delirium not otherwise specified.

- ✔ Is usually reversible if the patient recovers from the underlying illness, although symptoms may last for weeks or months.

- ✔ Is also referred to as an "acute confusional state" or "acute brain syndrome."

➤ Signs and symptoms of delirium can include:

- ✔ Sudden or rapid development of impaired consciousness.
- ✔ Reduced awareness of the surrounding environment.
- ✔ Diminished ability to sustain or purposefully shift attention.
- ✔ Fluctuating levels of consciousness over the course of the day (e.g., confused → lucid → confused).
- ✔ Cognitive impairment (i.e., loss of memory, loss of orientation to time and place [but less often to self], agnosia).

✔ Perceptual disturbances (e.g., misrepresentations, illusions, visual hallucinations).

✔ Suspiciousness or delusions.

✔ Mood lability (e.g., apathy, depression, hypomania).

✔ Changes in the sleep–wake cycle, often with increased confusion and insomnia at night ("sundowning").

➤ Physical changes reflecting the underlying cause(s) of the delirium include:

✔ Focal neurological signs (commonly seen in neurologically induced delirium, but less often in systemically induced delirium).

✔ Fever and tachycardia (systemic or central nervous system [CNS] infection).

✔ Asterixis (a flapping movement of the hyperextended hand, prominent in hepatic encephalopathy, often secondary to long-term alcohol abuse).

✔ Hypertension (e.g., malignant hypertension).

✔ Hyperthermia (e.g., malignant hyperthermia, neuroleptic malignant syndrome).

✔ Severe hypoglycemia (e.g., diabetes) or hyperglycemia (diabetic ketoacidosis).

✔ Electrolyte imbalance (e.g., hyponatremia, hypercalcemia).

✔ Seizure activity (e.g., seizure disorder, substance intoxication, alcohol withdrawal).

✔ Elevated serum creatinine (e.g., urinary tract infection, uremia, renal failure).

Etiological Considerations

➤ A mnemonic for remembering causes of delirium is:
I WATCH DEATH

✔ **I**nfections (e.g., urinary tract infection).

✔ **W**ithdrawal (e.g., alcohol).

✔ **A**cute metabolic (e.g., renal failure).

✔ **T**rauma (e.g., head injury).

✔ **C**NS pathology (e.g., seizure disorders).

✔ **H**ypoxia (e.g., pneumonia).

✔ **D**eficiencies (e.g., vitamin B_{12}, thiamine).

✔ **E**ndocrine pathology (e.g., hypothyroidism).

✔ **A**cute vascular (e.g., cerebral vascular accident).

✔ **T**oxins or drugs (e.g., hallucinogens).

✔ **H**eavy metals (e.g., mercury poisoning).

Risk Factors

➤ Advancing age (especially age greater than 65 years).

➤ Dementia.

➤ Prior episodes of delirium.

➤ Sensory deprivation (e.g., blindness, eye patches after cataract surgery, intensive care unit without a window). (Refer to description of Charles Bonnet syndrome in Chapter 1 ["Schizophrenia and Other Psychotic Disorders"].)

➤ Life-threatening medical or neurological illness.

➤ Surgical intervention (e.g., repair of a hip fracture, cataract surgery).

Epidemiology

➤ Highly prevalent in medical inpatients (10%–15%), specialty critical care inpatient units (50%), and terminally ill patients within the last few days of life (85%).

Differential Diagnosis of Non-Medically Induced Disorders (Nonexhaustive List)

➤ Dementia (DSM-IV-TR indicates that the most common diagnostic issue is to differentiate delirium from dementia or delirium superimposed on an existing dementia ("beclouded dementia"; Table 6–2).

➤ Psychotic disorders (e.g., schizophrenia, brief psychotic disorder).

➤ Mood disorders (e.g., mania, major depressive disorder with psychotic features).

➤ Acute stress disorder or exacerbation of posttraumatic stress disorder.

➤ Dissociative disorders (fugue states).

➤ Malingering and factitious disorder.

■ **Table 6–2   Comparison of delirium and dementia**

Function	Delirium	Dementia
Onset	Acute	Insidious
Course	Fluctuating	Progressive
Duration	Days to weeks	Months to years
Consciousness	Altered	Clear
Attention	Impaired	Normal (except for severe dementia)
Reversible	Usually	Much less often

Assessment

➤ Delirium represents a true medical emergency. Early detection and treatment of the underlying illness provides the most favorable prognosis.

➤ Always attempt to identify the underlying medical cause(s). Utilize consultants when appropriate.

   ✔ Order appropriate laboratory testing:

   ■ Blood chemistries (e.g., electrolytes, glucose, calcium, magnesium, thyroid function tests, renal function tests, creatinine, liver function tests, ammonia level).

   ■ Complete blood count (CBC) with differential (to help identify infection and anemia).

   ■ Vitamin B_{12} and folate levels.

   ■ Electroencephalogram (EEG):

   ● Increased fast-wave activity (delirium secondary to alcohol or sedative withdrawal).

   ● Diffuse electroencephalographic slowing (delirium secondary to hepatic encephalopathy).

   ■ Computed tomography (CT) or magnetic resonance imaging (MRI) scan of the head (to detect neurological insult).

   ■ Electrocardiogram (ECG; to detect ischemic and arrhythmic causes).

   ■ Chest X ray (to identify pneumonia or congestive heart failure).

   ■ Urinalysis (to detect urinary tract infections; catheter use can be associated with the development of delirium).

   ✔ Order additional laboratory tests as warranted by clinical condition:

   ■ Blood tests (e.g., HIV antibody titer, cardiac enzymes, venereal disease research laboratory [VDRL], vitamin B_{12} and folate, ammonia level [detects advanced hepatic disease], erythrocyte sedimentation rate [ESR]).

   ■ Urine culture and sensitivity (C&S).

   ■ Autoimmune antibody screen (e.g., systemic lupus erythematosus).

   ■ Drug screen (e.g., alcohol, cocaine).

   ■ Measurement of serum or plasma levels of prescribed medications (e.g., digoxin, theophylline, phenobarbital).

   ■ Blood cultures for systemic infections.

   ■ Blood gases (oxygen and carbon monoxide).

   ■ Lumbar puncture for cerebrospinal fluid (CSF) examination to detect a CNS infection (e.g., syphilis, meningitis)

➤ Testing can be helpful to establish the diagnosis and rate the degree of impairment (e.g., MMSE, Mini-Cog, Delirium Symptom Interview, Delirium Detection Scale).

Treatment Considerations

➤ Initiate acute interventions (e.g., monitor vital signs, sleep record, fluid intake/output, oxygenation level).

➤ Routinely assess and monitor mental status, especially rapidly fluctuating behavioral manifestations. Frequent administration of the MMSE is warranted.

➤ Monitor and ensure safety (self, others).

➤ Provide appropriate somatic treatments for the underlying medical condition. Table 6–3 presents a brief review of common somatic treatments to treat the associated delirium.

■ Table 6–3   Brief review of treatments to correct delirium

Medical condition	Initial treatment
Hypoxia	Oxygen
Dehydration	Fluids
Malnutrition	Calories
Hypoglycemia	Thiamine 100 mg intravenously, followed by 5 mL of 50% glucose
Hyperthermia	Rapid cooling
Hypertension	Antihypertensive medications intravenously
Alcohol withdrawal	Thiamine, benzodiazepines
Wernicke's encephalopathy	Thiamine
Anticholinergic-induced delirium	Physostigmine intravenously
Psychosis, confusion, agitation, aggression	Antipsychotic medications without significant cardiovascular or neurological side effects
Anxiety and mild agitation	Benzodiazepines without active metabolites (e.g., oxazepam, lorazepam)
Neuroleptic malignant syndrome and serotonin syndrome	See Chapter 1 ("Schizophrenia and Other Psychotic Disorders")

➤ Provide physical, sensory, and environmental supports:

✔ Encourage family visits (familiar faces).

✔ Promote reorientation with clocks, calendars, and pictures of family and friends.

✔ Optimize stimulation (e.g., avoid dark surroundings, avoid rooms without windows).

➤ Establish a sleep chart to document symptom progression or resolution.

➤ During periods of confusion, protect from self-injury, elopement, and leaving the hospital against medical advice (via civil commitment if necessary).

DEMENTIA

Diagnostic Issues (Based on DSM-IV-TR)

➤ Dementia is characterized by memory impairment and one or more of the following cognitive deficits:

✔ Aphasia (impaired ability to use language appropriately; language disturbance). Can be tested by asking the patient to name familiar objects in the room (e.g., chair, TV).

✔ Apraxia (impaired ability to carry out motor activities despite intact motor function). Can be tested by asking the patient to pantomime the use of a common object (e.g., a pencil, a cup).

✔ Agnosia (impaired ability to recognize or identify objects despite intact sensory function). Can be tested by blindfolding the patient, placing an object in his or her hand, and asking the patient to identify the object.

✔ Disturbance in executive functioning (impaired ability to sequence, plan, and organize; impaired ability to multitask; typically due to frontal/prefrontal lobe deficits). Can be tested by asking the patient to sequentially pick up a piece of paper, fold it in half, and place the folded paper on the floor.

➤ The onset of cognitive impairment may be gradual (e.g., dementia of the Alzheimer's type) or sudden (e.g., vascular dementia, dementia due to Creutzfeldt-Jakob disease).

➤ The dementia may be reversible (e.g., due to the effects of a medication, vitamin deficiency, nutritional deficits, or infection; pseudodementia) or irreversible (e.g., dementia of the Alzheimer's type, vascular dementia).

➤ Dementia may have associated psychotic features, typically involving paranoid delusions (e.g., accusations of theft of money or of infidelity of partner) and well-formed visual hallucinations.

➤ Dementia can be classified by the location of the neuronal damage:

✔ Cortical dementias:

■ Include dementia of the Alzheimer's type (AD), frontotemporal dementia (Pick's disease), Creutzfeldt-Jakob disease, and Binswanger's disease.

■ Present with cognitive impairment, impaired recall, impaired recognition, and aphasia but with preserved motor functioning until late in the disorder.

✔ Subcortical dementias:

- Include dementia due to Parkinson's disease, Huntington's disease, and AIDS.

- Present with personality changes, apathy, and motor changes (e.g., tremor, chorea, rigidity, dystonia). Language and memory are mostly preserved until late in the illness.

➤ The prevalence of dementia in persons over age 65 years is 6%–10%, with the prevalence increasing dramatically with increasing age.

➤ AD is the most common dementia (~70% of all dementias), followed in frequency by either vascular dementia or dementia due to Lewy body disease. However:

✔ In geographic areas with a greater incidence of diabetes, smoking, and cerebrovascular disease, the prevalences of AD and vascular dementia are approximately equal.

✔ There is increasing recognition of Lewy body dementia, which is likely more prominent than once thought. It is now estimated that up to 20% of patients diagnosed with AD actually have Lewy body dementia.

➤ Dementia can also be classified as reversible (e.g., dementia of depression; pseudodementia), potentially reversible (e.g., dementia due to normal-pressure hydrocephalus), or irreversible (e.g., AD, dementia due to Huntington's disease, vascular dementia).

Workup

➤ Assessment must be individualized (based on history and presentation). It is critically important to assess for potentially reversible (and therefore treatable) causes of dementia:

✔ Obtain a detailed medical and psychiatric history from reliable informants to include history of substance abuse, prescribed medications, and progression of cognitive, mood, and behavioral changes.

➤ Coordinate treatment with other clinicians with appropriate expertise (e.g., internist, neurologist, infectious-disease specialist, psychologist).

✔ Testing should include:

- Physical examination.

- Neurological examination (e.g., pupil size, light reflex, deep-tendon reflexes, Babinski sign, primitive reflexes [e.g., grasp, snout, suck]).

- Psychological testing, with emphasis on organic functioning (e.g., Alzheimer's Disease Assessment Scale—Cognitive Subscale [ADAS-Cog], Wechsler Adult Intelligence Scale (WAIS), Bender-Gestalt, Luria test, Halstead-Reitan batteries).

✔ Laboratory studies should include:

- ECG.
- CT/MRI.
- Chemistries, to include thyroid panel, calcium level, B_{12} and folate levels, liver function tests, renal function, complete blood count with differential, serum amylase, and hematology for syphilis and HIV.

✔ Consider additional laboratory testing as indicated by history and clinical presentation (e.g., sedimentation rate, chest X ray, EEG, drug screen).

✔ Genetic testing is still considered investigational. Testing for CSF-14-3-3 protein when Creutzfeldt-Jakob disease is suspected is an example of the future direction of genetic testing. Testing for apolipoprotein E (APOE) can provide assessment for a risk factor for AD.

Common or Important Dementias

Dementia of the Alzheimer's type:

Diagnostic criteria (adapted from DSM-IV-TR):

➤ The development of multiple cognitive deficits manifested as memory impairment and one or more of the following:

  ✔ Aphasia (language disturbance).

  ✔ Apraxia (impaired ability to carry out motor activities despite intact motor function).

  ✔ Agnosia (failure to recognize or identify objects despite intact sensory function).

  ✔ Disturbance in executive functioning (i.e., planning, organizing, sequencing, abstracting).

➤ The cognitive impairments cause significant social or occupational impairment and represent a significant decline from a previous level of functioning.

➤ The course is characterized by a gradual onset and continuing cognitive decline.

➤ The deficits are not attributable to other causes of dementia, a substance, or another Axis I diagnosis.

DSM-IV-TR subtypes:

➤ With early onset (onset age 65 years or younger)—accounts for approximately 5%–10% of AD cases, can rarely occur in individuals as young as age 30 years, usually progresses more rapidly than the late-onset type, and likely is genetically transmitted (e.g., may involve the protein presenilin 1 found on chromosome 14).

➤ With late onset (onset age greater than 65 years)—accounts for the majority of AD cases.

Diagnostic issues:

➤ Memory loss alone will not qualify for a diagnosis of AD. At least one additional cognitive impairment and significant social or occupational impairment must also be present. Therefore, memory loss, even if advanced, is not synonymous with AD.

➤ AD is described neurologically as a complex, progressive, nonreversible neurodegenerative disorder and in lay terms as "the long goodbye."

Neurological findings:

➤ Brain autopsy is the only definitive means for diagnosis. Therefore, until death, patients with a diagnosis of AD are "presumed" to have the disorder. With careful clinical assessment, a "presumptive diagnosis" of AD can be accurate 85% of the time. More recently, brain biopsies may provide clues to presence of dementia.

➤ Significant brain-imaging findings:

✔ Diffuse cortical atrophy (e.g., flattened cortical sulci and enlarged cerebral ventricles), initially affecting the temporal and parietal lobes. However, these findings may also be consistent with normal aging, although the rate of atrophy is much faster in AD. Thus, cortical atrophy is not conclusive for AD.

✔ Beta-amyloid (i.e., neuritic or "senile") plaques, intraneuronal neurofibrillary tangles, synaptic degeneration, and Tau protein dysregulation are hallmark microscopic findings.

✔ Parietal and temporal hypometabolism (seen on positron emission tomography [PET] scan).

✔ Marked loss of cerebral cholinergic function (provides the basis for treatment with acetylcholinesterase (AChE) inhibitors) .

✔ Glutamate-induced toxicity, possibly secondary to the effects of beta-amyloid. Glutamate is the principal excitatory neurotransmitter in the brain and provides the basis for treatment with memantine (Namenda).

Etiological considerations:

➤ Deficiency of acetylcholine (basis for use of AChE inhibitors).

➤ Buildup of beta-amyloid plaque, accumulating from beta-amyloid protein fragments.

➤ Buildup of neurofibrillary tangles consisting of insoluble twisted fibers of the tau protein.

➤ Free-radical damage—neurons are extremely vulnerable to attacks by destructive free radicals (basis for use of vitamin E and selegiline).

➤ Inflammatory process (basis for use of COX-2 inhibitors).

➤ Heavy metal poisoning (iron, copper, zinc, and aluminum are often present in damaged neuronal cells and may serve as catalysts to produce free radicals and subsequent cell death).

➤ Advanced glycation end products (AGEs)—glucose binds tightly to proteins to form AGEs, which in turn damage neuronal tissues. AGEs have been found in neurofibrillary tangles of AD.

➤ Cardiovascular disease and homocysteine elevation—elevated serum homocysteine can damage arteries and increase the risk of coronary artery disease and stroke. Some studies show an increase in serum homocysteine levels in patients with AD. Deficiencies of vitamin B_{12} and folate may also increase homocysteine levels.

➤ Nutritional deficiencies.

➤ Electromagnetic fields—exposure to intense electromagnetic fields may increase the risk for developing AD (not strongly supported).

➤ Head injury or repeated head injuries—a well appreciated risk factor.

➤ Educational level—lower educational training is associated with an increased risk for developing AD. On the other hand, increased "mental activities" reduce the risk and/or slow the progress of AD, possibly by stimulating the growth of new neurons ot neuronal tracks.

➤ Genetic factors—four chromosomal abnormalities are prominent:

  ✔ Chromosome 1—presenilin 2.

  ✔ Chromosome 14—presenilin 1.

  ✔ Chromosome 19—apolipoprotein E (APOE). Three alleles are recognized (e2, e3, and e4). e4 binds strongly to beta amyloid and increases the risk of late-onset AD.

  ✔ Chromosome 21—amyloid precursor protein (tied to trisomy 21 and Down's syndrome).

Risk factors:

➤ Universally accepted risk factors:

  ✔ Increasing age is the strongest risk factor. AD affects 2%–4% of the population at age 65 years, with the prevalence doubling every 5 years. The prevalence approaches 35%–50% in persons age 85 years or older.

  ✔ Family history of AD or Parkinson's disease, especially in first-degree relatives.

  ✔ APOE-e4 on chromosome 19 (genetic transmission of late-onset AD). APOE-e2 is protective.

  ✔ Down syndrome.

  ✔ Chromosomal 14 abnormalities (presenilin 1) is responsible for a rare form of genetically transmitted early-onset AD.

➤ Possible risk factors:

  ✔ Female gender.

  ✔ Lower educational achievement and/or lower IQ ("lack of cognitive reserve").

✔ Cigarrette smoking in persons age 55 years or older.

✔ Head injury, especially with loss of consciousness. Prizefighters (as well as football players) can develop *dementia pugilistica* ("punchdrunk syndrome") from repeated head trauma.

✔ Ethnicity (e.g., African Americans are four times more likely to develop AD than whites).

✔ Disorders imparting cardiovascular damage (e.g., diabetes, hypertension, coronary artery disease, hyperlipidemia, smoking, atrial fibrillation).

✔ Vitamins B_6, B_{12}, and folate deficiencies (leading to elevated homocysteine levels and subsequently to cardiovascular damage).

✔ Exposure to toxins (e.g., organic solvents, alcohol) and heavy metals (e.g., aluminum, copper, zinc).

✔ Mild cognitive impairment (MCI)—involves memory impairment without dementia. However, the risk of developing AD increases 10% each year for persons with MCI. Ultimately, 85% of individuals with MCI will develop AD within 5–10 years after diagnosis.

✔ Late-life depression (relatively new finding, controversial).

✔ Menopause or hormonal replacement therapy used after age 65 years.

Staging of AD (Table 6–4):

■ **Table 6–4   Stages of dementia of the Alzheimer's type**

Stage of illness	Duration in years	Memory	Personality changes	Physical changes	EEG and imaging findings
Stage I	1–3	New lost, old preserved	Subtle, with apathy, agitation, or lability of affect	Subtle, if any	Normal EEG, normal or near-normal CT/MRI findings
Stage II	2–10	Intermediate and remote lost	More pronounced, with complaints by family	Aphasia and apraxia present	Slowing on EEG, ventricular dilatation, sulcal enlargement, atrophy on CT/MRI
Stage III	8–12	Severe loss of new, intermediate, and old memory; language impairments become severe	Possibly severe, with frank aggressiveness, comorbid depression, poor insight, and poor judgment	Severe impairment in speech and movement, with patient becoming bedridden, followed by death	Further progression of EEG and CT/MRI changes

Note.   CT = computed tomography; EEG = electroencephalogram; MRI = magnetic resonance imaging.

Treatment:

➤ Loss of acetylcholine appears to mediate memory loss. AChE inhibitors modestly slow (but do not arrest) cognitive impairment by increasing cellular acetylcholine through inhibition of the enzyme AChE.

➤ Inhibition of the NMDA receptor with the glutamate inhibitor memantine slows the toxic effects of glutamate on cellular processes. Effectiveness is improved when memantine is combined with donepezil (Aricept).

➤ Table 6–5 lists the medications FDA-approved for the treatment of AD.

➤ Protective/preventative measures (not universally accepted) include estrogen, Mediterranean diet (rich in B vitamins, vitamin E, and omega-3 oils), nonsteroidal anti-inflammatory agents (e.g, COX-2 inhibitors), ginkgo biloba, huperzine (Chinese herb), curcumin, vaccination (research), lipid-lowering agents (controversial), moderate alcohol use, increased social interaction, and physical/mental exercise.

Caregiver issues:

➤ Caregivers have a high propensity for depression and anxiety. *The 36-Hour Day,* Fourth Edition, by Mace and Rabins (Johns Hopkins Press, 2006), is an excellent reference for caregivers. Antidepressants and anxiolytics may be of value.

Vascular dementia (multi-infarct dementia):

➤ Vascular dementia accounts for 10%–20% of dementias, with onset typically after age 60. Risk factors include hypertension, diabetes, increasing age, and cigarette smoking.

➤ Onset of clinical symptoms is either abrupt (e.g., with major strokes) or stepwise (e.g., with less-obvious ministrokes). Neuroimaging studies show vascular lesions.

➤ Vascular dementia can be cortical and/or subcortical, depending on the location of the infarcts.

➤ Focal neurological findings (e.g., increased deep tendon reflexes, weakness of extremities, gait abnormalities) or laboratory evidence of cerebrovascular disease is helpful to make the diagnosis.

➤ Apathy and depression are usually more pronounced in vascular dementia than in AD and are more prominent in left-sided strokes. Ministrokes (easily missed clinically) are frequently associated with depression.

➤ There is increasing evidence that AChE inhibitors can slow the progression of vascular dementia, especially if it is subcortical. The cellular damage from the CVA generates a cholinergic deficiency.

Table 6–5 Medications approved for the treatment of dementia of the Alzheimer's type

Medication	FDA approval	Mechanism of action	Daily dosage (start/highest), mg	Advantages	Side effects; considerations
Tacrine (Cognex)	Mild to moderate AD	Inhibits AChE	40/160	First available	GI qid dosing Impaired liver functioning
Donepezil (Aricept)	Mild to moderate AD	Inhibits AChE	5/10	Very selective inhibitor of AChE (reduces side effects) Once-daily dosing	GI Paroxetine can increase blood levels
Rivastigmine (Exelon)	Mild to moderate AD	Inhibits AChE and BChE	3/12	BChE inhibition may improve efficacy	GI bid dosing
Rivastigmine patch (Exelon)	Mild to moderate AD	Inhibits AChE	4.6/9.5	Patch	GI
Galantamine (Reminyl)	Mild to moderate AD	Inhibits AChE Nicotinic receptor modulation	8/24	Maintains functioning as well as cognition	GI bid dosing Highest doses are more effective but are poorly tolerated
Memantine (Namenda)	Moderate to severe AD	NMDA receptor antagonist	5/20	Only medication approved for advanced AD	Very mild; dizziness, mild GI distress

Note. AChE = acetylcholinesterase; AD = dementia of the Alzheimer's type; BChE = butyrylcholinesterase; FDA = U.S. Food and Drug Administration; GI = gastrointestinal; NMDA = N-methyl-D-aspartate.

Dementia due to head trauma:

➤ Dementia can develop from a single severe traumatic episode or from the accumulation of multiple traumatic episodes (e.g., *dementia pugilistica*).

➤ In addition to dementia, frontal lobe injury can result in a number of behavioral changes (e.g., affective instability, poor impulse control, apathy, intrusiveness, profanity, loud speech), colloquially termed "frontal lobe syndrome."

Dementia due to HIV infection:

➤ HIV infection can directly induce a subcortical dementia, with a prevalence of 4%–15% in HIV-infected patients.

➤ Early signs include apathy, social withdrawal, and MCI, followed in later stages with cognitive deficits (due to cortical atrophy) and motor signs consistent with a subcortical dementia. Further progression can lead to behavioral issues and psychosis.

➤ Stress associated with having a fatal illness can result in anxiety and depressive disorders.

Dementia due to Huntington's disease:

➤ Huntington's disease is an autosomal dominant disorder with complete penetrance. Initially, damage is principally subcortical in the caudate and putamen.

➤ Onset is usually insidious, starting in midlife with the development of choreoathetosis (involuntary jerky, dancelike ["dancing gait"] movements of the extremities) and milder muscle twitching of the face and limbs. Depression, apathy, poor motivation, and behavioral problems occur early in the illness (consistent with a subcortical dementia). In time, akinesia, rigidity, ophthalmoplegia (weakness of muscles controlling eye movement), confinement to bed, emaciation, and death occur.

➤ Dementia invariably develops and progresses uncontrollably, with executive functioning usually deteriorating before language skills.

Dementia due to Parkinson's disease:

➤ Classic physical findings of Parkinson's disease include muscular rigidity, postural abnormality, masklike facies, and resting tremor secondary to cell degeneration in the substantia nigra (located in the brain stem), leading to loss of dopamine.

➤ Dementia is subcortical and develops in approximately 30% of Parkinson's patients. Typically, motor symptoms precede cognitive deficits. Depression, anxiety, and psychosis are also prominent features.

Dementia due to Lewy body disease:

➤ Three core clinical features include:

✔ Motor features of Parkinson's disease.

✔ Fluctuating cognition and pronounced variations in attention and alertness.

✔ Well-formed visual hallucinations (often starting early in the illness) in 80% of patients. The hallucinations are often of people or animals and are not usually bothersome to the patient.

➤ Clinical presentation is a mix of Alzheimer's-type and Parkinson's-type symptoms. Symptom progression is faster than in AD. It is not clear if this is a distinct dementia or a variant of Parkinson's disease. Typically, dementia precedes motor deficits. On autopsy, Lewy bodies (eosinophilic inclusions) are found in the cortex.

➤ Notably, there is extreme adverse sensitivity to antipsychotic medications. Second-generation antipsychotics (especially olanzapine and quetiapine, but not risperidone) are preferred.

Frontotemporal lobar dementia (Pick's disease):

➤ Is characterized by insidious but progressive atrophy of the frontal and temporal lobes (whereas in Alzheimer's disease, there is progressive deterioration of the temporal and parietal lobes).

➤ Usually strikes individuals under age 65 years with early findings of deterioration in personality, insight, and social functioning followed by cognitive decline.

➤ Tau proteins accumulate into "Pick bodies."

➤ Results in deterioration of serotonergic and dopaminergic systems, with relative sparing of the cholinergic system. As a consequence, behavioral, language, and personality changes, rather than memory losses, are the most likely early presenting symptoms:

✔ Behavioral changes include obsessive-compulsive behaviors (e.g., repetitive counting), stealing, inappropriate sexual advances, and overeating.

✔ Language changes include singing, echolalia, and mutism.

✔ Personality changes include neglect of personal hygiene, social withdrawal, apathy, depression, and passivity.

Dementia due to Creutzfeldt-Jakob disease:

➤ Presents with the triad of dementia, myoclonus, and abnormal EEG.

➤ Typically progresses rapidly, often affecting individuals between the ages of 40 and 60 years.

➤ Is thought to be transmitted by a prion protein (also causes spongiform encephalopathies). Similar type illnesses include Kuru, "mad cow" disease, and scrapie in sheep.

Substance-induced persisting dementia:

➤ Includes alcohol-induced persisting dementia; inhalant-induced persisting dementia; and sedative-, hypnotic-, and anxiolytic-induced persisting dementia.

➤ The dementia may persist well after the person has stopped using the substance, and may continue to progress unabated.

➤ Alcohol-induced cortical dementia is a long-term consequence of alcohol dependence. Cortical damage is widespread (unlike in alcohol-induced persisting amnestic syndrome, where the damage is more focal). Cerebellar degeneration can induce gross motor gait disturbances and tremor and truncal ataxia.

Dementia due to normal-pressure hydrocephalus:

➤ Normal-pressure hydrocephalus presents with the triad of gait disturbance, urinary incontinence, and dementia; a potentially reversible cause of dementia.

Dementia due to Lyme disease and dementia due to neurosyphilis:

➤ Lyme disease initially develops from the bite of a deer tick.

➤ Neurosyphilis is the third stage of syphilitic infection spread through sexual contact.

➤ Both disorders are categorized as "the great imitators," in that symptoms are general and often nonspecific (e.g., malaise, arthralgias, depression, unexplained fevers, myalgias), making it difficult to diagnose the disorders without specific testing.

Dementia of depression (pseudodementia):

➤ Memory loss in individuals younger than 60 years is typically due to depression, substance abuse, adverse effects of prescribed or over-the-counter medications, anxiety ("the worried well"), or sleep deprivation.

➤ When memory loss occurs in depression, patients typically complain of memory deficits, indicate that they do not know the answers to questions, do not put much effort into answering questions, and present with depressed mood and affect. Patients typically show a positive response to antidepressant medications.

➤ Table 6–6 summarizes the salient features of the common dementias.

▓ Table 6–6 Salient features of the common dementias

Dementia	Salient clinical features
Dementia of the Alzheimer's type	Cognitive impairment accompanied by aphasia, apraxia, and/ or agnosia. The onset of the disease is gradual, with a slow progression. Usually, motor findings are not present until the middle or late stages of the disease.
Vascular dementia	Cognitive impairment develops in a stepwise fashion and is accompanied by focal neurological signs and symptoms. Onset is likely to be abrupt, occurring after either a major stroke or a ministroke.
Frontotemporal dementia	Cognitive impairment coupled with personality changes and deterioration of social skills. Onset usually is between the fifth and sixth decades. Frontal-release signs such as snout and grasp reflex are evident.
Dementia due to head trauma	Cognitive deficits, usually not progressive unless there is a history of repeated head injuries.
Dementia due to HIV infection	Progressive motor deficits due to subcortical involvement; cognitive deficits develop later, with associated psychiatric disorders (e.g., anxiety, depression).
Dementia due to Huntington's disease	Cognitive changes develop early (third to fourth decade), coupled with choreoathetosis.
Dementia due to Parkinson's disease	Cognitive changes coupled with extrapyramidal symptoms.
Dementia due to Lewy body disease	Cognitive impairment coupled with recurrent visual hallucinations and features of Parkinson's disease. The incidence of adverse reactions to antipsychotic medications is high.
Dementia due to Creutzfeldt-Jakob disease	Cognitive deficits developing between the fourth and sixth decades. Often associated with ataxia, seizures, and myoclonus. Progression is rapid. A prion-induced illness.
Dementia due to normal-pressure hydrocephalus	Triad of gait disturbance, urinary incontinence, and dementia. Possibly reversible.
Dementia due to Lyme disease and dementia due to neurosyphilis	Nonspecific symptoms (e.g., fatigue, arthralgias, myalgias) make diagnosis difficult from clinical observation alone.
Dementia of depression	Cognitive impairment, poor effort to answer questions, mood symptoms, positive response to antidepressant treatment.

AMNESTIC DISORDERS

DSM-IV-TR Diagnostic Criteria (Summary)

➤ Memory impairment as manifested by impairment in the ability to learn new information (anterograde amnesia) or the inability to recall previously learned information (retrograde amnesia).

➤ The memory impairment causes significant impairment in social or occupational functioning and represents a significant decline from a previous level of functioning.

➤ The memory impairment is not caused by a dementia or delirium.

➤ The disturbance is a direct physiological consequence of a general medical condition, physical trauma, or substance (classified as substance-induced persisting amnestic disorder).

Specifiers

➤ Amnestic disorder may be *transient,* with memory impairment lasting several hours to a few days (transient global amnesia), or *chronic,* with memory impairment lasting more than 1 month.

Clinical Considerations

➤ Amnestic disorders involve the loss of memory as a consequence of a medical disorder, trauma, or a substance. Criteria for delirium and dementia are not met.

➤ DSM-IV-TR differentiates the memory impairment of amnestic disorders by etiology. The three major categorizations are:

✔ Substance-induced persisting amnestic disorder (e.g., a substance of abuse, a medication, a toxin).

✔ Amnestic disorder due to a general medical condition (e.g., head injury, thiamine deficiency):

■ Transient amnestic disorder—memory impairment lasts for 1 month or less.

■ Chronic amnestic disorder—memory impairment lasts for more than 1 month.

✔ Amnestic disorder not otherwise specified (specific etiology for memory loss cannot be determined).

Important Amnestic Syndrome

➤ Alcohol-induced persisting amnestic syndrome (Korsakoff's syndrome):

✔ Thiamine deficiency leads to damage to the mammillary bodies, hypothalamus, diencephalon, and hippocampus.

✔ Anterograde amnesia is coupled with confabulation (nontruths) and is likely not to be recoverable.

✔ Treatment is supportive, as replenishing thiamine is unlikely to significantly improve memory or reverse the damage.

➤ Sedative-, hypnotic-, or anxiolytic-induced persisting amnestic disorder—amnesia develops from abuse of these substance. Unlike Korsakoff's syndrome, recovery from amnesia is typically good.

➤ Postictal stage of a seizure.

➤ Electroconvulsive therapy—retrograde and/or anterograde amnesia occurs around the time of treatment and typically fully resolves within 6–9 months.

COGNITIVE DISORDER NOT OTHERWISE SPECIFIED

DSM-IV-TR Diagnostic Criteria (Summary)

➤ Cognitive deficits that are secondary to a medical cause not better classified by a delirium, dementia, or amnestic disorder.

➤ Important disorders that may be classified under this designation include:

✔ Mild neurocognitive disorder (cognitive deficits must be secondary to a medical disorder or central nervous system dysfunction).

✔ Postconcussional disorder (cognitive deficits following a head injury).

7

VIOLENT BEHAVIOR

Principal Categories

Self-harming behavior
Assaultive behavior

Additional Issues

Contracting for safety

CLINICAL ISSUES RELATED TO VIOLENT BEHAVIOR

➤ In regard to this discussion, violent behavior is categorized as violence directed toward self (self-harming behavior) or others (assaultive behavior).

➤ Psychiatrists are not able to predict who will or will not become violent. The prediction of future events is best left to those who forecast the future with a crystal ball. However, the potential (i.e., risk) for violence can be assessed through knowledge of the risk factors that, historically, have been associated with violent behavior.

➤ The importance of accurately assessing the risk of violence is greatest for violent behavior that is deemed imminent:

✔ Most commitment statutes specify imminent danger of violence as a requirement for commitment.

✔ Hospitalization is unlikely to protect against the long-term risk of completed suicide.

✔ Published risk factors for suicide are usually formulated on medium- to long-term considerations. The imminent risk of suicide is much more difficult to accurately assess.

✔ The number of risk factors for violent behavior is so large that their usefulness for predicting the true risk of violence must be considered in light of the clinical circumstances. Published risk factors have a high sensitivity (they will identify almost all persons with increased suicide risk) but low specificity (few persons with a given risk factor actually attempt or complete suicide).

✔ When assessing for suicide risk, also assess for the potential for rescue. The "risk-to-rescue ratio" can help assess for the seriousness of the suicide attempt:

■ A suicide attempt in which the person does not tell anyone of his or her plan and uses a loaded gun has a dangerously high risk-to-rescue ratio.

■ A suicide attempt in which the person takes an overdose of five aspirin tablets in the presence of persons who are aware of this behavior has a low risk-to-rescue ratio.

➤ There are 8–25 suicide attempts for every completed suicide.

➤ Violent behavior has been studied from a wide variety of perspectives. The issues are complex and not well defined, as exemplified by the all-too-frequent reports of mass suicides, contagion-related suicides, assisted suicides, and individuals committing homicide in schools, colleges, and malls and then committing suicide.

Etiological Theories

Biological formulations:

➤ Low serotonin (5-hydroxytryptamine [5-HT]) levels, as measured by the serotonin metabolite 5-hydroxyindoleacetic acid (5-HIAA) in cerebrospinal fluid (CSF), correlate with an increased potential for violent behavior. Reduced levels of 5-HIAA have been found in persons who commit violent acts (e.g., arson, suicide attempts). It appears that a compensatory increase in 5-HT_{1A} and 5-HT_{2A} receptors in the prefrontal cortex develops in response to low 5-HT levels. It is proposed that the hyposerotonergic state ultimately results in a reduced ability to control impulsive and aggressive behavior.

➤ Norepinephrine, dopamine, glutamate, and gamma-aminobutyric acid (GABA) dysregulation may correlate with an increased potential for violent behavior.

➤ Genetics may determine vulnerability to express violent behavior:

✔ In males, an extra Y chromosome (YYX theory) has been correlated with lower levels of monoamine oxidase A (MAO-A) and a subsequent increased potential for violent behavior. However, it is generally accepted that an extra Y chromosome has only a minor impact on the potential for aggressive behavior. The XYY theory has been used to defend persons accused of murder who carry an extra Y chromosome ("murder gene").

✔ Genetic factors may influence the risk of suicide. Suicide rates are six times higher among identical twins than among fraternal twins, although other factors (e.g., concomitant psychiatric illness) may also play a role.

➤ A study of brain scans of violent offenders showed decreased prefrontal activity, leading to the hypothesis that damage to the prefrontal cortex can result in aggressive and impulsive behavior.

➤ Increased levels of testosterone in men correlate with an increase in the potential for violent behavior.

➤ Hyperfunction of the hypothalamic-pituitary-adrenal (HPA) axis, as demonstrated by elevated corticotropin-releasing factor (CRF) and increased cortisol, can lead to suicidal behavior.

➤ Declining cholesterol levels and the use of statin medications are likely not associated with an increased risk of aggression and violent behavior, as was once postulated (controversial).

➤ Lithium decreases impulsivity in prison inmates and reduces the risk of suicide in both bipolar and unipolar major depression.

➤ Antiseizure medications (e.g., divalproex, carbamazepine) have recently been endorsed as possibly increasing suicide risk.

➤ Antidepressants may increase the risk for suicidal thinking in adolescents and young adults. A black box warning was endorsed by the FDA in October 2004.

➤ Dysfunction in the emotion-controlling limbic system (includes amygdala and hippocampus) can result in aggressive behavior.

➤ Early exposure to lead (fetus, infancy, childhood) has been linked to poor impulse control.

Classical formulations:

➤ Losses can promote suicidal behavior (Humphrey) and can be ordered on the basis of their potential to result in suicide. Humphrey found that the death of a close relative, the death of a sibling, an arrest, and alcoholism were higher-ordered losses.

➤ The risk of suicide increases when individuals experience difficulty integrating into societal norms and are unable to cope with crisis and sudden disruption (Durkheim).

➤ Frustration leads to aggression (Palmer).

➤ Suicide is a possible ending when an individual is trying to cope with a loss. The loss becomes a narcissistic injury and rage develops toward the lost object because of its unavailability, with a subsequent desire to obliterate the object. Because the lost object resides within the ego, obliterating the object means obliterating self through suicide (Freud, *Mourning and Melancholia*).

➤ Excessive use of alcohol increases the risk of violent behavior secondary to its disinhibiting effects, in that alcohol "dissolves the superego" (extension of the concept of the id, ego, and superego as formulated by Freud).

➤ Suicide is a means of killing pain (psychological, physical) rather than a desire to kill oneself (paradigm concept).

SELF-HARMING BEHAVIOR

Risk Factors (Nonexhaustive List)

Suicide issues:

➤ Suicidal ideation (especially when accompanied by obsessive thoughts of dying or being dead).

➤ Prior suicide attempt (regardless of the degree of seriousness).

➤ Suicide planning (e.g., suicide note, giving away valued possessions, preparing a will, obtaining or investigating lethal means for suicide [e.g., rope, gun]). Sixty percent of suicides are by a gunshot wound.

➤ Family history of suicide.

➤ Having known a suicide victim, especially a parent, spouse, significant other, or close friend.

➤ Being a victim of abuse.

➤ Attraction to suicide.

➤ "Contagion-related suicide":

   ✔ Can be described as "imitative suicide."

   ✔ May increase in frequency as the result of extensive media coverage of suicides (the *Werther effect*).

Health issues:

Mental health considerations:

➤ Mood disorders:

   ✔ The risk of suicide increases significantly if the mood disorder is accompanied by substance abuse, hopelessness, and/or significant agitation.

   ✔ Depression (unipolar, bipolar) is considered one of the most important risk factors for suicide. Mixed bipolar states and manic episodes are also linked to self-harming behavior. Sixty percent to 80% of persons who commit suicide have a mood disorder.

➤ Psychosis from any cause (e.g., schizophrenia, schizoaffective disorder, brief psychotic disorder, substance-induced psychosis, postpartum psychosis), especially when accompanied by command hallucinations.

➤ Anxiety disorders (particularly panic disorder and posttraumatic stress disorder in Vietnam veterans). Abrupt discontinuation of anxiolytics can promote increased psychic anxiety and subsequent suicidal behavior.

➤ Anxiety (recurrent, ruminating) associated with major depression.

➤ Personality disorders (e.g., Cluster B personality disorders, schizotypal personality disorder).

➤ Hopelessness (a significant risk factor).

➤ Anhedonia.

➤ Conduct disorder.

➤ Anorexia nervosa and bulimia nervosa.

➤ Current inpatient psychiatric hospitalization.

➤ Attention-deficit/hyperactivity disorder.

➤ Global insomnia (initial insomnia, difficulty maintaining sleep, early-morning awakening).

➤ Conflict over being homosexual.

➤ Losses or stressors (e.g., bereavement, unemployed, recent separation, divorce, never married, social isolation).

➤ Dementia or delirium.

➤ Recent (within 6 months) discharge from a psychiatric facility.

➤ Decreased 5-HT levels in CSF.

Physical health considerations:

➤ Chronic medical illness (e.g., AIDS, renal failure, multiple sclerosis, seizure disorder, cardiovascular disease, porphyria, Klinefelter's syndrome, hemodialysis, cancer [especially breast and genital]).

➤ Chronic pain syndromes.

➤ Recent surgery.

➤ Recent childbirth.

➤ Seizure disorder.

Substance or medication issues:

➤ Substance-related disorders (e.g., abuse, dependence, intoxication, withdrawal).

➤ Substance-induced mood or substance-induced psychotic disorder (e.g., alcohol, cocaine, reserpine, pegylated interferon, mefloquine [Lariam], antidepressant use in adolescents).

➤ Akathisia as a side effect of antipsychotic medications and, rarely, as a side effect of antidepressant medications.

➤ Medications possibly associated with suicidal behavior unrelated to mood or psychotic changes (controversial):

✔ Antidepressants, antiseizure medications, isotretinoin (Accutane).

Behavioral issues:

➤ Impulsivity.

➤ Risk-taking behavior.

➤ Aggressive behavior.

➤ Emotional lability.

Demographic issues:

➤ Attempted suicide—female-to-male ratio is 3:1.

➤ Completed suicide—male-to-female ratio is 4:1.

➤ White male (21/100,000) >> African American male (11/100,000) > white female (5/100,000) > African American female (2/100,000).

➤ American Indian, Alaska Native > white, Asian, or Hispanic > African American.

➤ Advancing age (except for a high rate of suicides in teenagers). The suicide rate for white males 85 years or older is 65 per 100,000.

➤ Divorced/widowed > single > married > married woman with children.

➤ Protestant > Jew or Catholic.

➤ Isolated or living alone > strong social supports.

➤ Spring or fall > summer or winter.

➤ Lowest and highest socioeconomic classes > middle socioeconomic class.

➤ Presence of a firearm in the home > absence of a firearm in the home.

➤ Physicians (highest rates for psychiatrists, ophthalmologists, and anesthesiologists; lowest rates for pediatricians) and dentists.

➤ Barriers to or unavailability of mental health services.

➤ Incarceration, especially when detoxifying from alcohol.

Clinical Issues

➤ The risk factors for self-harming behavior are often interrelated. For example, chronic pain syndromes may impart a higher risk of suicide because of associated depression rather than because of the pain itself.

➤ Not all of the listed risk factors are fully established or accepted. For example, there is controversy surrounding the claims that isotretinoin (Accutane), antidepressants, falling cholesterol levels, antiseizure medications, and statins can increase the risk of suicide.

➤ The suicide rate in the United States is 11.3 per 100,000 population. Among European societies, Hungary has the highest rate (37.0 per 100,000) and Italy has the lowest rate (6.8 per 100,000).

➤ Women attempt suicide three times more often than men, but men are four times as successful in completing suicide. Men tend to use a more lethal means (e.g., guns, hanging) than do women (e.g., overdose, wrist cutting). The most common means of committing suicide is a gunshot.

➤ The most prominent age for suicide in white males is 85 years or older (65 per 100,000). The most prominent age for suicide in African American males is 20–24 years (21 per 100,000).

➤ Adolescent and young adult suicide rates have tripled over the past 30 years. Suicide rates among adolescent African American males have increased dramatically in recent years. With the advent of the FDA warning in 2004 for antidepressant-related suicidal behavior in adolescents and young adults, the suicide rate has begun to climb higher in that group.

➤ Although uncommon in children, self-harming behaviors, suicide attempts, and completed suicides do occur.

➤ A nonlethal suicide attempt more indicative of relief of tension or a cry for help than a desire to die is termed *parasuicide* or *self-injurious behavior.* This complicates research studies as to what constitutes a true suicide attempt as opposed to parasuicide.

➤ Tricyclic antidepressants (especially when combined with alcohol) and lithium are the most toxic of the common psychotropic medications in overdose.

➤ More than 90% of patients who commit suicide have a psychiatric diagnosis:

✔ Mood disorders:

■ Depression is the most highly correlated disorder associated with suicide. In the United States, about 60%–80% of all suicides occur in persons with a mood disorder.

✔ Schizophrenia and schizoaffective disorder: ~10% of individuals commit suicide.

✔ Borderline, antisocial, and schizotypal personality disorders: ~5%–10% of individuals commit suicide.

✔ Alcohol-related disorders: ~10%–15% of individuals commit suicide.

➤ Suicide is the eighth leading cause of death in the United States.

➤ The SAD PERSONAS scale (Patterson and colleagues; Campbell) is a mnemonic outlining the important risk factors for suicide:

✔ S   Sex

✔ A   Age

✔ D   Depression

✔ P   Previous suicide attempts

✔ E   Ethanol abuse

✔ R   Rational thinking loss (i.e., psychosis)

✔ S   Social supports lacking

✔ O   Organized plan

✔ N   No spouse

✔ A   Availability of lethal means to commit suicide

✔ S   Sickness

Hospital Management

➤ Safety and protection are the primary initial concerns, which may necessitate hospitalization with or without the patient's willingness to be admitted.

➤ If the patient is hospitalized, frequent suicide monitoring is mandated. The physician's note should reflect that the patient was asked to contract for safety.

➤ Be certain to ensure that firearms and other potentially lethal weapons are removed from the home.

➤ Provide strict instructions prior to discharge for emergency situations should they arise (e.g., doctor's phone number, hospital phone number).

➤ Outpatient follow-up immediately after discharge is mandated (1–2 days), with an appointment arranged prior to discharge and contact made with the outpatient treating physician before the patient leaves the hospital.

➤ If substance abuse is a primary factor prompting suicidal intent, additional treatment in a "rehab center" may be warranted.

➤ Prescribe a minimal quantity of medication that will carry the patient over to the outpatient appointment.

➤ Early discharge to satisfy managed care organizations can have deleterious results for both the patient and attending physician.

Outpatient Management

➤ Apply the same considerations outlined for the hospital management of self-harming behavior in the section above.

➤ Enlist family members and friends to provide increased observation, possibly to the level of 24-hour monitoring.

➤ Provide frequent visits with the patient, as mandated by clinical findings.

➤ Medications that may reduce the potential for self-harming behavior:

  ✔ Antidepressants (despite concerns about an increased risk of suicidal behavior in teenagers and young adults).

  ✔ Lithium (documented antisuicidal activity), when used for the treatment of bipolar disorder.

  ✔ Clozapine, when used for the treatment of schizophrenia and schizoaffective disorder.

  ✔ Olanzapine and risperidone.

ASSAULTIVE BEHAVIOR

Risk Factors

Aggressive, violent, or homicidal issues:

➤ Combination of fire setting, bed-wetting, and cruelty to animals (classic triad for prediction of future violent behavior).

➤ Assaultive or homicidal intentions.

➤ History of violence or rage.

➤ Stalking behaviors.

➤ Significant psychomotor agitation or anger.

➤ History of impulsive behaviors or fantasies of violence.

➤ History of childhood abuse.

➤ Frequently visualizing abuse.

➤ Weapons present or readily available.

➤ School failure, school truancy, and delinquency as an adolescent.

Health issues:

Mental health considerations:

➤ Psychiatric disorders:

✔ Manic or depressed phases of bipolar disorder.

✔ Major depressive disorder.

✔ Brief psychotic disorder.

✔ Schizophrenia (controversial, but likely true when actively paranoid).

✔ Anxiety disorders (e.g., panic disorder, posttraumatic stress disorder).

➤ Cognitive disorders (e.g., delirium, dementia).

➤ Psychosis from any cause (e.g., postpartum psychosis).

➤ First psychiatric hospitalization before 18 years of age.

➤ Substance-related disorders (e.g., abuse, dependence, intoxication, withdrawal) involving both licit and illicit substances.

➤ Personality disorders (e.g., antisocial personality disorder, narcissistic personality disorder, borderline personality disorder).

➤ Mental retardation.

➤ Intermittent explosive disorder.

➤ Physical or sexual abuse by a parent (possibly leading to parricide [killing of one's parents]).

Physical health considerations:

➤ Cortical and subcortical dementias.

➤ Delirium.

➤ Central nervous system infections.

➤ Ictal and postictal states.

➤ Head injury, particularly with damage to temporal or frontal lobes.

➤ Hypoglycemia and other endocrine disturbances.

➤ Acute intermittent porphyria.

➤ Low or falling cholesterol levels in men (controversial).

Medication issues:

➤ Pegulate interferon and mefloquine (Lariam).

➤ Akathisia from antipsychotic medications.

Demographic issues:

➤ Male > female.

➤ Young adult > older adult.

➤ Lower socioeconomic status > higher socioeconomic status.

➤ Few social supports > strong social supports.

Clinical Issues

➤ The claim of an increased risk of assaultive behavior in persons with major mental illnesses (particularly schizophrenia) is controversial. However, the literature is more supportive of a positive correlation between major mental illness and assaultive behavior.

➤ There is a high correlation between alcohol intoxication/alcohol withdrawal and an increased potential for assaultive behavior. During intoxication, disinhibition, poor insight, and poor judgment may be prominent. During alcohol withdrawal, agitation (hyperexcitability) may be prominent.

Management

Emergency department:

➤ Prevention and safety are the first considerations.

➤ Expose the fewest people possible to the violent person. Heroics (e.g., approaching a person who is pointing a gun while attempting to "talk him down") are never acceptable.

➤ Verbal communication can de-escalate the potential for violence and is a logical first choice, as long as emergent safety issues are first considered.

➤ A show of force (e.g., several safety officers) can reduce the potential for violence. Do not expose potentially violent persons to objects that can be used as weapons.

➤ Involuntary hospitalization should be used to reduce the potential for violent behavior. If needed, under strict guidelines, seclusion and restraints can be used.

➤ Antipsychotic medications (e.g., haloperidol, aripiprazole, olanzapine) and/or benzodiazepines (e.g., lorazepam) administered intramuscularly or orally can be very helpful on an acute basis.

➤ Medical disorders precipitant to assaultive behavior (e.g., seizure disorder) should be treated.

➤ The *Tarasoff* ruling mandates that when the threat of violence is imminent, the clinician should:

  ✔ Take action to prevent the patient from acting on the violent feelings. This is typically accomplished through psychiatric commitment or police action. The intended victim is referred to as the *third party*.

  ✔ Warn the intended victim(s) despite violating patient confidentiality.

Outpatient treatment:

General considerations:

➤ For patients not considered imminently dangerous, medications and psychotherapy can potentially be helpful.

➤ No medication is U.S. Food and Drug Administration–approved for the treatment of assaultive behavior, and no medication can be assumed or assured to be effective. Therefore, the choice of a medication is often empirical and based on clinical assessment (e.g., the presence of psychosis, depression, anxiety, or agitated states).

Medications that may reduce the potential for assaultive behavior:

➤ Antidepressants (sertraline, fluvoxamine, trazodone).

➤ Antipsychotic medications:

  ✔ The typical antipsychotic agents (e.g., haloperidol, fluphenazine) are widely used to treat aggressive behavior. However, they can cause a paradoxical increase in assaultive behavior secondary to extrapyramidal symptoms (akathisias).

  ✔ The atypical agent clozapine has antiaggression properties in patients with schizophrenia and schizoaffective disorder (as measured by a decrease in the use of restraints and need for seclusion in inpatient psychiatric settings). This effect may be distinct from its antipsychotic activity. Olanzapine and risperidone are demonstrating similar benefits in early studies.

➤ Anxiolytic agents:

  ✔ Benzodiazepines (with consideration for possible disinhibition and a subsequent increase in the potential for violence) and buspirone.

➤ Mood stabilizers:

  ✔ Include lithium, carbamazepine, divalproex sodium. Caution regarding recent FDA concerns for antiseizure medications increasing the potential for self-harming behavior.

➤ Other medications:

  ✔ Beta-blockers (e.g., propranolol). More recent studies do not support this conclusion.

  ✔ Conjugated estrogens, diethylstilbestrol, and medroxyprogesterone.

  ✔ Opiate antagonists.

  ✔ Acetylcholinesterase inhibitors (donepezil, tacrine, galantamine) can potentially reduce aggressive behavior associated with dementia of the Alzheimer's type.

Nonsomatic treatments:

➤ Behavior therapy (focusing on rewards for acceptable control) and psychotherapy (e.g., individual, group, marital, family) can be helpful for motivated patients.

CONTRACTING FOR SAFETY

➤ The effectiveness of the "contract for safety" has received mixed reviews in the literature.

➤ The following considerations apply:

  ✔ For patients without a therapeutic bond with the treatment provider (e.g., emergency setting, first interview), contracts for safety are virtually worthless.

  ✔ The more closely the treatment provider and patient have built a trusting relationship, the more likely the contract for safety may have merit (controversial).

  ✔ Be cautious in relying on a contract for safety to fulfill its intended purpose or to protect the treatment provider from malpractice claims should the patient commit suicide or harm someone else. There is much debate as to whether such contracts meet the established standard of care.

8

EATING DISORDERS

Principal DSM-IV-TR Eating Disorders

Anorexia nervosa
Bulimia nervosa
Binge-eating disorder (classified as an eating disorder
not otherwise specified)

Additional Issues

Anorexia nervosa and bulimia nervosa: a comparison
General considerations regarding eating disorders

ANOREXIA NERVOSA

DSM-IV-TR Diagnostic Criteria (Summary)—All 4 Criteria Must Be Met

➤ Refusal to maintain a body weight at or above a minimally normal weight for age and height (e.g., weight loss leading to maintenance of body weight less than 85% of that expected; failure to make expected weight gain during period of growth, leading to body weight less than 85% of that expected).

➤ Intense fear of gaining weight or becoming fat, even though underweight.

➤ Disturbance in the way in which one's body weight or shape is experienced, undue influence of body weight or shape on self-examination, or denial of the seriousness of the current low body weight.

➤ In postmenarcheal females, amenorrhea (i.e., the absence of at least three consecutive menstrual cycles). A woman is considered to have amenorrhea if her periods occur only following hormone (e.g., estrogen) administration.

Subtypes

➤ Restricting type:

✔ During the current episode of anorexia nervosa (AN), the person has not regularly engaged in binge-eating or purging behavior (i.e., self-induced vomiting or the misuse of laxatives, diuretics, or enemas).

➤ Binge-eating/purging type:

✔ During the current episode of AN, the person has regularly engaged in binge-eating or purging behavior (i.e., self-induced vomiting or the misuse of laxatives, diuretics, or enemas).

Clinical Issues

➤ Core findings in AN include:

✔ A refusal to maintain a minimally normal body weight.

✔ A profound disturbance of body image.

✔ A relentless pursuit of thinness.

✔ Menstrual irregularities in otherwise normally menstruating women. Amenorrhea is often an early presenting sign.

➤ Full diagnostic criteria may not be met early in AD, thereby leading to a failure to make an accurate diagnosis when treatment can be most valuable.

➤ Individuals purposefully restrict their diet, classically described as "willful starvation":

✔ Medical consequences become evident as weight loss becomes severe. Mortality is high, principally because of the medical consequences of starvation (e.g., emaciation, heart failure, cardiac arrhythmias, electrolyte imbalance) or suicide (5%–10% of individuals).

✔ Individuals typically have a normal appetite until the illness progresses to dangerous levels of emaciation, when true anorexia may develop.

✔ Fundamentally, food restriction represents a "drug of choice."

➤ Individuals have very unusual (but not deemed psychotic) attitudes regarding food and exercise, including:

✔ An intense fear of becoming fat.

✔ A distorted belief of being fat, despite profound thinness or emaciation.

✔ Compulsive eating behaviors (e.g., hoarding food, only eating alone, chewing food a fixed number of times before swallowing, always leaving food on the plate, eating at a fixed time that cannot be adjusted) and obsessions about food, body weight, and body shape.

✔ Exercise routines that often are intense, ritualistic, and excessive, even to the point of inflicting serious physical injury.

➤ Individuals have unusual characteristics regarding the nature of the illness, including:

✔ Denial of illness or lying about the presence of the illness.

✔ Lack of interest in or resistance to psychotherapy (often because of fear of being forced to gain weight).

➤ Self-worth often becomes tied to the ability to achieve and maintain an emaciated state.

➤ Alternation between the restricting and binge-eating/purging types is possible.

➤ Physical and laboratory findings are related to the consequences of self-induced malnutrition and an emaciated state (at times resembling concentration camp victims) and include:

✔ Vital sign changes:

■ Bradycardia, hypotension, dehydration, and hypothermia (cold, cyanotic extremities).

✔ Cardiovascular changes:

■ Electrocardiographic changes and arrhythmias, with possible sudden death (e.g., QTc interval widening on the electrocardiogram [ECG]).

■ Congestive heart failure with subsequent peripheral edema.

■ Dehydration.

■ Orthostatic hypotension.

■ Impaired peripheral circulation.

✔ Gastrointestinal changes:

■ Impaired motility, often with constipation.

■ Elevated liver function tests and serum amylase.

■ Vomiting-induced erosion of tooth enamel.

■ Vomiting/laxative/enema–induced electrolyte changes, possibly with dire consequences.

■ Mallory-Weiss syndrome (esophageal tear with massive bleeding) due to recurrent emesis (rare but life-threatening).

✔ Hematological changes (e.g., pancytopenia, leukopenia, anemia).

✔ Renal changes (e.g., renal calculi, elevated blood urea nitrogen from dehydration).

✔ Endocrine changes (e.g., decreased liothyronine [T_3], decreased estrogen in females and testosterone in males, increased cortisol).

✔ Musculoskeletal changes:

■ Osteoporosis or osteopenia (with resultant pathological fractures).

■ Muscle wasting, leading to emaciation.

✔ Dermatological changes:

■ Dry, yellowish skin with fine downy hair (lanugo hair).

■ Hair loss.

■ Calluses on the dorsum of the hand (Russell's sign) secondary to friction from self-induced vomiting.

✔ Nutritional changes:

■ Signs and symptoms of severe malnutrition (e.g., hypomagnesemia, decreased albumin, inadequate vitamin absorption with resultant deficiencies).

■ Electrolyte disturbances.

■ Parotid gland enlargement ("chipmunk face") secondary to recurrent emesis.

✔ Neurological changes:

■ Metabolic encephalopathy.

■ Cortical atrophy (possibly reversible with return of adequate nutrition).

■ Seizure activity.

■ Mild cognitive deficits or mental slowing.

■ Peripheral neuropathy.

Epidemiology

➤ Lifetime prevalence is 0.25%–1.0%, and point prevalence is 0.5%–1.0% in adolescent and young adult women.

➤ Females constitute 90% of the patient population.

➤ Mean age at onset is 17 years, with bimodal peaks at ages 12 and 18 years. Onset after age 40 years is uncommon.

➤ Rate of recovery is only 40% after 5–10 years. In 20% of persons, another major psychiatric disorder emerges (e.g., schizophrenia, mood disorder, personality disorder, substance abuse), further reducing the potential for recovery.

➤ Mortality (principally due to the consequences of electrolyte imbalance, heart failure, or suicide) is 0.5%–1.0% per observational year.

Etiological Formulations

➤ Genetic formulations:

✔ The risk of AN increases with closer genetic associations. The serotonin (5-hydroxytryptamine [5-HT]) transporter gene, which is under genetic influence, impacts the availability of 5-HT.

✔ Mood disorders and alcohol dependence are more prominent in family members of individuals with AN.

➤ Biological formulations:

✔ Norepinephrine, 5-HT, dopamine, hypothalamic dysfunction (altered release of gonadotropin, corticotropin-releasing hormone, and thyroid hormones), and release of beta-endorphins may be involved.

✔ Elevated 5-HT in the central nervous system (CNS) may be a strongly predisposing factor. High levels of 5-hydroxyindoleacetic acid (5-HIAA) (reduces appetite) in the CNS are found in recovering AN patients.

➤ Social and psychological considerations:

✔ Eating disorders reflect disturbances of the family system as a whole. Individuals often have troubled relationships with family members. This can include sexual abuse by family members or other individuals.

✔ Western societies promote a drive for thinness. This stress may prompt psychopathology, expressed as an eating disorder. "One can never be too rich or too thin."

✔ Participation in sports that emphasize weight restriction (e.g., ice-skating, gymnastics) can promote an eating disorder through behavioral conditioning.

✔ Individuals use obsessive eating behaviors as a replacement for normal adolescent pursuits of social and sexual functioning. As a consequence of continual conflicts regarding the transition from girl to woman, thinness becomes a means of staying prepubertal.

✔ Individuals feeling under excessive control of their parents rebel through starvation for autonomy and independence.

✔ Individuals are unable to interpret body hunger signals because of early experiences of inappropriate feeding.

Comorbidity (Percentage of Persons With the Designated Comorbid Disorder)

➤ Bulimia nervosa (BN; variable percentage, may change over time).

➤ Substance use disorders (26%).

➤ Major depression and dysthymia (50%–75%).

➤ Anxiety disorders (obsessive-compulsive disorder; posttraumatic stress disorder, often secondary to a history of childhood physical and/or sexual abuse; social phobia) (50%–75%).

➤ Personality disorders or traits (up to 50%).

Differential Diagnosis

➤ Medical causes of weight loss (e.g., malignancies, tuberculosis, chronic infections [e.g., hepatitis], malabsorption syndromes [e.g., inflammatory bowel disease], endocrine disorders [e.g., thyroid disease, diabetes], pituitary gland lesions) or emesis after eating.

➤ Mood disorders (e.g., major depressive disorder, dysthymic disorder).

➤ Substance abuse disorders.

➤ Psychotic disorders (e.g., schizophrenia, schizoaffective dsorder, delusional disorders).

➤ Anxiety disorders (e.g., obsessive-compulsive disorder, social phobia).

➤ Personality disorders.

➤ BN.

➤ Body dysmorphic disorder.

Workup

➤ Provide a complete physical and psychiatric examination (especially screening for suicidal ideation).

➤ Laboratory studies should include electrolytes, complete blood count, renal function tests, thyroid function tests, fasting blood glucose, serum amylase, beta-carotene levels, and ECG.

➤ Psychological testing can be helpful to confirm the diagnosis:

   ✔ Minnesota Multiphasic Personality Inventory–II.

   ✔ Eating Attitudes Test.

   ✔ Eating Disorder Inventory.

Treatment Considerations

➤ Treatment goals (address both physical and mental symptoms):

   ✔ Restore and maintain at least a minimally adequate body weight. Set reasonable expectations for eating and weight increases. All treatment protocols establish this criteria.

   ✔ Reduce complicating factors (e.g., depression, substance abuse, obsessive-compulsive behaviors, medical complications).

   ✔ Improve willingness to correct the anorexia through psychotherapy (success rates are low).

➤ Strongly consider hospitalization if weight is more than 20%–30% below normal or if other signs or symptoms (e.g., severe hypokalemia, severe anemia, hypoproteinemia, refusal to eat, cardiac arrhythmias, depression, psychosis, incapacitating obsessions or compulsions, family in crisis, suicidal ideation) are in the severe or dangerous range. For effective treatment, hospitalization will usually require 2–4 months and may not be supported by health insurance companies.

➤ Medications can help with ancillary symptoms (e.g., depression, anxiety), but will not reverse the core symptoms of AN, and none are U.S. Food and Drug Administration (FDA) approved.

   ✔ General considerations:

      ■ Purportedly, the poor response to antidepressants is due to impairment of 5-HT neurotransmission and low availability of the essential amino acid precursor to 5-HT (L-tryptophan) due to poor eating habits.

- AN can be associated with an increase in the QTc interval. Be especially cautious when adding medications that can further increase the QTc interval (e.g., thioridazine).

✔ Medication and electroconvulsive therapy (ECT) (anecdotal reports):

- Fluoxetine (Prozac) can be effective to prevent relapse after weight stabilization, reducing obsessive and compulsive behaviors, and treating underlying depression. It is not especially effective for underweight individuals.

- Chlorpromazine (Thorazine) 50 mg tid can help reduce uncontrollable behavioral rituals and improve the likelihood of some benefits from psychotherapy. Historically, chlorpromazine was widely used but is now mostly replaced with second-generation antipsychotics.

- Olanzapine (via antagonism of 5-HT$_2$) can increase appetite, induce weight gain, and reduce anxiety. However, patients may refuse to take the medication for fear of gaining weight.

- Cyproheptadine (Periactin), a 5-HT antagonist, 4–8 mg/day can increase appetite and induce weight gain.

- Naltrexone (ReVia) may be helpful for some patients to reduce bingeing via blockade of opioid receptors.

- ECT can be helpful for patients who are severely depressed or suicidal.

- Prokinetic medications (e.g., cisapride [Propulsid], metoclopramide [Reglan]) can be helpful for patients with delayed gastric emptying, to prevent bloating and the feeling of satiety that can further prompt reduced food intake.

➤ Nonpharmacological therapies (structured therapies with expected weight gains):

✔ Outpatient treatments include behavior modification (rewards for increasing weight), cognitive-behavioral therapy (correcting erroneous thinking about eating), systematic desensitization (gradual increases in caloric intake over time), individual or group psychotherapy, family therapy (referred to as the Maudsley method), and interpersonal therapy.

✔ Appreciate that patients are resistant to treatment and may be untruthful about their eating behaviors.

➤ Factors affecting a favorable treatment outcome include:

✔ Admission of hunger.

✔ Acknowledgment of having an illness (i.e., good insight).

✔ A greater level of maturity and self-esteem.

✔ Illness onset between ages 13 and 18 years.

BULIMIA NERVOSA

DSM-IV-TR Diagnostic Criteria (Summary)

➤ Recurrent episodes of binge eating. An episode of binge eating is characterized by both of the following:

  ✔ Eating, in a discrete period of time (e.g., within any 2-hour period), an amount of food that is definitely larger than most people would eat during a similar period of time and under similar circumstances.

  ✔ A sense of lack of control over eating during the period (e.g., a feeling that one cannot stop eating or control what or how much one is eating).

➤ Recurrent inappropriate compensatory behavior in order to prevent weight gain, such as self-induced vomiting; misuse of laxatives, diuretics, enemas, or medications; fasting; or excessive exercise.

➤ The binge eating and inappropriate compensatory behaviors both occur, on average, at least twice a week for 3 months.

➤ Self-evaluation is unduly influenced by body shape and weight.

➤ The disturbance does not occur exclusively during episodes of AN.

Subtypes

➤ Purging type:

  ✔ During the current episode of BN, the person has regularly engaged in self-induced vomiting or the misuse of laxatives, diuretics, or enemas.

➤ Nonpurging type:

  ✔ During the current episode of BN, the person has used other inappropriate compensatory behaviors, such as fasting or excessive exercise, but has not regularly engaged in self-induced vomiting or the misuse of laxatives, diuretics, or enemas.

Clinical Issues

➤ Cardinal findings include eating binges, followed by purging behaviors such as self-induced vomiting or laxative abuse.

➤ Purging, laxative abuse, and exercise (alone or together) are often used to compensate for binge-eating behaviors:

  ✔ There are few physical findings. Individuals are usually of normal or near-normal weight, most often with a history of obesity.

  ✔ Individuals typically choose foods that are sweet and high in caloric value (e.g., cakes, pastries, ice cream) and may eat secretly, compulsively, rapidly, and without chewing, at times far past the point of satiety. Guilt and shame often accompany binge-eating behaviors.

✔ Depression ("postbinge anguish") typically follows bingeing and is ameliorated (temporarily) by purging.

✔ Self-induced emesis is the most common purging technique (80%–90% of individuals).

✔ Excessive exercise is common to reduce the weight gain from binge eating. The exercise level may be to the point of exhaustion or injury.

➤ Individuals with BN, unlike those with AN, have an interest in physical attractiveness, sexual issues, and a greater interest in recovery.

➤ Medical complications of BN can include:

✔ Dehydration.

✔ Vomitus-induced swelling of the parotid gland.

✔ Mallory-Weiss syndrome (esophageal tears with potentially massive bleeding) due to recurrent emesis (rare but life-threatening).

✔ Dental caries and enamel erosion (due to recurrent purging).

✔ Electrolyte disturbances (due to purging).

✔ Mild elevations in serum amylase.

Epidemiology

➤ Lifetime prevalence ranges from 1% to 3%, with females accounting for 90%–95% of the patient population.

➤ Average age at onset is 18 years, with an age range of 12–40 years.

➤ Prognosis is significantly better than for AN. Within 2 years of treatment, 50%–70% of individuals are symptom free. After 10 years, 50% of individuals remain symptom free.

Comorbidity

➤ A prior history of mental health disorders is common, including:

✔ Major depression and bipolar disorder.

✔ Anxiety disorders (e.g., posttraumatic stress disorder [often secondary to a history of childhood sexual abuse], panic disorder, social phobia, obsessive-compulsive disorder).

✔ Substance abuse disorders (33%–60% of individuals).

✔ Borderline personality disorder (about 25%–48% of individuals).

✔ AN (may initially start with AN and then progress to BN).

Differential Diagnosis

➤ Medical causes of emesis (e.g., inflammatory bowel disease, hepatic dysfunction, gastrointestinal parasites, pancreatitis).

➤ Borderline personality disorder.

➤ AN with binge/purge cycle.

➤ Binge-eating disorder.

Treatment Considerations

➤ Hospitalization is rarely necessary, except for patients with severe electrolyte imbalance or with severe depression.

➤ Cognitive-behavioral therapy (CBT) is the best validated psychotherapeutic treatment for BN. Additionally, individual/group psychotherapy, family therapy, interpersonal therapy, support groups, and nutritional counseling can be very helpful.

➤ Antidepressants (especially when combined with CBT) can be very effective in reversing bulimic behaviors of bingeing/purging (unlike in AN). Medications shown to be effective in reducing bingeing behaviors include:

✔ Fluoxetine (the only FDA-approved medication). Higher dosages (40–80 mg/day) are likely needed.

✔ Topiramate—showing significant promise at dosages between 100 and 200 mg/day.

✔ Tricyclic antidepressants (especially amitriptyline, imipramine, and desipramine) and trazodone. May cause an increase in appetite and weight.

✔ Baclofen (a gamma-aminobutyric acid [GABA]$_B$ agonist).

✔ Ondansetron (Zofran)—an antiemetic medication.

✔ Naltrexone (ReVia) via blockade of opioid receptors.

➤ Several augmentation strategies can also be tried if monotherapy is not adequate:

✔ Add liothyronine sodium (T$_3$; Cytomel) 10–25 µg to the antidepressant.

✔ Add topiramate (Topamax) to the antidepressant. The additional benefit of decreased appetite is often welcome.

➤ Cautions:

✔ Poor response to antidepressants may well be secondary to poor compliance.

✔ Bupropion (Wellbutrin) is associated with an increased risk of grand mal seizures in persons who binge and therefore is contraindicated in this patient group. The risk is greatest with the immediate-release formulation.

✔ The usefulness of monoamine oxidase inhibitors (MAOIs) is limited with patients for whom control of eating is problematic; these agents are relatively contraindicated in this patient group.

BINGE-EATING DISORDER

Diagnostic Features

➤ Impaired control over repeated food binges and distress over this lack of control.

➤ Absence of compensatory mechanisms (e.g., vomiting, fasting, laxative abuse, excessive exercise).

Clinical Issues

➤ Essential features include the inability to control binge-eating episodes, but without compensatory mechanisms to control weight:

✔ Food consumption is rapid, and the typical caloric intake during a binge-eating episode is often between 2,000 and 4,000 calories, usually past the point of satiety. Cycling with weight gains and weight losses is common.

✔ Individuals often are overweight or obese (in many cases 100 pounds or more overweight), eat when not hungry, and frequently report self-loathing, disgust, or depression after a binge-eating episode.

✔ Individuals often hide their eating habits, typically eating small amounts of food in social settings, yet binge eating when they are alone.

✔ Despite their eating habits (at least two binge-eating episodes per week or at least 2 days a week), individuals have a fear of being fat, an intense preoccupation with body shape and size, and a preoccupation with thoughts of food, weight, and becoming thin.

✔ Individuals with binge-eating disorder are frequent participants in Overeaters Anonymous (~70% of patients) and seekers of bariatric surgery (up to 50% of patients).

✔ Binge-eating disorder is also described as "compulsive overeating."

✔ A variant of binge-eating disorder is night eating syndrome, in which more than half the daily calories are consumed at night with little daytime interest in eating. As opposed to binge eating disorder, eating is continuous over the evening and night rather than in short bursts of massive amounts of food.

Epidemiology

➤ Prevalence is 1.5%–3.0%.

Treatment Considerations

➤ No medications are FDA approved.

➤ CBT is considered the treatment of choice to reduce bingeing behaviors. Behavioral weight-loss treatments (focusing on diet and exercise) and interpersonal therapy (IPT) are also useful treatments.

➤ Fluvoxamine (Luvox), citalopram (Celexa), fluoxetine (Prozac), and sertraline (Zoloft) can be helpful (off-label use).

➤ Topiramate (Topamax), baclofen, and naltrexone (ReVia) can be helpful to reduce binge-eating episodes (as labeled).

➤ Sibutramine (Meridia), a 5-HT and norepinephrine reuptake inhibitor FDA approved for the management of obesity, can be helpful.

ANOREXIA NERVOSA AND BULIMIA NERVOSA: A COMPARISON

Similarities

➤ Distorted body image.

➤ Intense fear of gaining weight.

➤ Inability to de-emphasize the individual's preoccupation with physical appearance, even in the presence of serious medical consequences.

➤ Similar weight-control measures (purging, dieting, fasting, exercise).

➤ Comorbidity with each other and with mood, anxiety, substance abuse, and personality disorders.

➤ Significantly higher frequency in females.

Differences

➤ Individuals with BN are typically of normal body weight, whereas individuals with AN have very low body weight.

➤ BN is more prevalent and has a far better prognosis (in terms of morbidity and mortality) than AN.

➤ Individuals with BN show greater interest in physical attractiveness and sexuality than individuals with AN.

➤ Antidepressants may be of significant value for treating the core symptoms of BN but of little value for treating the core symptoms of AN.

GENERAL CONSIDERATIONS REGARDING EATING DISORDERS

Diagnostic Issues

➤ Be cautious in your labeling of a patient with an eating disorder without paying strict attention to diagnostic requirements. Individuals may have characteristics of AN, BN, or binge-eating disorder that do not fully satisfy diagnostic criteria or overlap with each other.

➤ DSM-IV-TR provides a diagnostic category (*eating disorder not otherwise specified*) to include variants that do not satisfy the criteria for another type of eating disorder. Binge-eating disorder falls into this category. Other examples of *eating disorder not otherwise specified* taken from DSM-IV-TR include:

✔ All of the criteria for AN are met except that the patient has regular menses.

✔ All of the criteria for AN are met except that despite weight loss, the patient has normal weight.

✔ All of the criteria for BN are met except that the binge eating and compensatory mechanisms occur at a frequency of less than twice a week or for a duration of less than 3 months.

✔ An individual of normal weight regularly uses inappropriate compensatory behavior after eating small amounts of food.

✔ The individual repeatedly chews and spits out large quantities of food but does not swallow.

Neurotransmitter Issues

➤ Low levels of endorphins stimulate hunger for fats.

➤ Low levels of serotonin stimulate hunger for carbohydrates.

➤ Exercise raises both endorphin and serotonin levels and can reduce food craving behaviors.

Compensatory Weight-Control Measures in Anorexia Nervosa and Bulimia Nervosa

Purging:

➤ Found in the binge-eating/purging type of AN and the purging type of BN. Types include:

✔ Self-induced vomiting:

■ Individuals use their fingers or another object to induce a gag reflex. Eventually, vomiting can be induced at will without any mechanical intervention. Scars and abrasions on the back of the hand (Russell's sign) and erosion of teeth are signs of chronic vomiting.

■ Syrup of ipecac is used to induce emesis but in excess can lead to cardiomyopathy (with reported deaths), tachycardia, prolonged QTc interval, and premature atrial and ventricular contractions.

- Recurrent vomiting can lead to electrolyte imbalance from loss of stomach acid, severe dental disease, hypokalemia, and Mallory-Weiss syndrome.
- Vomiting is the most common method of purging.

✔ Laxatives, diuretics, and enemas:

- General considerations:
  - Excessive use may lead to electrolyte imbalance.
  - Psychopathology is generally greater in individuals who use laxatives.
- Commonly used agents:
  - Phenolphthalein preparations (e.g., Ex-Lax, Feen-a-mint)—excessive use can lead to "cathartic colon" (resembles ulcerative colitis).
  - Mineral oil—excessive use can lead to lipid pneumonia secondary to aspiration.
  - Diuretics—excessive use can lead to dehydration and/or electrolyte imbalance (especially low potassium), possibly resulting in cardiac arrhythmias and sudden death.

Dieting and fasting:

➤ Extensively employed by individuals with AN (the primary mechanism of weight control).

➤ Often (but not always) employed by individuals with BN to compensate for binge-eating episodes.

Excessive exercise:

➤ Exercise is often (but not always) used by individuals with AN and BN to lose weight or to compensate for binge-eating episodes.

➤ Exercise may be ritualistic and compulsive to the point where bodily injury is ignored and many hours daily are devoted to intensive exercise.

Alternative methods:

➤ Self-administration of thyroid medications to speed metabolism (can lead to thyrotoxicosis and bone loss).

➤ Self-administration of insulin by nondiabetic persons (can lead to severe hypoglycemia or insulin coma).

9

MISCELLANEOUS TOPICS

Topics Reviewed

Differential diagnosis
Outcomes
Development of the DSM
Intelligence
Affect
Insight
Visual hallucinations
Brain imaging and electroencephalography
Clinical studies of particular importance
Somatoform disorders, malingering, and factitious disorder
Impulse-control disorders
Paraphilias
Adult attention-deficit/hyperactivity disorder
Psychiatric disorders over the female life span
Psychiatric manifestations of thyroid disorders
Psychiatric manifestations of HIV infection
Classification of involuntary abnormal movements
The glutamate–GABA connection
Pharmacotherapy for insomnia
Serotonin, norepinephrine, and dopamine metabolic pathways
Clinical indications for antidepressant medications
Clinical indications for antipsychotic medications
Metabolic syndrome
Cigarette smoking and psychotropic medications
Inhibitory effects of SSRIs, SNRIs, and atypical antidepressants
 on specific CYP isoenzymes
CYP isoenzymes substantially inhibited by antidepressant
 medications
Mnemonic for the major cytochrome P450 isoenzymes
 that have an impact on psychotropic medications
"STEPS" mnemonic for choosing a medication
Mnemonic for achieving a desired clinical response from a
 medication

Pharmacogenetic relevance to psychiatric disorders
Pharmacokinetic issues in the elderly
Death and dying (Elisabeth Kübler-Ross)
Selected neurological disorders with neuropsychiatric involvement
Pregnancy risk categories
Experimental drug testing phases
Ethical dilemmas in psychiatry
Malpractice issues in brief

DIFFERENTIAL DIAGNOSIS

➤ This section is perhaps one of the most important for improving your chances to pass the oral boards.

➤ For every patient, include in your differential diagnosis the possibility that the observed psychiatric symptoms could be due to:

✔ A medical illness (systemic, neurological).

✔ A substance (e.g., a prescribed medication, an over-the-counter medication, an herbal remedy, alcohol, an illicit substance).

➤ For every patient, consider (even if just for completeness) including in your differential diagnosis the possibility that the observed psychiatric symptoms could be due to:

✔ Factitious disorder or malingering (look for secondary-gain issues).

OUTCOMES

➤ Outcomes are of critical importance and take precedence over symptom reduction. For example, a response to an antidepressant is valued, but not nearly as much as is remission (recovery).

➤ Virtually all DSM-IV-TR diagnoses (with the exception of hypomania) require a dysfunctional course to satisfy diagnostic criteria. Therefore, when discussing treatment options (e.g., "I would add Lamictal"), also state that the purpose for this addition is not only for symptom reduction, but for an improved outcome with regards to functionality.

➤ Often, a balance must be achieved between symptom reduction and improved functioning. For example, a first-generation antipsychotic (FGA) medication dosage can be raised to further reduce auditory hallucinations, but if the patient is left overly sedated, work/school/relationships may suffer.

DEVELOPMENT OF THE DIAGNOSTIC AND STATISTICAL MANUAL OF MENTAL DISORDERS (DSM)

■ Table 9–1   Evolution of the Diagnostic and Statistical Manual of Mental Disorders, beginning with the U.S. Census

Year	Census or DSM edition	Examples of listing
1840	Census	Idiocy and insanity
1880	Census	Mania, melancholia, monomania, paresis, dementia, dipsomania, and epilepsy
1954	DSM-I	Gross stress reaction
1968	DSM-II	Manic-depressive psychosis, anxiety neurosis (included panic disorder and generalized anxiety disorder)
1980	DSM-III (first edition with diagnostic criteria)	Affective disorders, brief reactive psychosis, Axes designations.
1987	DSM-III-R (DSM-III, Revised)	Affective disorders
1994	DSM-IV	Affective disorders changed to mood disorders; brief reactive psychosis changed to brief psychotic disorder
2000	DSM-IV-TR (Text Revision)	Text revision, not a substantive revision; note that DSM-IV is now 14 years old and much out of date
2012	DSM-V due to be published	

INTELLIGENCE

➤ Intelligence can be measured by the Wechsler Adult Intelligence Scale (WAIS) as well as by other standardized tests. Category ranges vary by reporting agencies, but in general the following categories with corresponding intelligence quotient (IQ) ranges apply:

✔ Very superior (>130).

✔ Superior (120–130).

✔ Bright normal (110–119).

✔ Normal (90–109).

✔ Dull normal (80–89).

✔ Borderline intellectual functioning (71–79).

✔ Mild mental retardation (50/55–70).

✔ Moderate mental retardation (35/40–50/55).

✔ Severe mental retardation (20/25–35/40).

✔ Profound mental retardation (<20/25).

AFFECT

➤ Disturbances in affect include:

✔ Flat—absence or near absence of affective expression.

✔ Blunted—significant reduction in the intensity of emotional expression.

✔ Restricted or constricted—mild-to-moderate reduction in the range and intensity of emotional expression.

✔ Inappropriate—discordance between affective expression and the content of thinking or speech.

✔ Labile—abnormal variability in affect, with repeated, rapid, or abrupt shifts in affective expression.

INSIGHT

General Considerations

➤ *Insight* ("psychological mindedness") refers to the patient's awareness or understanding of the presence of a mental illness or psychopathology.

➤ Psychiatric disorders associated with poor insight include:

✔ Psychotic disorders (e.g., schizophrenia, schizoaffective disorder, delusional disorders, brief psychotic disorder).

✔ Mood disorders (e.g., major depression with or without psychotic features, bipolar disorder).

✔ Somatization disorders.

✔ Substance use disorders.

✔ Eating disorders.

✔ Personality disorders.

✔ Impulse-control disorders.

✔ Body dysmorphic disorder.

➤ Neurological disorders associated with poor insight include:

✔ Parietal lobe syndromes due to right hemisphere stroke:

■ May be associated with denial of left-sided paralysis and lack of recognition of the person's arms and legs.

✔ Dementias:

■ Individuals with cortical dementias may not recognize that they are suffering from a dementing process, whereas individuals with the subcortical dementias (e.g., Parkinson's disease) usually have awareness of their memory impairment.

✔ Frontal lobe impairments:

■ May be associated with lack of awareness of memory loss and of changes in personality and social behavior.

✔ Tardive dyskinesia:

■ Individuals may be unaware of or not bothered by their abnormal movements.

Clinical Issues

➤ *Anosognosia* refers to lack of awareness of a variety of impairments (e.g., memory, aphasia, physical changes) as a consequence of brain damage. Other terms used interchangeably are *unawareness, impaired awareness of deficits,* and *lack of insight.*

➤ A correlation between frontal lobe abnormalities in schizophrenia and lack of insight has been proposed as a possible etiological consideration.

➤ Lack of insight contributes to poor treatment compliance and poor outcome.

VISUAL HALLUCINATIONS

➤ Visual hallucinations, especially when they are the only perceptual psychotic manifestation, are suggestive (but not pathognomonic) of medical illness rather than a primary (i.e., functional) psychiatric disorder. Some disorders with prominent visual hallucinations include:

✔ Delirium.

✔ Dementias (e.g., Alzheimer's disease, Lewy body dementia ["well-formed and detailed visual hallucinations"]).

✔ Substance-induced disorders and substance withdrawal syndromes.

✔ Occipital and temporal lobe epilepsy (classic neurological disorders associated with visual hallucinations).

✔ Cerebrovascular accident.

✔ Migraine headache aura.

✔ Charles Bonnet syndrome (complex visual hallucinations in elderly visually impaired persons, often secondary to macular degeneration, but without major cognitive deficits). Occurs in approximately 14% of sight-impaired persons.

BRAIN IMAGING AND ELECTROENCEPHALOGRAPHY

➤ Brain imaging (neuroimaging) and electroencephalography (EEG) can help distinguish between "functional" and "organic" causes of psychiatric symptoms and are important tools to help elucidate the etiology of psychiatric disorders

✔ Computed tomography (CT) reveals brain structure. CT is helpful for detecting mass lesions, calcification (superior to magnetic resonance imaging [MRI] in this regard), intracranial bleeds, and cerebrovascular accidents. There are no consistent CT findings with regard to mood disorders or schizophrenia.

✔ MRI also measures brain structures but is much more sensitive than CT for soft tissue. Images can be weighted (e.g., T_1 and T_2). MRI is helpful for detecting tumors, intracranial bleeds (although not as helpful as CT), demyelinization (e.g., multiple sclerosis), atrophy, and subcortical disorders (e.g., Parkinson's disease, Huntington's disease). Unlike CT, MRI can distinguish between gray and white matter, and it is of great utility in studies of brain changes in psychiatric disorders.

✔ Functional MRI (fMRI) is an imaging technique in which the patient performs a particular task and the corresponding area where the brain process is functioning can be visualized because of increased *blood flow* to that area. This technique is valuable in surgery to locate specific lesions and in neuropsychiatry as a research tool.

✔ Positron emission tomography (PET) uses radioactively labeled compounds (e.g., glucose) to assess blood flow, oxygen utilization, and glucose metabolism in the brain. This technique shows promise to help elucidate the etiology of a number of psychiatric disorders, including schizophrenia, mood disorders, dementias, anxiety disorders (particularly obsessive-compulsive disorder [OCD]), and substance use disorders.

✔ Single photon emission computed tomography (SPECT) measures regional blood flow much like that of PET. It provides a more rapid picture of blood flow but is of poorer resolution than PET. This technique is helpful in assessing for cerebrovascular accidents, focal seizures, and brain tumors and in discriminating between dementia of the Alzheimer's type and vascular dementia. It shows promise in helping to elucidate the etiology of a number of psychiatric disorders, including schizophrenia, mood disorders, and anxiety disorders (particularly OCD).

✔ EEG measures electrical activity in the brain. This technique is helpful in detecting seizure activity with characteristic spike-and-wave formation (e.g., temporal lobe epilepsy, complex partial seizures), drug-induced toxic states (increase in alpha activity), toxic metabolic states, tumors (focal slowing), delirium (generalized slowing and irregular high-voltage delta activity), and dementias (increase in slow-wave activity).

CLINICAL STUDIES OF PARTICULAR IMPORTANCE (CONCLUSIONS ARE OFTEN DEBATED AND NOT UNIVERSALLY ACCEPTED)

➤ Clinical Antipsychotic Trials of Intervention Effectiveness (CATIE 1 and 2):

✔ Several second-generation antipsychotics (SGAs; olanzapine, risperidone, quetiapine, ziprasidone) were compared to the FGA perphenazine. The primary outcome measure in both phases was the time to stopping treatment for any reason (efficacy, side effects):

■ Sixty to 80% of all patients discontinued their antipsychotic medication over the 18-month trial period for any reason (Phase 1 or 2).

■ Lack of efficacy was the primary reason for medication discontinuation followed by discontinuation due to medication side effects (except for olanzapine, which was reversed).

■ Olanzapine, despite a higher side-effect profile, was continued for a longer period of time than other antipsychotic medications.

■ Efficacy of perphenazine was equal to quetiapine, risperidone, and ziprasidone over the 18-month trial period.

■ Olanzapine had the highest weight gain and increases in glucose and lipids. Ziprasidone was effectively weight neutral.

■ In phase 2, Clozaril was found to be the most effective agent, followed by olanzapine and risperidone. Perphenazine was not used in Phase 2. Other than switching to Clozaril, there is little guidance from the study as to switching between the regularly used antipsychotic agents.

- Cost savings was considerable if perphenazine was used rather than an SGA.

✔ Analyzing the raw data in different ways produces somewhat different results, sufficient to provide a robust debate as to the true conclusions of the study.

➤ Sequenced Treatment Alternatives to Relieve Depression (STAR*D):

✔ Varying treatment strategies were compared for the treatment of clinical unipolar depression.

- Switching between various treatment protocols can be effective if one trial is not effective. However, if additional protocols are needed, the potential for improvement or recovery diminishes with each successive change. The best results occurred with the first treatment protocol.

- Level one started with citalopram (30% recovery rate). If the patient did not substantially improve, he or she could switch to another medication (sertraline, venlafaxine XR, bupropion) or another medication could be added (bupropion, buspirone).

- Additional levels provided mirtazapine, tricyclic antidepressants (TCAs), monoamine oxidase inhibitors, and augmentation with liothyronine (T_3).

➤ Systematic Treatment Enhancement Program for Bipolar Disorder (STEP-BD):

✔ The goal of the study was to determine the best practice treatment options for bipolar disorder (mood-stabilizing medications, antidepressants, atypical antipsychotics, and psychosocial interventions).

- Intensive psychotherapy along with medications provided the most robust response for the treatment of bipolar depression.

- Antidepressants added to a mood stabilizer did not seem to help with recovery from bipolar depression and may worsen bipolar mania.

➤ Combined Pharmacotherapies and Behavioral Interventions for Alcohol Dependence (COMBINE Study):

✔ The goal of the study was to assess the extent of abstinence from drinking utilizing medication (naltrexone, acamprosate) or therapy (combined behavioral intervention [CBI]).

- Naltrexone and CBI (alone or together) were more effective than placebo, but acamprosate did not provide benefit beyond placebo, even when combined with CBI.

- Naltrexone treatment alone can be effective when prescribed from a primary care office.

SOMATOFORM DISORDERS, MALINGERING, AND FACTITIOUS DISORDER

➤ Patients with *somatoform disorders* present with physical symptoms not fully explained by physical tests, substance abuse, medications, or other psychiatric disorders. The symptoms are not intentionally produced and cause significant impairment in social, occupational, or other important areas of functioning. Classically, the disorder satisfies the patient's need for primary gain (e.g., subconscious needs or expression of subconscious frustrations). Somatoform disorder is a diagnosis of exclusion. Clinically, a patient may be given a diagnosis of somatoform disorder, only later to have the diagnosis reversed when physical testing finally demonstrates medical pathology. A somatoform disorder referenced by DSM-IV-TR is pseudocyesis. A review of the somatoform disorders is presented in Table 9–2.

➤ *Malingering* and *factitious disorder* involve the intentional feigning of physical and/or psychiatric symptoms for secondary gain (e.g., to obtain financial reward, to avoid working, to avoid legal consequences, to maintain a sick role). Malingering and factitious disorder are reviewed in Table 9–3.

➤ For purposes of the oral board examination, somatoform disorders, malingering, and factitious disorder would require a longer period of assessment. A workup would include physical, laboratory, and psychological testing, with extensive interviews with the patient and, if possible, ancillary sources. When appropriate, these disorders should be included in your differential diagnosis.

IMPULSE-CONTROL DISORDERS

➤ Impulse-control disorders involve a failure or inability to resist an impulse or temptation to perform an act that is harmful to the person or to others (Table 9–4). Typical features include:
  ✔ Tension or anxiety prior to the act.
  ✔ Relief, pleasure, or excitement during the act.
  ✔ Guilt or depression after the act.
➤ Treatment:
  ✔ Impulse-control disorders may be partially responsive to antidepressant medications and mood stabilizers.

■ Table 9–2   Somatoform disorders (symptoms are not intentionally produced)

Disorder	Clinical findings not explained by a physical cause (adapted from DSM-IV-TR)	Additional considerations
Somatization disorder (Briquet's syndrome, "hysteria")	Multiple physical symptoms, including at least four pain symptoms, two gastrointestinal symptoms, one sexual symptom, and one pseudoneurological symptom (e.g., conversion symptoms, loss of consciousness).	Characterized by multiple and clinically significant somatic complaints beginning before age 30 years. A chronic disorder with a waxing and waning course. Multiple physicians are usually consulted over the course of the illness. Although the disorder is psychological in nature, surgeries or other diagnostic procedures can produce medical impairments (e.g., adhesions from exploratory surgeries).
Conversion disorder	One or more symptoms or deficits affecting voluntary motor or sensory function that suggest a neurological or other general medical condition.	Typically, symptoms do not conform to anatomic pathways (e.g., paralysis of the left hand and right foot). Often, a stressor is present (e.g., loss of the use of a hand after a child is accidentally burned by spilling hot liquid on the child with the involved hand). Characteristically, the individual is not overly bothered by the impairment (*la belle indifférence*). Impairments can involve motor, sensory, or neurological (i.e., seizure) deficits.
Pain disorder (chronic pain syndrome)	Pain in one or more anatomic sites sufficient to warrant clinical attention. Psychological factors are judged to have an important role in the onset, severity, exacerbation, or maintenance of the pain. Not diagnosed if the pain is better accounted for by a mood, anxiety, or psychotic disorder.	Pain may develop after an injury, but psychological factors play a primary role in the pain syndrome. Common disorders associated with pain disorder are musculoskeletal conditions (e.g., disc herniation, osteoporosis, arthritis, myofascial pain syndromes), neuropathies (e.g., diabetic neuropathy, postherpetic neuralgia), and malignancies. Examples of effects include inability to work or attend school, frequent use of the health care system, pain becoming a major focus of the person's life, and substantial use of medications. Medical treatments (e.g., exploratory surgeries) can create more pain.

Table 9–2 Somatoform disorders (symptoms are not intentionally produced) (continued)

Disorder	Clinical findings not explained by a physical cause (adapted from DSM-IV-TR)	Additional considerations
Hypochondriasis	Preoccupation with fears of developing, or that one may contract, a serious disease based on the person's misrepresentation of bodily symptoms, persisting despite appropriate medical evaluation and reassurance.	The disorder is frustrating to the patient and medical community. Patients typically "doctor-shop" when they refuse to accept the medical opinion that nothing serious is wrong. Negative countertransference is common, further exacerbating the overall problem.
Body dysmorphic disorder	Preoccupation with an imagined defect in appearance. If a slight physical anomaly is present, the person's concern is markedly excessive.	Significant distress over the imagined "ugliness" leads to requests for plastic surgeries or other "repairs." Common areas of focus are flaws (e.g., thinning hair, wrinkles, acne), "defects" of the face or head, or the size of body parts related to sexual attractiveness (e.g., breasts, hips, buttocks, penis). Individuals may go to extremes to identify or hide the defects (e.g., use magnifying glasses to visualize the defect, grow a beard, or wear a hat).
Somatoform disorder not otherwise specified	Somatoform symptoms that do not meet the criteria for other somatoform disorders.	DSM-IV-TR provides the example of pseudocyesis, characterized by a false belief of being pregnant with objective signs of being pregnant, such as abdominal enlargement, breast engorgement, reduced or absent menstrual flow, endocrine changes not explained by a medical cause, and labor pains.

■ Table 9–3   Malingering and factitious disorder (symptoms are intentionally produced)

Disorder	Clinical findings (adapted from DSM-IV-TR)	Additional considerations
Malingering	Intentional production of false or grossly exaggerated physical or psychological symptoms. The motivation involves external incentives such as avoiding military duty, avoiding work, obtaining financial compensation, evading criminal prosecution, or obtaining drugs. Thus, feigning mental illness to seek food and shelter in a hospital would be classified as malingering.	Malingering is suspected when: • There are marked discrepancies between the patient's complaints and the observed findings. • The person does not cooperate with the evaluation and treatment. • Complaints intensify when the patient is being observed. • There are "cues" to suspect malingering (e.g., attempting to obtain Social Security benefits, legal issues are at stake). • A positive Waddell's sign (orthopedic test) is indicative of nonorganic pain. Malingering is common among individuals with antisocial personality disorder.
Factitious disorder	Intentional production or feigning of physical or psychological signs or symptoms. The motivation involves assumption of the sick role rather than the tangible external incentives described under Malingering. Types include: • Total fabrication (e.g., claiming nonexistent chronic pain, claiming nonexistent anxiety to receive benzodiazepines). • Simulations (e.g., grimacing in response to inducing very mild pain). • Exaggeration (e.g., reporting occasional back pain as chronic back pain). • Aggravation (e.g., deliberately not using prescribed treatments that would ameliorate the illness). • Self-induction (e.g., purposefully taking insulin to induce a coma).	Patients often are knowledgeable about medical routines and use that knowledge to feign symptoms (e.g., put a drop of their blood in a urine specimen). Lying is common. Patients may go from doctor to doctor to propagate their sick role. Symptoms typically exceed objective findings. A very large number of tests and procedures have been undertaken. In Munchausen syndrome, the most severe form of factitious disorder, the patient's lifestyle is centered around medical assessments and unnecessary medical procedures. Classically, patients with Munchausen syndrome present with predominantly physical signs and symptoms. A "checkerboard abdomen" secondary to repeated exploratory surgeries may be evident. Major symptoms include 1) purposefully feigning illness, including inducing illness; 2) pathological lying (pseudologia fantastica), presenting their medical history in a dramatic manner; and 3) peregrination (i.e., changing names and living locations) to continue fostering the fake symptoms). Additionally, the person often has medical training and comorbid borderline or antisocial personality disorder. When the focus of the feigned illness is a child or another person under the care of the perpetrator, factitious disorder by proxy (Munchausen syndrome by proxy) is diagnosed.

Table 9–3   Malingering and factitious disorder (symptoms are intentionally produced) *(continued)*

Disorder	Clinical findings (adapted from DSM-IV-TR)	Additional considerations
Factitious disorder *(continued)*		In Ganser syndrome, the person makes absurd statements, complains of psychotic symptoms that are incongruent, or gives approximate answers (known as *vorbeireden*). In dermatitis artefacta, the person intentionally creates skin lesions to assume the sick role. Psychotherapy is the treatment of choice for factitious disorders.

■ **Table 9–4 Impulse-control disorders**

Disorder	Clinical findings (adapted from DSM-IV-TR)	Additional considerations
Intermittent explosive disorder	Several discrete episodes of failure to resist aggressive impulses that result in serious assaultive acts or destruction of property. The degree of aggressiveness expressed during the episode is grossly out of proportion to the precipitating psychosocial stressor.	Behavior can be explosive and damaging.
Kleptomania	Recurrent failure to resist impulses to steal objects that are not needed for personal use or monetary value.	Stealing for personal need or monetary gain does not qualify as kleptomania.
Pyromania	Deliberate and purposeful fire setting on more than one occasion. There is fascination, curiosity, or attraction with regard to the fire and its situational context (e.g., fire-setting paraphernalia, watching the burning).	A risk factor for violent behavior.
Pathological gambling	Preoccupation with gambling, with similarities to an addiction process (e.g., increasing pattern of gambling, inability to stop, involvement in illegal activities to finance the gambling).	Some authorities consider this disorder an addiction, such as with a substance. Gamblers Anonymous has a 12-step program like that of Alcoholics Anonymous. May be classified as part of an obsessive-compulsive spectrum disorder.
Trichotillomania	Recurrent pulling out of one's hair, resulting in noticeable hair loss.	May be classified as part of an obsessive-compulsive spectrum disorder.

PARAPHILIAS

➤ Essential features include recurrent, intense sexual arousing fantasies, sexual urges, or behaviors (i.e., sexual gratification) that cause clinically significant distress or functional impairment and that generally involve:

✔ Nonhuman objects.

✔ The suffering or humiliation of oneself or one's partner.

✔ Children (over a period of at least 6 months).

➤ Types:

✔ *Exhibitionism*—sexual gratification from exposure of one's genitals to a stranger.

✔ *Fetishism*—sexual gratification by using a nonliving object (e.g., masturbating into a pair of women's underpants).

✔ *Frotteurism*—sexual gratification from touching or rubbing against a nonconsenting person.

✔ *Pedophilia*—sexual gratification through sexual activity (the act itself) with a prepubescent child by a person who is at least age 16 years or at least 5 years older than the child.

✔ *Sexual masochism*—sexual gratification from being humiliated, beaten, bound, or made to suffer.

✔ *Sexual sadism*—sexual gratification from the psychological or physical suffering or humiliation of another person.

✔ *Voyeurism*—sexual gratification from observing an unsuspecting person naked, disrobing, or engaging in sexual activity.

✔ *Transvestic fetishism*—sexual gratification from cross-dressing.

ADULT ATTENTION-DEFICIT/ HYPERACTIVITY DISORDER

General Considerations

➤ Although it is unlikely to see a patient with a primary diagnosis of ADHD, the high comorbidity of ADHD (~75%–87%) with other psychiatric disorders (especially mood, anxiety, and substance use disorders) should be appreciated.

➤ ADHD is typically thought of as a disorder of childhood that usually dissipates as the child moves into adulthood. Actually, approximately 70% of children continue to experience symptoms in adulthood. The prevalence in adults is 4.4%.

➤ Typical symptoms in adults include poor ability to organize and prioritize tasks, poor tolerance of delays, procrastination, lack of motivation, poor sense of time constraints, forgetfulness, and temper outbursts. Functional consequences (often underappreciated) include difficulties at work (with frequent job changes or failure to advance) and marital difficulties (e.g., separation, divorce).

➤ ADHD is a risk factor for bipolar disorder and is often comorbid with bipolar disorder.

➤ The diagnosis is based on the criterion that symptoms must have been present in childhood. Thus, emergence of ADHD symptoms starting in adulthood does not satisfy DSM-IV-TR diagnostic criteria for ADHD, although some psychiatrists maintain a broader definition with fewer diagnostic requirements.

➤ The potential to develop ADHD is strongly influenced by genetic factors and multiple "candidate" genes have been identified (e.g., *DAT1, DRD5, DBH*).

➤ Neuroimaging studies (e.g., fMRI) demonstrate frontal, temporal, and parietal cortex involvement.

➤ A "comprehensive" assessment through inteview (patient, others) and testing (e.g., Conners, Brown, Barkley) is always recommended and is considered a prerequisite for diagnosing ADHD.

Treatment

➤ Treatment includes pharmacotherapy often coupled with psychotherapy (e.g., cognitive-behavioral therapy, individual):

✔ Stimulants (e.g., methylphenidate, dextroamphetamine)—not all are U.S. Food and Drug Administration (FDA) approved in adults.

■ Principally inhibit reuptake of dopamine and norepinephrine from the synapse.

■ Are formulated as an immediate release (methylphenidate, amphetamine, amphetamine salts), extended release (amphetamine salts, methylphenidate), lisdexamfetamine (D-amphetamine prodrug [Vyvanse]) and methylphenidate patch (Daytrana).

■ Side effects include appetite suppression, potentially leading to weight loss, and insomnia. Tics are uncommon but can be irreversible.

■ Are designed to provide a more smoothly delivered response when formulated as sustained-release formulations, lisdexamfetamine, and the methylphenidate patch.

■ When used inappropriately, can lead to dependence.

- Have minimal serious cardiovascular risks when taken properly, although increased warnings may be forthcoming.

✔ Atomoxetine (Strattera)—FDA approved in adults:

- Selectively blocks norepinephrine reuptake and increases dopamine in the prefrontal cortex.

- May require 2–6 weeks to become optimally effective but carries no abuse potential.

- Provides 24-hour coverage with once-daily dosing.

- Should initially be dosed at 40 mg/day, titrating upward as indicated to a maximum of 120 mg/day.

- Carries a black box warning regarding rare suicidal ideations in adolescents and young adults.

- Side effects typically include nausea and dizziness. Rare reports of hepatic damage.

✔ Alternative (non-FDA-approved) medications:

- Bupropion (Wellbutrin).

- Clonidine (Catapres) and guanfacine (Tenex).

- Selegiline (Eldepryl).

- Venlafaxine (Effexor-XR).

- Modafinil (Provigil).

- Estrogen supplementation.

- Nicotinic analogues.

PSYCHIATRIC DISORDERS OVER THE FEMALE LIFE SPAN

Gender Differences in Prevalence and Risk

➤ Most anxiety disorders, unipolar depression, bipolar II disorder, cyclothymic disorder, dysthymic disorder, mixed manic episodes, and rapid cycling are more prevalent (by at least a factor of 2) in females than in males. However, there are no gender differences for bipolar I disorder and schizophrenia.

➤ Although the risk of depression stays relatively constant in males over the adult life span, the risk in females increases at puberty, premenstrually, perimenopausally, and during the postpartum period but decreases postmenopausally.

➤ The reasons for the increased prevalence of mood disorders in females are not firmly established. Although hormonal changes throughout the life cycle (e.g., prepubescent, premenstrual, perimenopausal, postmenopausal, and postpartum) seem to be the most plausible explanation, research findings are not definitive. Other possible reasons include genetic, environmental, and developmental factors. Most of the research has focused on hormonal changes:

✔ Cyclic changes in estrogen, progesterone, and thyroid hormones over the life cycle are thought to play a role in the development of mood disorders in women.

✔ The general consensus is that loss of estrogen or an increase in progesterone can cause or exacerbate depression:

■ Birth control pills with a high progesterone-to-estrogen ratio are more likely to induce mood symptoms or depression.

■ Adding estrogen with progesterone can be effective for treating depression induced by estrogen loss (i.e., postmenopausally). However, the adverse risks (breast cancer, cardiovascular disease, pulmonary emboli) are of significant concern and may well offset the usefulness of estrogen in this population.

➤ Thyroid and autoimmune disorders are more frequent in females and are commonly associated with mood disorders.

General Considerations Regarding Depression

➤ There is an increased risk of depression beginning with puberty and ending postmenopausally.

➤ There is no increased risk of depression prior to puberty or after menopause.

➤ In addition to antidepressants, estrogen + progesterone has been advocated as a treatment for depression when falling estrogen levels are thought to be responsible for the depression.

➤ Selective serotonin reuptake inhibitors (SSRIs) appear to be more effective than TCAs in premenopausal women.

➤ SSRIs and TCAs appear to be equally effective in postmenopausal women (when the risk of depression is closer to that of men).

Prepubescent phase:

➤ No increased risk of mood disorders in comparison to men.

Puberty:

➤ Associated with fluctuating levels of estrogen and progesterone and an increased risk of depression in comparison to men or prepubescent/postmenopausal females.

Premenstrual phase:

➤ Sixty percent of women experience some change in mood premenstrually, whereas 5%–7% experience more severe symptoms (e.g., premenstrual syndrome, premenstrual dysphoric disorder):

✔ Premenstrual syndrome (PMS)—usually develops during the late luteal phase and resolves during menses (follicular phase). In addition to affective and mood symptoms, breast tenderness, headache, swollen extremities, and abdominal bloating are common findings. These symptoms may be due to estrogen "withdrawal" and/or progesterone increase. Antidepressants are commonly used to treat PMS (but are not FDA approved). Most often, these medications are prescribed either continuously throughout the month or during the luteal phase.

✔ Premenstrual dysphoric disorder (PMDD)—is more severe and causes more dysfunction than PMS. There is marked impairment in work, school, or social activities. Signs and symptoms include depressed mood, affective lability, anger, irritability, poor concentration, changes in appetite, changes in sleep, anxiety, decreased interest in activities, breast tenderness, headache, joint or muscle pain, a sensation of bloating, and weight gain. These signs and symptoms occur during the last week of the luteal phase and begin to resolve within a few days after the onset of the follicular phase. Fluoxetine (as Sarafem), paroxetine CR, and sertraline are FDA approved for the treatment of PMDD. They reduce both physical and psychiatric symptoms and are usually administered daily throughout the monthly cycle.

Perimenopausal phase (irregular menstrual periods, rising follicle-stimulating hormone levels, with patient typically between ages 45–49 years):

➤ Associated with a significantly increased risk of new-onset and recurrent major depression, possibly due to loss of estrogen. The risk is greatest in women with a prior history of postpartum depression or premenstrual syndrome.

➤ Estrogen alone has not been consistently shown to be helpful in reducing depressive symtoms. Estrogen augmentation with an SSRI does have merit. Adding progesterone can help protect from uterine cancer but can exacerbate depression.

Pregnancy:

➤ Pregnancy is not typically protective against the development or exacerbation of mood disorders, especially for persons with a history of bipolar disorder. A history of bipolar depression further predisposes to postpartum depression and postpartum psychosis.

➤ Depression during pregnancy has been linked to an increased likelihood for miscarriage, low birth weight, and preterm delivery.

➤ Psychotropic medication use during pregnancy can beneficially improve the underlying mental health disorder but can increase the risk of teratogenicity, obstetrical complications at birth, short-term adverse effects in the neonate at birth, and, possibly, long-term adverse effects (e.g., learning disabilities).

➤ On a statistical basis, TCAs and SSRIs (except for paroxetine and doxepin) are not felt to *significantly* increase the risk of teratogenicity. However, each patient must be assessed individually and the risk–benefit equation reviewed and understood by the patient.

Postpartum period:

Maternity blues:

➤ Occur in approximately 50% of women postpartum, with short-term depressive symptoms coupled with mood lability.

➤ Develop 3–10 days after delivery and last about 2 weeks.

➤ Risk factors include a history of PMS, prior history of depression, and family history of depression.

➤ Are likely caused by a combination of the rapid loss of estrogen after delivery, sleep disturbances from night feeding, and the realization of the tremendous added responsibility that comes with caring for a newborn child. No specific treatment other than reassurance and family support is usually required, and the blues should resolve within a short period of time.

Postpartum depression:

➤ Occurs in 10%–15% of women after delivery. Develops within 4 weeks postpartum (DSM-IV-TR) and is due, at least in part, to the massive drop in estrogen level after delivery. Additionally, the overwhelming requirement to care for a new infant can also contribute to the development of postpartum depression.

➤ Presents with more prominent and more sustained depressive symptoms than maternity blues and may be accompanied by hopelessness, a sense of failure as a parent, and suicidal or homicidal ideations or behaviors.

➤ Risk factors include a history of a mood disorder (e.g., major depressive disorder, bipolar disorder, prior history of postpartum depression), a family history of depression, a history of thyroid dysfunction, and various social factors (e.g., single, ambivalence about motherhood, low socioeconomic status).

➤ Is typically treated with a combination of psychotherapeutic and somatic therapies.

Postpartum psychosis:

➤ Is an uncommon disorder (0.1%–0.2% of women postpartum), typically occurring within the first few days or weeks after childbirth and then again 1–3 months after delivery. Coded as *psychotic disorder not otherwise specified.*

➤ Risk factors include bipolar disorder, schizophrenia, and thyroid disorders.

➤ Symptoms can vary greatly and change quickly, with periods of manic-like symptoms, depressive symptoms, florid psychotic symptoms, rage attacks, and lucid intervals.

➤ Is a psychiatric emergency because of the potential dangerousness to the infant and/or self (occurs in about 5% of mothers diagnosed with postpartum psychosis).

➤ A protective environment (inpatient psychiatric hospitalization) and antipsychotic medications are often needed.

Treatment considerations regarding the postpartum period:

➤ Estrogen replacement has been recommended as a treatment for mild depression in women whose depression seems related to lack of estrogen. Estrogen may also be added to augment antidepressants and may permit a dosage reduction of the antidepressant. To protect against possible uterine cancer, a combination estrogen/progesterone preparation should be considered. However, progesterone can induce dysphoria or depression. Who is best suited (i.e., primary care physician, gynecologist, or psychiatrist) to prescribe and monitor the estrogen remains unsettled.

Postmenopausal period:

➤ No increased risk of mood disorders in comparison to men.

PSYCHIATRIC MANIFESTATIONS OF THYROID DISORDERS

Risk Factors for Development of a Thyroid Disorder

➤ Female gender.

➤ Elderly.

➤ Premenopausal.

➤ History of a mood disorder.

➤ History of treatment with lithium, carbamazepine (Tegretol), phenytoin (Dilantin), or phenobarbital.

➤ Personal or family history of thyroid disease.

➤ Excess dietary iodine intake (leading to autoimmune hypothyroidism) or deficiency in iodine intake (leading to hyperthyroidism secondary to toxic nodular goiter).

➤ History of alcohol abuse.

Clinical Issues

➤ Thyroid disorders are one of the most prominent physical disorders with psychiatric manifestations (Table 9–5):

✔ Depressive disorders:

■ *Hypothyroidism* is a prominent medical cause of depression. Physical symptoms include fatigue (most common physical symptom), hair loss/hair brittleness, weight gain, dry skin, difficulty sweating, cold intolerance, constipation, muscle cramps, menstrual irregularities in females, and joint pain.

■ Onset of physical signs and symptoms of hypothyroidism typically occurs prior to observable mood changes.

■ *Hyperthyroidism* is most likely to cause emotional lability, anxiety, restlessness, and possibly mania. However, depression ("apathetic hyperthyroidism") has also been reported. Physical symptoms of hyperthyroidism include fatigue, unexplained weight loss, insomnia, diarrhea, heat intolerance, muscle weakness, tachycardia, hypertension, and atrial fibrillation.

■ The hypothalamic-pituitary-thyroid (HPT) axis is likely involved in the development of depression.

■ Liothyronine sodium (Cytomel; T_3) is a useful augmenting agent for the treatment of medication-refractory depression and medication-refractory bipolar disorder.

✔ Anxiety disorders:

■ Hyperthyroidism is a common finding in generalized anxiety disorder and panic disorder.

✔ Psychotic disorders:

■ Both hypothyroidism ("myxedema madness") and hyperthyroidism can lead to psychosis.

✔ Postpartum disorders:

■ Thyroid abnormalities have been associated with the development of both postpartum depression and postpartum psychosis.

Laboratory Considerations

➤ Thyroid-stimulating hormone (TSH) is the most useful and sensitive screening tool to assess for thyroid disease. An abnormal TSH suggests thyroid dysfunction.

Table 9–5   Common thyroid abnormalities with psychiatric manifestations

Condition or disorder	TSH	Free T$_4$	Free T$_3$	Physical symptoms related to thyroid disease	Psychiatric symptoms possibly related to thyroid disease
Euthyroid	Normal	Normal	Normal	No	None
Primary hypothyroidism	Increased	Decreased	Decreased or normal	Yes	Depression, anxiety, rarely psychosis
Subclinical hypothyroidism	Increased	Normal	Normal	No	Depression, anxiety
Hyperthyroidism	Decreased	Increased	Increased or normal	Yes	Mood lability, mania, anxiety, psychosis, rarely depression
Subclinical hyperthyroidism	Decreased	Normal	Normal	No	Mood lability, anxiety, hypomania

Note.   T$_3$ = liothyronine; T$_4$ = thyroxine; TSH = thyroid-stimulating hormone.

➤ To assess for subclinical thyroid disorders, additionally measure free thyroxine (T_4) and free liothyronine (T_3).

➤ Treatment of the underlying thyroid disorder is, of course, recommended. Adding an antidepressant at the start of treatment or waiting for the thyroid disorder to resolve or stabilize prior to initiating antidepressant medications is a physician choice.

PSYCHIATRIC MANIFESTATIONS OF HIV INFECTION

General Considerations

➤ HIV penetrates the blood–brain barrier early in the infectious process, leading to a wide range of psychiatric manifestations. These manifestations are additive secondary to the realities associated with contracting a potentially fatal disease.

➤ HIV is usually spread by unprotected homosexual and heterosexual sex, injecting drugs with "dirty" needles and/or syringes, perinatal transmission, and receiving contaminated blood and blood products from transfusions.

➤ Psychiatric manifestations of HIV infection include:

✔ Adjustment disorders.

✔ Mood symptoms or disorders (e.g., depressive symptoms, major depressive disorder, hypomania, mania). HIV infection is a significant risk factor for suicide.

✔ Anxiety symptoms or disorders (e.g., generalized anxiety disorder, panic attacks, avoidance behaviors).

✔ Personality changes.

✔ Psychotic symptoms (e.g., hallucinations, delusions).

✔ Cognitive impairment progressing to dementia (i.e., HIV-related dementia) and/or delirium.

Treatment

➤ Treatment of the psychiatric manifestations of HIV infection is multifactorial. In particular, keep anticholinergic side effects to a minimum and watch for drug interactions involving medications utilized to treat HIV infection:

✔ Psychotherapy can be an effective treatment.

✔ Depression can be treated with antidepressants. Choose medications with minimal anticholinergic side effects (e.g., SSRIs, selective norepinephrine reuptake inhibitors [SNRIs], and atypical antidepressants [AtypANs]) to avoid inducing additional cognitive impairment.

✔ Anxiety can be treated with buspirone (BuSpar) or benzodiazepines (in patients without a history of drug abuse). Panic attacks can be treated with SSRIs/SNRIs or benzodiazepines.

✔ Psychosis and delirium can be treated with antipsychotic medications with a low potential to induce anticholinergic side effects (e.g., avoid chlorpromazine).

CLASSIFICATION OF INVOLUNTARY ABNORMAL MOVEMENTS

➤ General considerations:

  ✔ Tardive = late onset.

  ✔ Dyskinesia = abnormal involuntary movement.

➤ Types of movements:

  ✔ Chorea—irregular, unpredictable, brief jerky movements.

  ✔ Athetosis—slow, writhing movements of distal parts of limbs.

  ✔ Choreoathetosis—movements are slow, writhing, and uncontrollable, but they may also be abrupt and jerky. Often involve fingers, hands, arms, and feet. Choreoathetosis is the most commonly observed movement of tardive dyskinesia.

  ✔ Ballismus—wild flinging or throwing movements of the extremities.

  ✔ Dystonia—involuntary muscle contraction causing a sustained, twisted, or abnormal posture. Patients with dystonia may also have superimposed movements that are slow (athetosis), rapid (myoclonic), or rhythmic (tremor). Tardive dystonia may be a subset of tardive dyskinesia or may be a distinct entity (controversial).

  ✔ Motor tics—involuntary, rapid, recurrent sudden movements that serve no apparent purpose.

  ✔ Tardive dyskinesias—abnormal, hyperkinetic, involuntary movements characterized by some combination of orofacial movements, tics, chorea, and/or athetosis. Orofacial dyskinesia is the most characteristic early feature of tardive dyskinesia. It may begin as mild fasciculations of the tongue, followed by exaggerated movements of the tongue and lips. Bulging of the cheeks, chewing movements, blinking, blepharospasm, grimacing, and arching of the eyebrows can also occur. Movements of the extremities and trunk are also noted in some persons. These include choreoathetoid-like movements. Truncal involvement may produce rocking and swaying and rotational pelvic movements.

✔ Tardive dystonia—late-onset spasms that may persist despite stopping the medication.

✔ Tardive akathisia—late-onset internal restlessness (anxiety) and/or physical inability to remain still that may persist despite stopping the medication.

➤ Medications that can cause tardive dyskinesia (nonexhaustive list):

✔ FGA medications.

✔ SGA medications (much lower potential than the first-generation antipsychotic medications).

✔ Metoclopramide (Reglan).

✔ Prochlorperazine (Compazine).

✔ Promethazine (Phenergan).

✔ Amoxapine (Asendin).

✔ Perphenazine/amitriptyline (Triavil).

➤ Time frame of antipsychotic-induced movement disorders:

✔ Acute (early; acute extrapyramidal side effects [EPS])—can occur within minutes or hours after administration of an antipsychotic medication but usually occur within less than 48 hours. Resolve with discontinuation of the antipsychotic medication or the administration of an anticholinergic medication.

✔ Tardive (late-appearing). Can take the form of tardive dyskinesia, tardive dystonia, tardive akathisia, and tardive tics—usually do not begin until after 3 months or more of antipsychotic use (sooner in the elderly). May or may not resolve with discontinuation of the antipsychotic medication. Tardive dyskinesia is the most common antipsychotic-induced tardive movement disorder. However, tardive dystonia (involving the neck and trunk) and tardive akathisia (nonresolving akathisia) have also been reported:

■ Anticholinergic medications can help to temporarily relieve tardive dystonia. Low-dose anticholinergic agents may worsen tardive dyskinesia, whereas high-dose agents can improve symptoms. However, anticholinergic agents are not believed to cause tardive dyskinesia.

■ Beta-blockers (propranolol) can help relieve tardive akathisia.

THE GLUTAMATE–GABA CONNECTION

➤ Glutamate and gamma-aminobutyric acid (GABA) are structurally and functionally related, in that GABA is synthesized from glutamate. GABA is the major inhibitory neurotransmitter, and glutamate is the major excitatory neurotransmitter. Both are widely distributed in the brain.

➤ Benzodiazepines augment the activity of GABA (i.e., GABAergic activity) at the $GABA_A$ receptor complex.

➤ Glutamate acts on multiple receptors localized on neurons, the most widely studied being the *N*-methyl-D-aspartate (NMDA) receptor.

➤ The glutamate–GABA connection has been implicated as playing a role in the etiology and treatment of schizophrenia, major depression, bipolar disorder, anxiety disorders (e.g., generalized anxiety disorder, panic disorder, PTSD), dementias, and substance abuse disorders (the "glutamate pathway" is activated during alcohol withdrawal). The impact of the excitatory–inhibitory balance is far-reaching and likely affects the majority of—if not all—brain cells. Recently, it has been proposed that the monoamine basis of antidepressant activity is ultimately mediated through glutamate activity.

➤ Hyperexcitability (e.g., mania, alcohol withdrawal) may in part be secondary to low GABAergic activity or increased glutamate activity.

➤ Importantly, many candidate medications now being studied affect GABA or glutamate receptors and show great promise as a direction for the development of novel medications:

  ✔ Lamotrigine, carbamazepine, topiramate, valproate, gabapentin, tiagabine, olanzapine, lithium, benzodiazepines, and memantine are proposed to impart at least some of their activity through the glutamate–GABA pathways.

PHARMACOTHERAPY FOR INSOMNIA

➤ All FDA-approved agents are GABAergic except ramelteon (Rozerem).

➤ There are five true benzodiazepine (BDZ) receptor agonists, three non-BDZ receptor agonists, and one selective melatonin receptor agonist.

➤ Prior to the BDZs, bromide salts (produced horrific skin lesions), chloral hydrate (a "Micky Finn" when combined with alcohol), paraldehyde, barbiturates, and meprobamate (extremely lethal in overdose) were classified as anxiolytics or hypnotics.

➤ Initially, consider insomnia as a symptom rather than a disorder. Evaluate for psychiatric (e.g., depression, anxiety), medical (e.g., hyperthyroidism, restless legs syndrome, sleep apnea), and substance-induced (e.g., corticosteroids, cocaine, alcohol) or substance withdrawal (e.g., alcohol, BDZs) causes.

➤ Other commonly used non-FDA-approved treatments include promoting good sleep hygiene (e.g., limit caffeine, promote a regular pattern for sleep) and medications such as melatonin and trazodone, sedating TCAs, diphenhydramine, and quetiapine (a poor choice).

➤ The FDA has cautioned that hypnotics can rarely cause sleep-related activities (e.g., sleep driving, sleep eating), severe allergic reactions (e.g., anaphylaxis), and severe facial swelling (e.g., angioedema).

➤ Eszopiclone (Lunesta) and ramelteon (Rozerem) are FDA approved for the maintenance treatment of insomnia. See Table 9–6 for FDA-approved medications for the treatment of insomnia.

■ **Table 9–6   FDA-approved medications for the treatment of insomnia**

Medication	Recommended dosage (mg/day)	Elimination half-life (hours)
Selective melatonin receptor agonist		
ramelteon (Rozerem)	8	1.0–2.6
Immediate-release nonbenzodiazepines		
zolpidem (Ambien)	5–10	1.5–2.5
zaleplon (Sonata)	5–20	1
eszopiclone (Lunesta)	1–3	5–7
Extended-release nonbenzodiazepines		
zolpidem ER (Ambien CR)	6.25–12.5	~3
Immediate-release benzodiazepines		
temazepam (Restoril)	7.5–30	8–20
triazolam (Halcion)	0.125–0.25	2–4
quazepam (Doral)	7.5–15	50–120
estazolam (ProSom)	1–2	8–24
flurazepam (Dalmane)	15–30	50–120

SEROTONIN, NOREPINEPHRINE, AND DOPAMINE METABOLIC PATHWAYS

➤ Figure 9–1 illustrates the serotonin, norepinephrine, and dopamine metabolic pathways.

Tryptophan ⟶ 5-HTP ⟶ **5-HT** ⟶ 5-HIAA

⟶ DOPAC + HVA

Phenylalanine ⟶ L-Tyrosine ⟶ L-DOPA ⟶ **DA** ⟶ **NE** ⟶ MHPG and VMA

Figure 9–1   Serotonin, norepinephrine, and dopamine metabolic pathways.
Note. 5-HIAA = 5-hydroxyindoleacetic acid; 5-HT = 5-hydroxytryptamine (serotonin); 5-HTP = 5-hydroxytryptophan; DA = dopamine; DOPAC = 3,4-dihydroxyphenylacetic acid; HVA = homovanillic acid; L-DOPA = L-dihydroxyphenylalanine; MHPG = 3-methoxy-4-hydroxyphenylglycol; NE = norepinephrine; VMA = vanillyl mandelic acid.

CLINICAL INDICATIONS FOR ANTIDEPRESSANT MEDICATIONS

Purported Uses of Antidepressant Medications (FDA Approved and Unapproved)

➤ Mood disorders (e.g., major depression, dysthymic disorder, "double depression," bipolar depression, atypical depression, melancholic depression, postpartum depression, chronic depression, recurrent depression, minor depressive disorder, seasonal affective disorder, pseudodementia).

➤ Depression inherently associated with schizophrenia, schizoaffective disorder, and schizophreniform disorder.

➤ Anxiety disorders (e.g., generalized anxiety disorder, panic disorder, posttraumatic stress disorder [PTSD], social phobia, OCD, obsessive-compulsive spectrum disorders).

➤ Impulse-control disorders (e.g., intermittent explosive disorder, pathological gambling, kleptomania).

➤ Personality disorders (to reduce impulsive and aggressive behavior and treat comorbid depression).

➤ Eating disorders (anorexia nervosa, bulimia nervosa, and binge-eating disorder) and obesity.

➤ Substance-related disorders (especially when comorbid with depression or anxiety).

➤ Attention-deficit/hyperactivity disorder (ADHD) (bupropion, imipramine).

➤ Narcolepsy (imipramine).

➤ Insomnia (amitriptyline, doxepin).

➤ Enuresis (imipramine).

➤ Smoking cessation (bupropion).

➤ Tourette's disorder (when accompanied by depression).

➤ Paraphilias (SSRIs/SNRIs/AtypANs).

➤ PMS and PMDD (fluoxetine, sertraline, paroxetine).

➤ Pain disorders (TCAs [especially amitriptyline] and SNRIs with both 5-hydroxytryptamine [5-HT] and norepinephrine agonism):

  ✔ Neuropathic pain (e.g., postherpetic neuralgia, diabetic neuropathy).

  ✔ Chronic back pain.

  ✔ Poststroke pain.

  ✔ Irritable bowel syndrome.

  ✔ Temporomandibular joint (TMJ) dysfunction.

  ✔ Atypical facial pain.

  ✔ Fibromyalgia.

  ✔ Vulvodynia (vulvar pain).

  ✔ Migraine headache.

➤ Premature ejaculation (paroxetine).

➤ Pruritis (doxepin [Zonalon] cream is FDA approved).

➤ Chronic fatigue syndrome (SSRIs/SNRIs/AtypANs, TCAs).

➤ Agitation, aggression, and violence (SSRIs).

FDA-Approved Indications for Antidepressants in Adults

➤ Table 9–7 lists FDA-approved indications for antidepressants in adults.

Table 9–7 FDA-approved indications for antidepressants in adults

Medication	Acute treatment of MDD	MDD with psychotic features	GAD	Social anxiety disorder (social phobia)	Maintenance of MDD	OCD	Panic disorder	PTSD	BN	PMDD	Pregnancy risk category	Smoking cessation
Tricyclic/heterocyclic antidepressants[a]	Yes				Yes						C	
Amoxapine	Yes	Yes			Yes						C	
Clomipramine	Yes					Yes					C	
MAOIs	Yes										Safety not established	
Fluoxetine	Yes				Yes[b]	Yes	Yes		Yes	Yes	C	
Paroxetine	Yes		Yes	Yes	Yes	Yes	Yes	Yes			C	
Paroxetine CR	Yes			Yes	Yes	Yes	Yes			Yes	C	
Sertraline	Yes			Yes	Yes	Yes	Yes	Yes		Yes	C	
Fluvoxamine						Yes					C	
Citalopram	Yes				Yes						C	
Escitalopram	Yes		Yes		Yes						C	
Bupropion SR	Yes				Yes						B	Yes (Zyban)
Bupropion IR/XL	Yes				Yes						B	
Duloxetine	Yes		Yes		Yes						C	
Venlafaxine XR	Yes		Yes	Yes	Yes						C	
Nefazodone	Yes				Yes						C	
Mirtazapine	Yes				Yes						C	

Note. BN = bulimia nervosa; FDA = U.S. Food and Drug Administration; GAD = generalized anxiety disorder; MAOI = monoamine oxidase inhibitor; MDD = major depressive disorder; OCD = obsessive-compulsive disorder; PMDD = premenstrual dysphoric disorder; PTSD = posttraumatic stress disorder. [a]Other than clomipramine and amoxapine. [b]Including pediatric.

CLINICAL INDICATIONS FOR ANTIPSYCHOTIC MEDICATIONS

Purported Uses of Antipsychotic Medications (FDA Approved and Unapproved)

➤ Psychotic disorders (e.g., schizophrenia, schizoaffective disorder, brief psychotic disorder, schizophreniform disorder, delusional disorder).

➤ Mood disorders:

  ✔ Major depressive disorder with psychotic features.

  ✔ Mania (chlorpromazine, olanzapine, quetiapine, risperidone, aripiprazole, ziprasidone).

  ✔ Maintenance phase of bipolar disorder (olanzapine, aripiprazole).

  ✔ Depressed phase of bipolar disorder (olanzapine + fluoxetine [Symbyax], quetiapine).

➤ Psychosis due to a general medical condition.

➤ Substance-induced psychosis (e.g., Cushing's disease, cocaine), or substance withdrawal with excessive agitation or hallucinations (e.g., benzodiazepine withdrawal).

➤ Personality disorders, during periods of regression (especially borderline, schizotypal, and obsessive-compulsive personality disorders).

➤ Severe agitation, especially with the concern for violent behavior (e.g., impulse-control disorders, PTSD, delirium, dementia).

➤ Tics and Tourette's disorder (haloperidol [Haldol], pimozide [Orap]).

➤ Nausea and vomiting (e.g., prochlorperazine [Compazine]).

➤ Gastroesophageal reflux (e.g., metoclopramide [Reglan]).

➤ Adjunctive use in anesthesia for medical and surgical procedures (e.g., droperidol [Inapsine]).

FDA-Approved Indications for Antipsychotics in Adults

➤ Table 9–8 lists FDA-approved indications for selected typical and all atypical antipsychotic medications in adults.

Table 9–8 FDA-approved indications for selected typical and all atypical antipsychotic medications in adults

Medication	Treatment of psychotic disorders	Maintenance treatment of schizophrenia	Treatment of mania associated with bipolar disorder	Treatment of depression associated with bipolar disorder	Maintenance of bipolar disorder	Other	Pregnancy risk category
Haloperidol (Haldol, Haldol Decanoate)	Yes					Tourette's disorder	C
Pimozide[a] (Orap)		Yes (when not accompanied by excitement, agitation, or hyperactivity)				Motor and phonic tics in patients with Tourette's disorder	C
Fluphenazine (Prolixin, Prolixin Decanoate)	Yes						Not known
Loxitane (Loxapine)		Yes					Not known
Molindone (Moban)	Yes						Not known
Trifluoperazine (Stelazine)	Yes						Not known
Chlorpromazine (Thorazine)	Yes		Yes				Not known

■ Table 9–8   FDA-approved indications for selected typical and all atypical antipsychotic medications in adults (continued)

Medication	Treatment of psychotic disorders	Maintenance treatment of schizophrenia	Treatment of mania associated with bipolar disorder	Treatment of depression associated with bipolar disorder	Maintenance of bipolar disorder	Other	Pregnancy risk category
Thioridazine[a] (Mellaril) and mesoridazine[a] (Serentil)		Yes (when refractory or intolerant to other antipsychotic medications)					Not known
Thiothixene (Navane)		Yes					Not known
Clozapine (Clozaril)		Yes (and schizoaffective disorder when accompanied by suicidal behavior)					B
Olanzapine (Zyprexa)		Yes	Yes	Yes (combined with fluoxetine)	Yes		C
Zyprexa IM		Yes (when accompanied by acute agitation)	Yes				C
Risperidone (Risperdal)		Yes	Yes				C
Risperdal Consta		Yes					C

Table 9–8 FDA-approved indications for selected typical and all atypical antipsychotic medications in adults (continued)

Medication	Treatment of psychotic disorders	Maintenance treatment of schizophrenia	Treatment of mania associated with bipolar disorder	Treatment of depression associated with bipolar disorder	Maintenance of bipolar disorder	Other	Pregnancy risk category
Paliperidone extended release (Invega)	Yes						
Quetiapine (Seroquel)	Yes		Yes	Yes	Yes		C
Quetiapine extended release (Seroquel XR)	Yes		Yes				C
Ziprasidone (Geodon)	Yes		Yes				C
Ziprasidone IM	Yes (when accompanied by acute agitation)						C
Aripiprazole (Abilify)	Yes		Yes			Augmentation of SSRIs	C

Note. SSRI = selective serotonin reuptake inhibitor.

[a]Pimozide, thioridazine, and mesoridazine can significantly increase the QTc interval. Escitalopram (Lexapro) can increase pimozide levels, further increasing the QTc interval.

METABOLIC SYNDROME

➤ The recognition that increased appetite leading to increased weight can foster the development of type 2 diabetes has been appreciated since well before SGAs were first used. However, it is clear that some of the SGAs represent an additional risk factor for the devlopment of cardiovascular disease and type 2 diabetes through their propensity to stimulate appetite with resultant weight gain and perhaps through a direct effect on the endocrine system.

➤ Not all risk factors for metabolic syndrome are universally accepted. The first four risk factors listed below are universally accepted. The first two represent the highest risk factors:

✔ Abdominal obesity.

✔ Insulin resistance or glucose intolerance.

✔ Atherogenic dyslipidemia (high triglycerides, low HDL cholesterol and high LDL cholesterol).

✔ Hypertension.

✔ Prothrombotic state (e.g., high fibrinogen or plasminogen activator inhibitor-1 in the blood).

✔ Proinflammatory state (e.g., elevated C-reactive protein in the blood).

➤ Diabetes is defined as a fasting blood glucose of 126 mg/dL or above or a random blood glucose level of 200 mg/dL or above.

CIGARETTE SMOKING AND PSYCHOTROPIC MEDICATIONS

➤ Cigarette smoking is ubiquitous among psychiatric patients, with the highest comorbidity (approaching 90%) in schizophrenia and opioid dependency.

➤ Smoking cessation is of utmost importance. Nicotine replacement therapy, varenicline (Chantix), clonidine, and bupropion (Zyban) are all helpful to reduce cravings, especially when combined with psychotherapy and/or a 12-step program. Recent concerns for depression with varenicline is of clinical significance.

➤ In terms of drug interactions, the polycyclic aromatic hydrocarbons found in cigarette smoke are potent inducers of cytochrome P450 (CYP) 1A2 and can dramatically reduce blood levels of numerous medications. As a consequence, smokers may require higher doses of medications to achieve the desired therapeutic effect.

➤ With smoking cessation, enzyme induction slowly reverses, and serum levels of these medications can subsequently increase dramatically, potentially resulting in toxicities (e.g., clozapine toxicity after smoking cessation).

➤ Selected common medications susceptible to clinically important induction from cigarette smoking are shown in Table 9–9.

■ **Table 9–9   Selected medications susceptible to clinically important CYP 1A2 induction secondary to cigarette smoking**

Antidepressants	Anxiolytics
Amitriptyline	Diazepam
Nortriptyline	
Imipramine	
Clomipramine	
Fluvoxamine	**Other medications**
Trazodone	Acetaminophen
Mirtazapine (Remeron)	Propranolol
Duloxetine	Propoxyphene (Darvon)
Antipsychotics	Pentazocine (Talwin)
Clozapine	Theophylline
Olanzapine	Aspirin
Quetiapine	Codeine
Haloperidol	Insulin
Fluphenazine	Heparin
Chlorpromazine	

INHIBITORY EFFECTS OF SSRIs, SNRIs, AND ATYPICAL ANTIDEPRESSANTS ON SPECIFIC CYP ISOENZYMES

➤ The CYP isoenzyme system is involved in Phase I metabolism (primarily oxidative) and is strongly influenced by genetics (i.e., fast metabolizers, slow metabolizers).

➤ Table 9–10 summarizes the CYP isoenzyme inhibitory effects of selective serotonin reuptake inhibitors (SSRIs) and second-generation mixed-mechanism antidepressants (SNRIs, AtypANs).

■ **Table 9–10   CYP isoenzyme inhibition profiles of antidepressants**

Medication	Mild inhibition[a]	Moderate inhibition[a]	Substantial (clinically meaningful) inhibition[a]
Tricyclic antidepressants	—	—	—
Fluoxetine	3A3/4	1A2	2D6[b,c] 2C9/19
Paroxetine	3A3/4	1A2	2D6[b,c]
Sertraline	2D6 (low dose), 2C, 3A3/4	—	2D6 (high dose)[d]
Fluvoxamine	—	—	1A2[e] 3A3/4[f] 2C9/19[g]
Citalopram	2D6	—	—
Escitalopram	2D6	—	—
Venlafaxine	2D6	—	—
Nefazodone	—	—	3A3/4[f]
Duloxetine	1A2, 2D6	—	—
Mirtazapine	—	—	—
Bupropion	—	—	2D6
Selegiline transdermal	—	—	—

Note. — = not significant or minimal for cytochrome P450 (CYP) 3A3/4, 2C, 2D6, and 1A2 isoenzymes.
[a]Findings vary from different studies.
[b]Inhibition of amitriptyline, amphetamine, clomipramine, desipramine, fluoxetine, haloperidol, imipramine, nortriptyline, paroxetine, thioridazine, risperidone, and others.
[c]Fluoxetine and paroxetine inhibit their own metabolism via the 2D6 pathway.
[d]Questionable.
[e]Inhibition of a wide variety of medications, including antipsychotic medications, SSRIs, diazepam, warfarin, propranolol, and verapamil.
[f]Inhibition of a very wide variety of medications, including nefazodone, sertraline, trazodone, alprazolam, buspirone, carbamazepine, diazepam, estradiol, progesterone, verapamil, and codeine. Grapefruit juice is a 3A4 enzyme inhibitor. Carbamazepine, phenobarbital, and St. John's wort are 3A4 enzyme inducers. Cardiotoxicity can result from 3A4 enzyme inhibition of terfenadine (Seldane) by erythromycin and ketoconazole.
[g]Inhibition of citalopram, clomipramine, amitriptyline, imipramine, diazepam, phenytoin, tolbutamide, propranolol, and others.

CYP ISOENZYMES SUBSTANTIALLY INHIBITED BY ANTIDEPRESSANT MEDICATIONS

➤ **CYP 1A2**—inhibited by fluvoxamine.

➤ **CYP 2C9/19**—inhibited by fluoxetine, fluvoxamine.

➤ **CYP 2D6**—inhibited by fluoxetine, paroxetine, bupropion, sertraline (high dose).

➤ **CYP 3A3/4**—nefazodone, fluvoxamine.

➤ **No or minimal enzyme inhibition**—mirtazapine, sertraline (low dose), venlafaxine, duloxetine, citalopram, escitalopram, TCAs, selegiline.

MNEMONIC FOR THE MAJOR CYTOCHROME P450 ISOENZYMES THAT HAVE AN IMPACT ON PSYCHOTROPIC MEDICATIONS

1 = 1A2

➤ **Inhibitors**—caffeine, fluvoxamine, grapefruit juice.

➤ **Inducers**—carbamazepine, cigarette smoke.

2 = 2D6

➤ **Inhibitors**—fluoxetine, paroxetine, high-dose sertraline, bupropion, amitriptyline, imipramine, haloperidol.

➤ **Inducers**—none prominent.

2 = 2C9/19

➤ **Inhibitors**—fluoxetine, fluvoxamine.

➤ **Inducers**—carbamazepine, secobarbital, rifampin.

3 = 3A4

➤ **Inducers**—fluoxetine, sertraline, nefazodone, quetiapine, risperidone, barbiturates, carbamazepine, phenytoin.

➤ **Inhibitors**—ketoconazole, erythromycin.

"STEPS" MNEMONIC FOR CHOOSING A MEDICATION

➤ **S**   safety (e.g., drug interactions, protein binding, potential for hepatic/cardiovascular damage, safety in pregnancy).
➤ **T**   tolerability (side effects).
➤ **E**   efficacy.
➤ **P**   price.
➤ **S**   simplicity (e.g., once-daily dosing).

MNEMONIC FOR ACHIEVING A DESIRED CLINICAL RESPONSE FROM A MEDICATION

➤ Right **d**rug.
➤ Right **d**iagnosis.
➤ Right **d**osage.
➤ Right **d**uration.

PHARMACOGENETIC RELEVANCE TO PSYCHIATRIC DISORDERS

➤ *Pharmacogenetics* refers to the utilization of an individual's gene phenotype (variability) to predict the effectiveness of a medication prior to its use in the patient.
➤ Usually, the variability relates to changes in metabolism that involve the CYP isoenzyme system. Slowed metabolism can result in toxicity, and faster metabolism can result in lack of effectiveness.
➤ It is impossible to list the known phenotypic expressions, as the list is almost endless and rapidly expanding. Some examples:
    ✔ Variability in ethnic groups is well appreciated. Caucasian and African populations are more likely to be slow metabolizers of medications requiring CYP 2D6, whereas Asians are more likely to be slow metabolizers of medications requiring CYP 2C19.

✔ The potential to develop tardive dyskinesia may, in part, be dependent on genetic variability of CYP 1A2, which is responsible for the metabolism of some of the antipsychotic medications.

✔ The value of clozapine as an antipsychotic medication is undeniable, but serious side effects limit broad-based clinical use. If genetic polymorphism could predict who would or would not have an adverse reaction to the medication, its utility could dramatically increase. Genetic polymorphism is thought to play a role in the risk-to-benefit ratio.

➤ Although the clinical relevance of testing is not fully known (or appreciated), the AmpliChip CYP 450 genotyping test will assess for CYP 2D6 and CYP 2C19 genotypes.

PHARMACOKINETIC ISSUES IN THE ELDERLY

General Considerations

➤ Elderly patients present with significant functional changes that can alter the absorption, distribution, metabolism, and excretion of prescribed medications:

✔ The total amount of an oral dose of medication absorbed remains relatively intact, although the speed of absorption may slow, especially if the patient is taking anticholinergic medications (can slow gastrointestinal motility). With advancing age, the absorption of nutrients requiring active transport (e.g., iron, calcium, folic acid, vitamin B_{12}) can slow or diminish. Decreased levels of folic acid and vitamin B_{12} are implicated in depressive disorders and dementia.

✔ Oxidative metabolism involving the CYP isoenzyme system slows, both on the "first pass" during the absorption from the gastrointestinal tract and from blood perfusing the liver. The net effect of this slowing is higher-than-expected blood levels, which can potentially translate into toxicity and/or longer-than-normal duration of drug activity.

✔ Renal excretion of intact drugs is slowed. Medications eliminated principally by renal excretion (e.g., lithium, gabapentin, lamotrigine) can have higher-than-normal or toxic blood levels.

✔ The elderly tend to lose lean muscle mass at the expense of increased body fat, resulting in a net decrease in available total body water. Therefore, for fat-soluble medications (e.g., most prescribed psychiatric medications) elimination is slowed, potentially prolonging the activity. For water-soluble medications (e.g., lithium, digoxin, aminoglycosides) or alcohol, the decrease in total body water can result in higher-than-normal blood levels.

✔ Protein stores and serum albumin usually decrease in the elderly. Because many psychiatric medications are highly protein bound, lack of sequestration by serum proteins can result in increased blood levels.

Treatment Guidelines

➤ The net effect of these changes is that elderly patients can have higher-than-normal medication serum levels when "usual" doses are utilized. For psychotropic medications, one-third to one-half of the normal adult dose is often adequate. These considerations give validation to the statement "Start low, go slow, keep it as low as possible, and keep it simple" (i.e., avoid polypharmacy).

➤ When treating psychosis, use antipsychotic medications that have a low potential for EPS and anticholinergic side effects:

✔ Quetiapine, olanzapine, ziprasidone, and aripiprazole provide the best characteristics to satisfy this requirement. Clozapine has significant anticholinergic activity, and risperidone can have dose-dependent EPS.

➤ When treating depression, higher doses may ultimately be needed. Depression in the elderly tends to be more treatment resistant than in younger individuals. Avoid TCAs (with the possible exception of desipramine).

➤ When treating anxiety and sleep disorders, caution is advised when using benzodiazepines, which can cause undesirable side effects in the elderly (e.g., disinhibition, impairment in mechanical performance, memory loss, dependency). Do not forget that alcohol abuse in the elderly remains largely unrecognized.

DEATH AND DYING (ELISABETH KÜBLER-ROSS)

➤ Elisabeth Kübler-Ross described five sequential stages a person typically goes through after learning that his or her death is inevitable and will likely occur sooner than later:

✔ Denial of the inevitability of death.

✔ Anger over the loss or what the loss will mean to others.

✔ Bargaining to live longer (prayer, good deeds).

✔ Depression when there is finally realization that dying is now inevitable.

✔ Acceptance of the finality, perhaps completion of the grieving process.

SELECTED NEUROLOGICAL DISORDERS WITH NEUROPSYCHIATRIC INVOLVEMENT

➤ Table 9–11 lists neurological disorders with neuropsychological involvement.

■ **Table 9–11   Selected neurological disorders with neuropsychiatric involvement**

Disorder	Location of injury	Nonpsychiatric symptoms	Psychiatric symptoms
Normal-pressure hydrocephalus	Ventricular system	Ataxia, urinary incontinence	Dementia Anterograde amnesia
Anton's syndrome	Occipital cortex	Blindness	Anosognosia (denial of loss of function)
Klüver-Bucy syndrome	Temporal lobes		Placidity, hyper-sexuality, visual agnosia, obsessive-compulsive features
Fahr's syndrome	Basal ganglia	Parkinsonism, chorea, seizures	Depression, cognitive impairment, obsessive-compulsive disorder
Amyotrophic lateral sclerosis	Motor cortex, corticospinal tracts, temporal lobe, other subcortical structures	Progressive motor weakness	Pathological crying or laughing, dementia
Systemic lupus erythematosus (with central nervous system involvement)	Broad-based	Seizures, strokes, headache	Multiple (e.g., anxiety, depression, mania, psychosis, cognitive impairment)
Neurosyphilis	Broad-based, including frontal lobes and ascending posterior columns (tabes dorsalis)	Meningovascular involvement is the most common neuropsychiatric complication	Mood disorders, psychosis, dementia
Sydenham's chorea	Basal ganglia	Complication of rheumatic fever or streptococcal infection Chorea (St. Vitus' dance)	"Maniacal chorea" (agitation, delirium, obsessive-compulsive symptoms or disorder, psychosis)

PREGNANCY RISK CATEGORIES

➤ **Category A**—no adverse fetal effects in the first trimester of pregnancy and no evidence of adverse fetal effects in later trimesters (e.g., folic acid, levothyroxine).

➤ **Category B**—adverse fetal effects are observed in animals but are not observed in humans, or animal studies show no adverse fetal effects but human studies have not been done (e.g., buspirone, clozapine [Clozaril], bupropion, diphenhydramine [Benadryl]).

➤ **Category C**—adverse fetal effects in animals but no human studies. The benefits of the drug in pregnant women may be acceptable despite the potential risks (e.g., some TCAs, monoamine oxidase inhibitors, SSRIs, SNRIs, AtypANs [except bupropion], SGMMAs, typical and atypical antipsychotic medications [except clozapine], benztropine).

➤ **Category D**—evidence of human fetal risk, but the potential benefits from the use of the drug may be acceptable despite its potential risks (e.g., benzodiazepines, some TCAs, lithium, divalproex sodium, carbamazepine).

➤ **Category X (high risk)**—animal and human studies demonstrate fetal abnormalities, or adverse-reaction reports indicate evidence of fetal risk. The risk of use in pregnant women clearly outweighs any possible benefit (e.g., thalidomide, warfarin, isotretinoin [Accutane]).

➤ **Category NR**—not rated (e.g., acetaminophen).

EXPERIMENTAL DRUG TESTING PHASES

➤ **Phase I**—high-dose testing in fewer than 100 volunteers to test for safety; mandatory.

➤ **Phase II**—medication compared with placebo in several hundred patients to test for efficacy; mandatory.

➤ **Phase III**—safety and efficacy testing (as in Phase I and Phase II) on a larger scale, involving several hundred to several thousand patients; at least 2 trials are mandatory.

➤ **Phases IIIB and IV**—similar to Phase III testing, for medications that treat life-threatening illnesses that lack other treatments.

➤ **Postmarketing surveillance**—monitoring of rare or unusual side effects, long-term effectiveness, and cost effectiveness on a continual and long-term basis, among patients treated by physicians in ordinary clinical settings.

ETHICAL DILEMMAS IN PSYCHIATRY

Ethical issues are at times posed during the oral boards, not to elicit a right or wrong answer but to test your ability to weigh the pros and cons of an issue. Some ethical matters are clear-cut (e.g., issues related to having sex with a patient), although nuances of these issues might be considered an ethical dilemma (e.g., developing a relationship with and eventually marrying a patient you have not treated for 20 years). Your ability to weigh the issues and present both sides of the argument is what the examiners are looking for. The breadth of ethical dilemmas spans the entire field of psychiatry. Examples are provided to demonstrate how one might approach a question regarding an ethical dilemma.

Ethical Dilemma 1

➤ The identical-twin sister of a patient you treat for bipolar disorder calls after reading a newspaper article about the genetic transmission of the illness. The woman has called your office several times in the past hour, sounding frantic and possibly manic, wanting to know if she or her children could also develop the disorder.

Ethical considerations:

✔ Despite the panicked nature of the call, confidentiality issues related to your patient must not be compromised unless an emergent situation develops.

✔ You should be careful about even acknowledging that her sister is your patient.

✔ You should be cautious about counseling the patient on the telephone (e.g., "Why are you panicking?"), in that you might inadvertently develop a new doctor–patient relationship that might compromise or jeopardize the current working relationship with your bipolar patient and inadvertently develop a duty (treatment and legal) to the caller.

✔ Treating a relative of a current patient can be ethically problematic.

✔ You might consider referring the caller to another psychiatrist who is experienced with issues related to the genetic transmission of mental illnesses.

Ethical Dilemma 2

➤ A patient you are treating psychiatrically asks you to write a prescription for an antibiotic to treat his sore throat.

✔ Ethical considerations:

Unless you examine the patient, you should not prescribe an antibiotic. Also, this treatment is outside your field of expertise. Should a significant adverse reaction develop, your lack of expertise, correctness of diagnosis, etc., could lead to a viable malpractice claim.

Ethical Dilemma 3

➤ A patient you are treating psychiatrically asks you to write a prescription for a double dose of the medication to save him money on his insurance plan by having the prescription last twice as long.

✔ **Ethical considerations:**
Inappropriate action on your part (insurance fraud). Also, if your action is pursued by the medical board, your license to practice medicine could be in jeopardy.

Ethical Dilemma 4

➤ A patient you are treating psychiatrically asks you to write a prescription for her "heart medicine" to "hold her over" until she can see her regular medical doctor to obtain a refill.

✔ **Ethical considerations:**
Basic medical expectations require examination and assessment prior to treatment. Yet this action is commonly done.

Ethical Dilemma 5

➤ A patient you are treating psychiatrically asks you to write a prescription in his name for his spouse because of insurance savings.

✔ **Ethical considerations:**
Basic medical expectations require examination and assessment prior to treatment. This action is both medically and legally inappropriate.

MALPRACTICE ISSUES IN BRIEF

➤ This section touches on the basis for malpractice, which requires all four of the following criteria to be met (the four D's: **d**ereliction of **d**uty **d**etermining **d**amages):

✔ Dereliction—the doctor must have errored in a way that other doctors in his profession, his practice location, and his type of practice would not have.

✔ Duty—the doctor must have a valid connection to the patient, most often (but not always) as the treating physician.

✔ Determining—the doctor's error, despite duty and dereliction, must have been the proximate cause for the injury (i.e., but for the actions of the doctor, the damage would not have occurred).

✔ Damages—the doctor's error produced damage to the patient in terms of loss, pain, and/or suffering.

INDEX

*Page numbers printed in **boldface** type refer to tables or figures.*